Sociology a
Psychology
for the Dental Team

Sociology and Psychology for the Dental Team

An Introduction to Key Topics

Sasha Scambler, Suzanne E. Scott
and Koula Asimakopoulou

polity

The right of Sasha Scambler, Suzanne E. Scott and Koula Asimakopoulou to be identified as Authors of this Work has been asserted in accordance with the UK Copyright, Designs and Patents Act 1988.

First published in 2016 by Polity Press

Polity Press
65 Bridge Street
Cambridge CB2 1UR, UK

Polity Press
350 Main Street
Malden, MA 02148, USA

ISBN-13: 978-0-7456-5433-1
ISBN-13: 978-0-7456-5434-8(pb)

Library of Congress Cataloging-in-Publication Data

Scambler, Sasha Jane.
  Sociology and psychology for the dental team : an introduction to key topics / Sasha Scambler, Suzanne Scott, Koula Asimakopoulou.
      pages cm
  Includes bibliographical references and index.
  ISBN 978-0-7456-5433-1 (hardback : alk. paper) – ISBN 978-0-7456-5434-8 (pbk. : alk. paper)
1. Dentistry–Social aspects. 2. Dentistry–Psychological aspects.
I. Asimakopoulou, Koula. II. Scott, Suzanne. III. Title.
  RK53.S33 2016
  617.6001'9--dc23
2015025828

A catalogue record for this book is available from the British Library.

Typeset in 10.5 on 13pt Minion Pro by
Servis Filmsetting Ltd, Stockport, Cheshire
Printed and bound in the UK by Clays Ltd, St Ives PLC

For further information on Polity, visit our website:
politybooks.com

Contents

Figures, Tables and Images

Figures

Tables

Images

Acknowledgements

As with all work of this kind, we owe a debt of thanks to a large number of people. The team at Polity have been extremely helpful and supportive and we are grateful for their patience and advice. We would like to thank our co-authors for working with us to make this book possible, and to friends and colleagues at King's College London Dental Institute and beyond for their support, advice and feedback throughout the process. Our thanks also go to successive years of undergraduate dental students at KCL who have challenged us to explain the relevance of our work to the dental team and in doing so have created the basis for this book.

Finally we would like to thank our families for their ongoing love and support without which this book would never have been completed. Our love and thanks go to our respective husbands: Darren, Will and Dave, and to our children: Elliot, Jamie, Dominic, Nell, George and Anne-Marie.

Sasha, Suzanne and Koula

Introduction: the Sociology and Psychology of Dentistry

Sasha Scambler and Koula Asimakopoulou

The social and behavioural sciences are a relatively recent addition to the dental curriculum, introduced initially in the 1980s, and it is an area that will be new to most dental students. This book aims to introduce key topics and theories from sociology and psychology to dentists, dental students and allied health professionals with an interest in the relationship between individuals, society and oral health. In doing so, we are hoping to show how and why modern dental practice should benefit from current thinking in the behavioural sciences.

The social and behavioural sciences, incorporating both sociology and psychology, are an essential part of dental training, providing ways of understanding the complex interactions between health, illness, the person and society. Together, these two disciplines give an insight into the 'human side' of dentistry and as such help dentists see patients as people rather than mouths. The main driving force behind writing this textbook has been precisely the need to show the dental trainee the many complexities inherent in practising dentistry on people rather than on sets of teeth. Whilst the main dental curriculum is focused on the technical aspects of preventing and treating oral pathologies, this textbook is designed to identify those opportunities seen in the dental surgery, which lend themselves to understanding oral health and disease more holistically.

In particular, this textbook aims to explain: how patients approach the dental setting and dentistry both from an individual and a wider social level; the impact that constructs such as ethnicity, gender and disability might have on the dental team's interaction with patients; how a consultation might support patients to change their behaviour to adhere to dental recommendations; broad principles that shape people's behaviour within and outside the dental surgery. Whilst there was a plethora of topics available to us to demonstrate the human side of dentistry here, we have chosen, deliberately, topics that we feel lend themselves particularly well to demonstrating the complex relationship that exists between the person, society, social systems and oral health. As such, this text neither aspires to be, nor purports to be, a complete compendium of all psychosocial issues that a member of the dental team might encounter in their day-to-day clinical practice. Rather, the textbook presents a carefully selected range of mainstream sociological and health psychological issues to demonstrate the need to see and treat oral health within the broader psychosocial setting that people find themselves in.

Why should I study sociology when training to become a member of the dental team?

The dental team is situated, works and functions within society rather than in isolation. Sociology, like the other social sciences, is interested in people and how they behave in different circumstances and when faced with different experiences and environments. As such, an understanding of sociology is imperative when trying to understand the society in which the dental team is placed. Sociologists study the way in which behaviour and experiences are shaped by the environment in which individuals live and act.

The type of questions sociologists ask relate to how the environment and people's place within it shape people's opportunities and experiences in general. For example, if all people are equal, and social class no longer exists, why is it that your life expectancy is linked to the type of job that you choose to do? Why is it that children from deprived areas are twice as likely to be diagnosed with a mental disorder? How do gender or age or ethnicity shape your life? If men and women are equal, then why is there still a pay gap between men and women? In the UK, why are 70 per cent of the Members of Parliament male? Why are men twice as likely to die from alcohol-related disease than women? Within this context, health, oral health and healthcare are areas in which the individual and society interact and as such are of interest to sociologists. Within dentistry, the environment and societal structures within which readers of this book are expected to practise dentistry are going to influence how such practice is delivered. For example, where members of the dental team practise in a government-subsidized health system such as the UK's National Health Service (NHS), the care options, materials and time they have available to offer to patients may differ from a situation where no such constraints exist. So, the book explores the relationship between oral health, individuals, groups and the wider social environment, presenting cutting-edge sociological theory where appropriate. Using broad sociological constructs such as ethnicity, disability, sex and gender, we systematically explore how these influence patients' and dental practitioners' experiences in the dental surgery. We then present the reader with common dilemmas and case studies that demonstrate the sorts of issues they might face in daily practice and how sociology as a behavioural science would propose addressing these. A critique of the ideas is presented throughout, making it clear that these issues are still debated and constantly changing, just as society changes.

Why should I study psychology when training to become a member of the dental team?

The dental team interacts, engages with and seeks to understand the behaviour of human patients and human healthcare professionals. Psychology is the science of human behaviour. Health Psychology, in particular, is the application of mainstream psychological thinking to health, illness, healthcare systems and healthcare settings. Psychologists are interested in how people behave under different circumstances and using scientific, reliable and valid methods, set out to understand, predict and modify people's behaviour. An understanding of the principles of psychology is thus useful when one considers patient, but also healthcare professional, behaviour.

These are some of the questions that dentists often ask us:

- 'Why do my patients always leave it until they are in pain before arranging a visit?'
- 'This person has not seen a dentist in 25 years. They say they are terrified of dentists. How can I persuade them to come and see me?'
- 'I have told this person they need to floss and brush twice a day. They agreed they would do it. Their plaque and gingival scores are telling me that they have not. Why have they not been doing as they agreed?'

Psychologists can help answer these questions and, in doing so, rely on and create theory that shapes and underpins their advice to clinicians. Theory is always evidence-based and it is the use of evidence that makes scientific psychology different from popular psychology. As readers of this book are probably getting trained to practise evidence-based dentistry, an understanding of psychological and sociological theory is essential in this journey of understanding and reflecting on current evidence. So, just as there are better ways to deal with caries, there are better ways to help patients learn to floss. Just like it takes practice to administer topical anaesthetic through injection, it takes practice to learn how to communicate in a way that patients will find helpful. This book gives the reader a taste of some psychological theories and explains their relevance to everyday clinical work in the dental practice. The theories are introduced, described in detail using dental examples, are related to dental settings and their advantages and shortcomings are critically pointed out.

How to read this book

As we have alluded to already, this text is not meant to be a comprehensive guide to all sociological and psychological topics that the dental team will ever meet in their day-to-day practice. Rather, we have selected topics that we believe are good exemplars of key psychosocial issues that might permeate the practice of dentistry in modern society. At the same time, although all chapters follow the same structure, where a topic is introduced, put into practice through a case study, explored in depth through discussion points and summarized at the end of each section, the style in which each chapter is delivered differs. There is a purpose behind this; just as the environment and the patients the dental team see are unique, where no two dental practices and no two patients are going to be identical, the people who research the areas we have written about, the progress made in each, the style in which such information is made available, and the overall conclusions are inherently different. It is for this reason that we have chosen a range of styles to present the material in this text.

Finally, although we expect that readers will find the material interesting and engaging, there will be occasions where what we discuss does not apply universally to all settings and all people. Some of the ideas that are presented here will appear more challenging than others and might be more readily questioned; this, again, is intended to replicate the diversity of thought found in the psychosocial fields at the moment. In many cases, we have invited the reader to critique, with us, these ideas. In other cases, we expect readers to question the ideas we discuss; this is fine and thoroughly appropriate and expected in the social sciences.

Concluding thoughts

Our hope in putting this book together is that the sociology and psychology of dentistry can be made accessible to dental students and professionals who have little or no background in these disciplines. This will foster a better understanding of the context in which dentists and allied professionals work and of the patients with whom they work, and will provide an evidence base for a new way of thinking about and practising dentistry.

Finally, we see this book as an invitation to learn and think about dentistry in a holistic way. In giving dental trainees a chance to think about the social and psychological context of dentistry, and the role of the dentist in society, we hope that their day-to-day practice will benefit from the evidence base that the social and behavioural sciences have to offer.

The Social Context of Oral Health and Disease

Sasha Scambler

IN THIS CHAPTER YOU WILL LEARN ABOUT:

▶ Definitions of health, illness and disease
▶ The social patterning of disease and death across time
▶ The social patterning of oral disease across time
▶ Models of disease causation
  ▶ The Germ Theory
  ▶ The Epidemiological Triangle
  ▶ The Web of Causation
  ▶ The Theory of General Susceptibility
  ▶ The Socio-Environmental Approach

Introduction

The aim of this chapter is to explore the relationship between our health and the society in which we live. Increasingly, health policy is focusing on the social context of health, the need for holistic care and an understanding of the social determinants of health and illness as well as the provision of clinical or biomedical care. This ties in with calls for integrated packages of health and social care and the integration of public and patient voices into health research. There is a widening understanding of the importance of social context when looking not just at health but also at patterns of disease, and it is this that is addressed in this chapter, drawing on a large body of social research across medicine and dentistry.

The excerpt in box 1.1 is from a blog posted on the *British Medical Journal* website and written by Richard Smith.

Box 1.1: The end of disease and the beginning of health

'I think I'm healthy, but am I right? I'm tubby. My hair is white and thin and gone altogether from some parts of my head. I'm short sighted and astigmatic. My Achilles tendon aches at times, and when I get out of bed in the morning I hobble. I haven't had my blood pressure measured for a while; nor my blood lipids. My prostate is, I suspect, large, but I haven't had it examined. Nor have I had my prostate-specific antigen measured. And my bowel has not been sigmoidoscoped. My genes have not been examined, but I suspect something dreadful lurks there. My mother is dementing as her mother did before her. I often can't remember names. I don't smoke, but I drink more alcohol than the Royal College of Physicians thinks wise – and I'm rather too fond of pies. I walk a lot, cycle often, and run occasionally, but I don't exercise as much as I should.

So as I complete this paragraph I'm convinced that I can't be healthy: I'm a mass of imperfections, and I've not bothered to discover the hypertension or latent cancer that may be about to carry me off [. . .]

Consider a patient called Lucy. She has heart failure, diabetes, asthma, and osteoarthritis. Her cardiologist treats her heart failure, her diabetologist her diabetes, her chest physician her asthma, and her rheumatologist her osteoarthritis. Her general practitioner holds the ring and writes her prescriptions.

But actually she's not much interested in her diseases, and she's not worried about dying. Indeed, if she could get to see her son in Australia one more time she'd welcome death: life has never been the same since her husband died. She needs a travel agent, not five doctors, but doctors are supplied on the NHS and travel agents aren't.

I'm coming close to flippancy, but in a world where most of medicine is concerned with people with multiple chronic conditions combined with social and family problems, health care must be person not disease centred.'

Excerpt from Smith (2008) The end of disease and the beginning of health. Blog post. http://blogs.bmj.com/bmj/2008/07/08/richard-smith-the-end-of-disease-and-the-beginning-of-health/

This excerpt highlights some of the issues that we will be addressing in this chapter, relating to the relationship between society and health and between health and disease. What do we mean when we talk about health and disease? Are these concepts understood in the same way by everyone? How does our understanding of health and disease affect the way that we treat people who are ill? What is the link between the social environment in which we live and the levels of health and illness that we experience throughout our lives? These questions and many more will be answered in this chapter, starting with the definition of key terms and moving on to explore different models that can help us to understand the relationship between disease and the body.

Defining health, illness and disease

The terms health, illness and disease are used frequently and often without distinguishing clearly between them. It is worth noting, not only that these terms have distinct meanings but that they are also 'ideal types' representing diverse categories or groups of conditions, experiences or symptoms. In basic terms disease can be defined as a biomedically defined pathology within the human system, which may or may not be apparent to the individual, whilst illness refers to the lay interpretation of bodily or mental signs or symptoms as somehow abnormal. Following this logic, disease is defined by others whilst illness relies on the subjective self-analysis of what is or is not normal.

Defining disease

Disease is seen ostensibly as an objective view of signs and symptoms. Medical and dental approaches use a range of scientific tests and indices to interpret signs as the presence or absence of disease regardless of whether the patient is feeling any discomfort or symptoms. Medicine and dentistry are based on the 'biomedical model', the key components of which are:

- *Scientific rationality*: Scientific knowledge and methods are the means through which we can understand disease and seek to eradicate it.
- *Emphasis on objective numerical measures*: 'Normal' parameters for the functioning of the body have been set and are used to make objective comparisons with data from the patient.
- *Emphasis on physico-chemical data*: Physical signs within the body are sought and analysed through laboratory tests in the search for a diagnosis.
- *Mind–body dualism*: Building on work of Descartes (1596–1650), the biomedical model is based on knowledge of anatomy derived from post-mortem examination of bodies. This only became acceptable with the belief that the soul/mind existed outside the physical body.
- *Views of diseases as entities*: This allows for the exploration of how these entities can be eradicated.

The main advantages of the biomedical model are that it is clear, objective and focused in its aim. There are, however, a number of disadvantages that also need to be considered. The biomedical model ignores subjective reactions and meanings. This can lead to downplaying the experiences of patients in relation to the results of, for example, physico-chemical tests. At the most extreme level, this can lead to the branding of some syndromes that exhibit very real and distressing symptoms for sufferers as psychosomatic. The second disadvantage is that the biomedical model focuses on pathology and yet it is possible to feel ill without having a disease. Thirdly, the biomedical model also makes no allowance for the fact that disease can be present with no outward symptoms such as pain.

Defining illness

Illness, in contrast, relates to the lay or subjective interpretation of signs or symptoms as a problem that is perceived as health-related. Illness, therefore, can be described as a subjective reaction to feelings of pain or discomfort. The ways in which signs and symptoms are interpreted can vary across cultures and across times, and so illness can be seen as a socially constructed category. At the most basic level, a patient enters the clinic with an illness and leaves with a disease. Only a doctor or dentist can diagnose someone as having a disease; thus you only have a disease if a doctor or dentist gives you one. For example, you may visit the dentist with a 'toothache' and return home with a 'diseased molar'. The relationship between illness and disease is not always clear, however. You can experience symptoms without having a disease (e.g. if you have sensitive teeth), or you can have a disease whilst experiencing no symptoms (e.g. with caries).

When symptoms are experienced without apparent pathology, they are sometimes described in medicine as 'psychosomatic'. This can lead to the illness being taken less seriously by medical professionals, regardless of the severity of symptoms experienced by the patient. Whilst there appears to be more awareness within dentistry of the importance of patients' perceptions, primarily due to variability of pain experienced by individuals, the variability of pain experiences has been acknowledged for over five decades (Zborowski 1952; Melzack & Wall 1965; Locker 1989). There are, however, syndromes within dentistry that cause similar confusion, such as 'temporomandibular joint disorder', 'burning mouth syndrome' or 'non-specific facial pain', which involve a range of symptoms but no obvious pathological cause. Such syndromes are regarded as 'psychosomatic' by some dentists, despite the very real distress caused to patients.

As previously stated, it is important to note that these definitions of illness and disease are ideal types. In practice, doctors and dentists do not behave exactly like medical or dental textbooks and will incorporate their own understandings about symptom experience into their diagnosis (Humphrey 1999). Similarly, and increasingly due to the plethora of medical information now available to the general population, patients are no longer reliant solely on lay understandings of symptoms and may well incorporate medical models of disease into their understanding of the symptoms being experienced. This is particularly the case for patients with chronic or long-term conditions, where they experience symptoms over an extended period of time and often develop sophisticated biomedical understanding of both the disease and the various treatment options available to them. For examples, see Scambler and Hopkins (1986) and Robinson (1989) or Scambler (2005). On a cautionary note, Mishler (1981), however, suggests that the assumptions inherent in the medical model of disease have become so entrenched in our way of thinking about medicine that health professionals may forget that it is merely a conceptual model, and treat it as the representation of reality rather than as one of a number of possible representations.

The problem of defining normality

The concept of illness is inherent in an understanding of what is and is not 'normal' with regard to the experience of symptoms. The concept of normality is difficult to establish in relation to health, however, as evidence suggests that understandings of health, and experiences of and reactions to phenomenon such as pain, are socially and culturally variable. An interesting example of this was presented by Ackernecht in 1947. He described the skin disease diachronic spirochetosis. This disease was so common in some South American tribes that it was considered abnormal not to have the disease, to the extent that men without it were not allowed to marry. Whilst the condition is objectively classified as a disease according to biomedicine, the tribes clearly did not see it as such.

Our understanding of normality is shaped not just by place but also by time. The ways that we see certain conditions and the social acceptability of them change according to historical context. For example, in the 1940s decayed teeth were very common and were considered 'normal', and in the 1970s smoking was widespread and the smokers' cough was considered 'normal'. To take a more recent example, it is only now that it is becoming 'normal' to retain teeth into old age; up to this point edentulism in later life was seen as 'normal'. Thus the concept of normality is a socially constructed one that varies across time and space, making assumptions about what is and is not normal in relation to our health problematic. These problems become even more apparent when the concept of normality is explored in relation to mental illness or disability.

> **In summary**, illness and disease exist in a social framework and indices of disease produced by dental and medical professionals do not always make sense to the lay population. Understandings of health and illness are constructed through the interplay between the symptom experience and the social and cultural framework within which this experience occurs.

Defining health

The definition of health that is most commonly used is that of the World Health Organization:

> Health is a state of complete physical, mental and social well-being and not merely the absence of disease or infirmity. (WHO 1948)

This definition was written in 1948 and has not been amended since. It is still held as the gold standard definition by many. Five decades later, Ewles and Symnett (1999) suggested that there are six dimensions of health that take it beyond the physicality of the body and set health firmly within the realm of the social. These are:

1 **Physical health** – concerned with the functioning of the body.
2 **Mental health** – the ability to think clearly and coherently.
3 **Emotional health** – to recognize and express emotions such as fear, joy or grief.
4 **Social health** – to form and maintain relationships.
5 **Spiritual health** – concerned with either religious beliefs and practices or personal creeds and principles of behaviour.
6 **Societal health** – a person's health is closely linked to the environment he or she lives in.

(modified from Ewles & Simnett 1999)

What is clear from this is that health is a multifaceted concept that can be experienced in different ways by different people at different times and in different places. It has also been suggested that health has moral connotations and that people feel a duty to be healthy and consider illness as a failure (Crawford 1987). This is a theme commonly found within the public health and political literature, where individuals are seen to have a responsibility to safeguard their own health by eating sensibly, exercising regularly, not smoking and not drinking to excess. Moral judgements are made about people who do not conform to this pattern of behaviour and, as we shall see in the next chapter, these immoral behaviours are often linked to poverty and deprivation. Further to this, certain diseases are ascribed negative moral connotations (often by the media), the most obvious examples being HIV/AIDS, lung cancer and cirrhosis of the liver.

In her seminal work on life in the East End of London, Cornwell (1984) explored attitudes towards health. She found that her respondents wanted to think of themselves as healthy and that having the 'right' attitude was deemed important in avoiding illness and maintaining health. Cornwell found that, in an attempt to prove the legitimacy of their illnesses, respondents categorized illnesses as 'normal', 'real' or as 'health problems that are not illnesses'. In this context, normal illnesses were common conditions such as chickenpox and real illnesses were major and potentially life-threatening such as cancer. Health problems that were seen as naturally occurring, such as those linked to reproduction or ageing, were not categorized as illnesses. Health has been defined in a range of other ways, including as negative, positive or functional (Schulman & Smith 1963) or as having the potential to satisfy the demands of life (Bircher 2005).

Discussion Point

• In the excerpt presented at the start of the chapter, is the author healthy according to the definitions outlined above? Can his health be determined objectively?

Defining oral health

Definitions of oral health also take us beyond the physical existence of illness or disease, to explore the social dimensions of the functioning of the mouth. Following on from the World Health Organization's idealized definition of health, Daly et al. (2002) suggest the following definition for oral health:

> Complete healthy dentition (with 32 sound straight teeth and no periodontal or other soft tissue lesions) which results in a state of physical, mental and social well-being. (Daly et al. 2002)

Clearly this is an ideal, but as such it is for most people unobtainable. A more practical definition might be that presented by Dolan (1993). He suggests that oral health is:

> A comfortable and functional dentition that allows individuals to continue their social role. (Dolan 1993)

A similar definition has been offered by the Department of Health who state:

> Oral health is the standard of health of the oral and related tissues which enables an individual to eat, speak and socialise without active disease, discomfort or embarrassment and which contributes to general well-being. (Department of Health 1994)

The focus of these definitions is on social functioning and not the presence or absence of disease. This suggests that the presence or absence of disease does not have to play an active role in health, i.e. you can be healthy and have a disease as the two are not mutually exclusive.

Discussion Point

- Is it possible to achieve Daly's definition of oral health? How useful is this definition for members of the dental team?

Challenging definitions of health and the place of disease in healthcare

In his *British Medical Journal* blog, Richard Smith (2008) suggests that it is health rather than disease that has the most significant affect on our daily lives, but that existing definitions of health are neither accurate nor helpful. Further to this, he makes the case that, if a medical model is followed, then there is no such thing as health. When subjected to a full battery of medical tests, the vast majority of people would have some part of their body that does not work as it should or is not performing to optimum capacity. Thus, for medicine, 'health' is a misnomer when

1

defined as 'the absence of disease'. Smith suggests that the main focus of daily life, even for those living with diagnosed diseases, is on living regardless of, or despite, the disease. Health, he suggests, needs to be redefined along the lines of Freud as 'the capacity to love and work' (cited in Smith 2008).

From the other side of the argument, there are calls for a debate about the relevance and importance of disease in the modern era, leading to calls for a wider focus within medicine and dentistry. Tinetti and Fried (2004) state that the focus on disease is no longer a helpful one for medicine or practitioners and is at best a partial solution and at worst harmful to the overall condition of the patient. They suggest that the growth of chronic conditions, the ageing population and recognition of the range of risk conditions affecting our daily lives over and above any disease that we might have, result in the need for an approach to medicine which is broader than a disease-based or biomedical approach.

> Clinical decision-making for all patients should be predicated on the attainment of individual goals and the identification and treatment of all modifiable biological and nonbiological factors, rather than solely on the diagnosis, treatment, or prevention of individual diseases. (Tinetti & Fried 2004: 179)

Tinetti and Fried advocate the adoption of an individually tailored model of healthcare that looks beyond the disease at the individual in their social context, and focuses on areas of lifestyle that are modifiable alongside the treatment of disease. This is an approach in line with public health thinking but tailored to individual needs.

Social patterning of disease and death

Knowledge about the body, disease and medicine itself are products of their time; they are socially constructed by what is 'known' or thought to be 'known' at any point in time. Patterns of disease also change over time, both in relation to how common a disease is and who is affected by it and also in relation to the nature of disease itself. This is not to suggest that diseases are unchanging entities and that it is only patterns that change. Rather, it is proposed that diseases themselves are socially constructed and can change over time.

Over the past 150 or more years there has been a dramatic change in both health and life expectancy, and the annual death rate in the UK has halved:

1851   22.7 per 1,000 of the population
1990   11.9 per 1,000 of the population
2008   9.4 per 1,000 of the population

At the same time life expectancy has almost doubled:

1840 Men 40 years, Women 43 years
1990 Men 72 years, Women 77 years
2011 Men 77.7 years, Women 81.9 years

The biggest change in this time has occurred amongst infants and children. In the mid-1800s it was amongst these groups, the very young, that the majority of deaths occurred. It is worth bearing in mind, however, that in many developing countries death rates are still very high and in some cases resemble the rates found in the UK in the mid-nineteenth century. In addition, life expectancy is variable and UN statistics suggest that life expectancy at birth between 2005 and 2010 varied from 82.6 years in Japan to 39.2 years in Mozambique with a world average of 67.2 years (United Nations 2007: table A.17 for 2005–2010).

Charting disease patterns across human history

The statistics presented above show changes in death rates and life expectancy across time and space. Historical patterns can also be seen when looking at diseases. There have been three major disease patterns in human history (Fitzpatrick 2008) and these have been tied into and created by the social context in which people were living in each era. It has been suggested that we are now moving into a fourth distinct era. The three historical eras (adapted from Fitzpatrick 2008) are the pre-agricultural era (8000–10,000 BC), the agricultural era (10,000 BC–1850 AD) and the modern industrial era (from circa 1850).

The pre-agricultural era (8000–10,000 BC)

In this period humans were predominantly living as forest dwellers or hunter-gatherers. They lived in small, often familial, groups. There was no settled agriculture and little in the way of communal living as life was predominantly nomadic with small groups moving across open grassland. The main causes of death at this time were exposure and hunting accidents. Diseases were passed to humans through animal vectors and included parasitic invasion, mites and malaria. Malnutrition, starvation and trauma were also common.

The agricultural era (10,000 BC–1850 AD)

The agricultural era covers by far the largest section of human history and is characterized by the development of farming. The ability to grow crops and raise domestic animals led to changes in living patterns and population density, changes in diet, and a growth in social patterns of health and disease and of stress. The major cause of death at this time was infectious disease. The growth in farming allowed people to stay in one place and develop permanent settlements with shelter and a food source. This led to a decrease in the number of deaths from exposure and hunting accidents but led to a dramatic rise in population density as people congregated around farms.

The period between 1340 and 1448 is called 'The Golden Age of Bacteria'. Four forms of infectious disease were prevalent at this time:

- airborne diseases, e.g. measles, mumps, smallpox, tuberculosis, diphtheria
- waterborne diseases, e.g. cholera
- food-borne diseases, e.g. dysentery
- vector-borne diseases, e.g. plague, malaria

The most significant cause of death in Europe at this time was plague.

Towards the end of this era there was a revolution in agricultural techniques with the development of crop rotation, seed drills and land enclosure. This was followed, from 1750, by the Industrial Revolution. The Agricultural Revolution meant that food production could meet the needs of the population increase necessary for the Industrial Revolution. Crude death rates began to decline as there were fewer deaths from starvation and, by the end of the era, infection rates were also beginning to fall.

The modern industrial era (from circa 1850)

The period from 1850 onwards saw a dramatic and unprecedented decline in mortality that has continued right through to the present day. This era was characterized by a decline in farming and a massive explosion in industry and urbanization. Through this period there was a huge drop in mortality from infections and it is suggested that up to 74 per cent of the mortality decline in this period was due to the decline in deaths from infectious diseases. The seminal work on the decline of infectious diseases from a social perspective was carried out by Thomas McKeown between 1950 and 1980. He suggested that it was broad economic and social changes affecting standards of living that best accounted for the decline in mortality from infectious diseases and the population growth experienced from 1700 onwards. Airborne diseases such as pneumonia were first to be affected. This thesis was deemed controversial amongst both medical professionals and public health professionals as it downplayed the roles of both medicine and targeted public health programmes. The debate about the implications of the McKeown thesis is still going on today (see Colgrove 2002).

McKeown (1976) suggested three reasons for the decline in infectious diseases that created a watershed of resistance to infectious diseases. Improvements in nutrition, personal hygiene and public health measures and medical interventions were all seen as important factors but precedence was given to the role of nutrition. There was a significant increase in the amount of food available along with new crops such as carrots, parsnips and potatoes. In addition, the real value of wages was rising, as was the general standard of living. Personal hygiene and public health measures were seen as of secondary importance to nutrition but, nevertheless, sanitation helped to lower the rates of water- and food-borne infections. Housing standards also improved and there was a greater awareness of the role of social factors in disease and in hygiene generally. McKeown saw medical measures and intervention as a minor explanation for the decline in deaths from infectious diseases. Mortality rates were declining for almost all the major infectious diseases before the causes of most diseases were discovered, let alone the development of inoculations or antibiotics (e.g. pulmonary TB, bronchitis, pneumonia, influenza). McKeown did, however, acknowledge the important role played by biomedicine in controlling smallpox (vaccine), respiratory TB (chemotherapy) and diphtheria (widespread immunization).

Diseases in the mid to late twentieth century

It can be suggested that a fourth era in disease patterns can now be identified. As infectious diseases lost importance as a cause of death, degenerative diseases took hold and circulatory disease and cancer are now the major causes of death in Europe. This pattern is illustrated in table 1.1. The overall decrease in death rates through the industrial era and into the late twentieth century can clearly be seen when standardized mortality ratios for selected causes of death are examined. Table 1.1 shows the decrease in deaths by selected causes using the standardized mortality ratio (Registrar General 1990).

What can be seen from this is that across the 100-year period, death rates declined for all causes of death except cancer. There has been a steady increase in the number of both men and women dying from cancer over the past 30 years. The same pattern can be seen when looking at death rates with ischaemic heart disease, neoplasms and cerebrovascular diseases, accounting for almost 40 per cent deaths in 2009 and other top causes including Alzheimer's/dementia and heart failure (Office for National Statistics 2009b). In addition, although survival rates for both circulatory disease and cancer are improving, they remain the most significant causes of death in England and Wales.

The growth in degenerative disease experienced more recently includes conditions that are chronic, with long-term morbidity and quality of life implications. These include cardiovascular disease, cancer, Alzheimer's disease, arthritis and diabetes. The causes of these types of diseases are often social and environmental and include standard of living. Factors such as poor diet have been identified as key risk factors; for example, obesity is a risk factor for a range of conditions including diabetes, bowel cancer has been linked to a lack of dietary fibre, and respiratory disease has been linked to deprivation and poor housing.

Table 1.1 Standardized mortality ratios for selected causes of death between 1890 and 1990 in England and Wales

Cause of Death	1891–1895	1921–1925	1946–1950	1961–1965	1986–1990
Tuberculosis	867	393	157	20	4
Influenza	514	359	57	36	7
Digestive Diseases	750	263	114	75	79
Diseases of the Respiratory System	526	250	93	94	60
Diseases of the Genito-Urinary System	309	226	113	60	35
Diseases of the skin, subcutaneous tissue, musculoskeletal system and connective tissue	671	381	127	97	182
Malignant Neoplasms	–	–	96	103	115
Diseases of the Heart	–	–	93	89	63
Cerebrovascular Disease	–	100	92	95	60
Suicide	137	125	106	112	74

Source: Registrar General's Mortality Statistics, HMSO, 1990.

Discussion Point

• How have our ideas about health, and our expectations about how healthy our lives should be, changed over time? Are people more or less healthy now than they were 100 years ago?

Changing patterns of oral disease

Historical records relating to general health are systematic, although both terminology and methods of reporting have changed over time, making it difficult, although not impossible as we have seen, to chart historical changes in disease. The situation is more complex when trying to chart patterns in oral health and disease over time. There is some data available dating back to the mid nineteenth century that coincides with the period when infectious diseases declined rapidly. The first systematic data were not collected until the 1920s, followed by the big population studies that were carried out in the 1950s and 1960s. When looking at the earlier eras, there is little data on factors such as social status. This said, patterns of oral health can still be distinguished when focusing on the three eras explored within general health (pre-agricultural, agricultural and industrial) (Scambler 2002).

The pre-agricultural era (8000–10,000 BC)

There is some archaeological evidence that both caries and periodontal were present in this era. Caries was found to be minimal, however, due to the non-carcinogenic diet of the time.

The agricultural era (10,000 BC–circa 1850 AD)

In the agricultural era non-refined grains were introduced into the diet, causing early period scoring of occlusal surfaces. Coronal caries was very rare in this time period and evidence of a small number of lesions has been found, mostly in the neck and roots of teeth. After 1500 diets became more refined, which led to increased evidence of pit and fissure caries and decay in inter-proximal surfaces.

The modern industrial era (circa 1850 onwards)

From 1850 onwards there was a dramatic increase in caries. This occurred at the same time as deaths from infectious diseases declined. There was also a big increase in per capita sugar consumption, with rates of consumption rising from 19 lbs per person in 1850 to 100 lbs in 1960. By the end of the nineteenth century caries was endemic and rates of tooth loss were very high (adapted from Scambler 2002).

Contemporary dental health and dental healthcare

From the mid twentieth century onwards tooth loss has steadily declined, and the main focus for the dental profession is now caries and prevention. There has been a big decline in caries since the 1970s and this trend is most significant in young children. As with general health, there have been significant changes in both dental theory and practice over the past century. In simplistic terms there has been a move from:

Extraction	to	Restoration	to	Prevention
(1900–50)		(1950 onwards)		(1970 onwards)

The high rate of extractions from 1918 to 1951 was fuelled by the Focal Infection Theory. This theory stated that both heavily decayed teeth and mildly decayed teeth and gums could cause infection and widespread systemic disorders. This theory is similar to the theories of balance or equilibrium that we saw in general health. Even small amounts of decay could upset the balance of the mouth (Locker 1989).

The shift from extraction to restoration was deemed to be the result of a combination of factors including:

- the demise of the Focal Infection Theory;
- the development of high-speed rotary cutting instruments, enabling crown and bridgework to be done;
- developments in materials and technology to replace even significantly decayed teeth;
- the growth in the size of the dental workforce, reducing dentist/ patient ratios and enabling more time for complex procedures.

1

Alongside these factors there was a growth in the general standard of living, accompanied by higher levels of disposable income. It has been suggested that higher affluence results in more restorations and fewer extractions (Locker 1989). Data from the Dental Estimates Board (1980, cited in Locker 1989) showed that in the ten years between 1970 and 1980, extractions fell by 40 per cent, crowns rose by 380 per cent and deep scaling and periodontal surgery rose by 160 per cent.

If you look at tooth loss you can see changes in both disease prevalence and dental practice. The highest rates can be found amongst older people, many of whom lost teeth in the years prior to the end of the 1940s when extraction was the main treatment mode. For adults, the number of people retaining their natural teeth is a useful indicator of dental health. Between 1978 and 2009 the proportion of edentate adults fell from 22 per cent to 6 per cent and the proportion halved from 12 per cent to 6 per cent between 1998 and 2009 (Adult Dental Health Survey 2009). In addition, people are losing their teeth later, with 1 per cent of edentate 45–54 years olds rising to 47 per cent of those aged 85+. From the 1960s onwards there was also a significant, and largely unanticipated, reduction in the amount of dental caries being experienced across a number of developed countries. There have been significant drops in the rates of decay found in both adults and children and decay in children can be seen to vary by region. Not only are caries rates falling, they are falling faster in the most affluent areas. It has been suggested that the disease is becoming concentrated in diminishing numbers of socially deprived children who are experiencing higher levels of disease (Scambler 2002). Suggested causes for the decline in caries include water fluoridation, more widespread use of fluoridated toothpaste, changes in the levels of sugar consumption, improved levels of oral hygiene and ecological changes and adaptation.

In addition, there has been a growth in the number of cosmetic treatments being offered. This is an area that has already seen marked growth that is likely to continue for the foreseeable future with the rapid development of implant technologies, whitening products and the widespread use of crowns and orthodontic treatments. It has been suggested that this trend will continue, and that as dentists become more successful at treating and eradicating oral diseases they, like doctors, will develop more ways to 'fill' their time.

Discussion Point

- How might the growth of available treatments in dentistry such as those highlighted above affect peoples' perceptions of their oral health? What are the possible implications of this for the provision of dental care in the future?

Models of disease causation

Before outlining the main theories of disease causation that have been developed and followed in Western biomedicine, it is worth reiterating the point that it is not only *patterns* of disease that change across time but *diseases themselves*. Disease categories emerged as social constructions from social categories based on ideas of what is and is not normal. They were based on underlying theoretical models, the two most significant being monism and the localization of pathology. The theory of monism suggested that all disease is due to one underlying cause – usually one of balance – in the solid or fluid parts of the body. If the balance is disturbed, illness will occur. A restoration of balance would then effect a cure and the illness would be eradicated. After monism, medical science developed the theory of localization of pathology. Cases were studied with the aim of constructing diseases out of symptoms and underlying pathologies. *Through this method, one disease became many diseases, each with different causes, and the biomedical paradigm was born.* This, with its reductionist techniques, fragmented the whole (body) into its constituent parts and, with its pathological determinism, focused attention away from the social sphere towards the individual biological body of the newly-created 'patient'. This illustrates the fact that definitions of illness and disease are not self-evident. They emerge in a socio-historical context and need to be understood in relation to that context.

When looking at the main theories or models of disease causation that have been followed since the development of biomedicine, five distinct models can be distinguished:

- The Germ Theory
- The Epidemiological Triangle
- The Web of Causation
- The Theory of General Susceptibility
- The Socio-Environmental Approach

It is worth noting that these reflect a Western, male, approach and are presented chronologically.

The Germ Theory

This is a monocausal theory based on the idea that there is one germ responsible for causing each disease and that if this germ is identified and eradicated then the disease will be wiped out. This theory led to the isolation, identification and eradication of the germs responsible for causing a number of the major infectious diseases including tuberculosis (Koch 1882). In total, the bacilli for 22 further major infectious diseases were identified between 1897 and 1900 (Locker 2008). The Germ Theory was challenged by the fact that certain groups exposed to germs did not go on to develop diseases. In addition, the monocausal theory does not adequately explain the cause of degenerative or chronic conditions.

The Epidemiological Triangle

The Epidemiological Triangle model is a multicausal explanation that looks at the relationship between the agent, the host and the environment. It suggests that the environment can either act as a buffer protecting the host from the agent and thus preventing disease, or that the environment can be the cause of the agent coming into contact with the host and thus can aid the development of the disease. The Epidemiological Triangle model was the first to acknowledge the role played by the environment in which people live in their likelihood of developing disease. Royce et al. (1997), for example, outlined the epidemiological triangle in relation to HIV transmission. Agent factors included the HIV subtype, and phenotypic and genotypic differences, whilst host factors included stage of infection, antiretroviral therapy, host genetics and the presence of male circumcision. Environmental factors included social norms, average rates of sex partner changes and social and economic determinants of risk behaviours such as unsafe sex. Again, the epidemiological triangle is useful as a means of explaining the development of infectious diseases but is less useful when looking at chronic conditions that are more complex.

The Web of Causation

This is a multicausal model suggesting that a range of factors may influence the likelihood of a person developing a disease. The Web of Causation approach suggests there are 'promoters' or factors that make it more likely the disease will develop, and 'inhibitors', factors which protect a person from developing the disease. For coronary heart disease, for example, promoters include diets high in unsaturated fat, high salt intake and obesity, whilst inhibitors include physical activity and polyunsaturated fats (Mausner & Kramer 1985). Many of these 'promoter' factors can be modified. This suggests that prevention may be a more appropriate option than cure in this case. In addition, many of the 'promoters' for coronary heart disease are also risk factors for other diseases. This means that moves to prevent coronary heart disease could have a positive knock-on effect on other diseases such as stroke or cancer (Locker 2008).

The Theory of General Susceptibility

The fourth approach follows neither a monocausal nor a multicausal explanatory path. Rather, the Theory of General Susceptibility explores why some groups are more susceptible than others to a range of diseases. They may look, for example, at what it is about poverty and deprivation that make those living in areas of low deprivation less susceptible to a whole range of diseases. The aim is to discover and isolate protective factors that can then be made available to those communities or populations at higher risk of developing disease.

The Socio-Environmental Approach

The Socio-Environmental Approach was developed in the 1980s and grew out of the Theory of General Susceptibility. This approach is based on the identification of risk factors from the social and physical environments. Thus the focus of the Socio-Environmental Approach is the identification of factors which keep people healthy or put them at risk of developing disease, rather than looking at disease itself. A range of factors has been identified as social and environmental determinants of health. These include:

- *Income and social status.* There is a close association between income and health so that health improves at each step up the income and social hierarchy. In addition, societies with a high standard of living, in which wealth is more equally distributed, are healthier, irrespective of the amount spent on health services.
- *Social support networks.* Support from family, friends and social organizations is associated with better health. Moreover, people living in communities with higher levels of social cohesion tend to be healthier.
- *Education.* Higher levels of education are associated with better health. Education increases opportunities for income and job security and equips people with the means to exert control over their life.
- *Employment and working conditions.* Hazardous physical working environments and the injuries they induce are important causes of health problems. Moreover, those with more control over their work and jobs which involve fewer stress-inducing demands are healthier. However, unemployment, particularly if long term, is associated with poorer health.
- *Physical environments.* The quality of air and water influence the health of populations. So do features of the constructed physical environment, such as housing, roads and community design.
- *Personal health practices and coping skills.* Social environments which encourage health choices and healthy lifestyles are key influences on health as are the knowledge, behaviours and skills which influence how people cope with challenging life issues and circumstances.
- *Healthy child development.* Prenatal and early childhood experiences can have a powerful effect on development and health throughout the lifespan.

- *Health services.* Although not a major determinant of population health, health services can, if appropriately organized and delivered, prevent disease and help promote and maintain health.

(Federal, Provincial and Territorial Advisory Committee on Population Health 1994, in Locker 2008)

These factors can be seen as 'risk conditions' (Labonté 1993) that make a person more likely to develop a range of diseases or to experience poor general health. In addition, behavioural, psychosocial and physiological risk factors have also been identified and are presented in figure 1.1.

The range of factors presented here illustrates the development of what Armstrong (1995) termed 'surveillance medicine'. If medicine is involved as mitigating in all of these circumstances, then the gaze of medicine is focused firmly on the healthy as well as on those with diagnosed disease. The focus of the public health branch of medicine is on those who might potentially become ill or develop a disease at some point in the future. The aim is thus to prevent disease development by mitigating risks. Again it is worth reiterating here that the idea of the influence of social and environmental factors on health is not a new one. Whilst it is relatively recent within the biomedical sphere, it reflects the more holistic approach taken in the Hygeian tradition of the Graeco-Roman approach to medicine, or to forms of Chinese

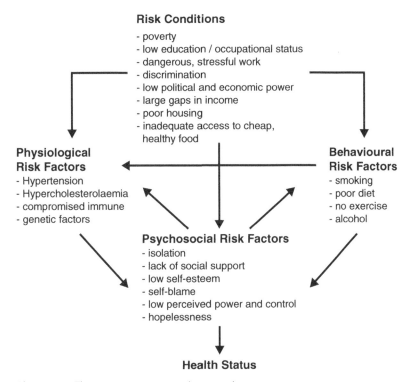

Figure 1.1 The socio-environmental approach
Source: Labonté (1993)

or Ayurvedic medicine, which are more holistic in vision and their approach to ill-health.

Discussion Point

- How might the models presented here be used to explain the concept of 'disease-centred' care as mentioned by Richard in the excerpt at the start of the chapter? Is this a useful model of care?

Conclusion

The argument made in this chapter is not that biological factors are unimportant when looking at oral health and illness, nor that they are less important than social factors. The important point is that patterns of oral health and illness cannot be separated from the social context in which they occur. Thus, if we want to understand patterns of oral health and illness or understand oral health and illness behaviour within populations, we need an understanding of the social context in which these patterns are occurring. Dahlgren and Whitehead (1991) developed a model of the main determinants of health, which is widely used by medical and dental professionals to contextualize the patient body. The model illustrates the importance of social context on many levels, from individual lifestyle factors through to social structures such as socio-economic conditions or environmental conditions. This suggests not only that social context is important but there are many different social factors which act together to affect the likelihood of a person living a healthy life or developing a disease.

Poverty, Inequality and Oral Health

Sasha Scambler

Introduction

There is a wealth of evidence linking poverty with poor general and oral health. A recent statement from the World Health Organization finds that as many as 1.2 billion people across the world live in extreme poverty, and many more live in relative poverty. They state that 'Poverty creates ill-health because it forces people to live in environments that make them sick, without decent shelter, clean water or adequate sanitation' (World Health Organization 2015). Whilst extreme poverty is relatively uncommon in the developed world, the link between poverty and poor oral and general health remains. The

UK-based Health Poverty Action group identifies income levels, where people live, social status and social exclusion as key factors influencing health alongside a variety of social determinants including education levels, access to nutritious food, access to and use of health services, and health behaviours (Health Poverty Action Group 2014). The concepts of poverty and social class or socio-economic status are relational and can be understood through the comparison of different groups of people in society. Thus, fundamental to discussions about poverty and health are the notions of equality and inequality.

The following case study of the Barringdon Estate in North-East England highlights some of the social factors that can be used to think about the relationship between poverty and health.

Box 2.1: The Barringdon Estate

The Barringdon Estate was built in the mid-1960s on the edge of a large town in the North-East of England. The estate has a population of approximately 6,000 people living in low-rise houses, maisonettes and blocks of flats up to eight storeys high. The rate of unemployment in Barringdon is above the national average and average wages are below the national average with the majority of available jobs being low paid and zero-hour contracts. There is a run-down parade of shops in the middle of the estate with a couple of small independent supermarkets. The nearest large supermarket is about 4 miles from the estate.

Most of the children from the estate go to one of the two local primary schools and then on to the large secondary school which also draws from neighbouring estates. The secondary school is currently without a head teacher and does not have a good reputation amongst parents or children for pupil attainment or behaviour. Residents complain of a growing problem of anti-social behaviour with young people – mostly aged between 11 and 15 – 'hanging out' around the parade of shops, making noise and displaying aggressive, threatening behaviour. Some of the older residents on the estate are reluctant to venture out to the shops for fear of abuse: young people on the estate complain about a lack of social venues or activities to engage in locally. Local police statistics suggest that significant numbers of Barringdon residents report being the victims of crime over the past 3 years.

The health needs of the estate are served by the community clinic which accommodates a GP service, a single-handed NHS dental practice and a children's centre. Mortality rates are above the national average in Barringdon, as are the number of people claiming incapacity benefits. Children in the two primary schools in Barringdon have higher rates of tooth decay than children attending schools in less deprived areas of town, and there are low rates of dental attendance across all age groups on the estate.

This case study illustrates some of the social factors identified by the Health Poverty Action Group.

A number of these factors will be explored in this chapter in relation to levels of general and oral health in the community and the provision and use of health services, as well as more generally in relation to life chances and the cycle of deprivation.

The chapter starts with a brief overview of equality and inequality in the UK and beyond in relation to income and wealth, before moving on to highlight some of the different ways in which societies have been stratified across time. The relationship between poverty, inequality and health/oral health are then explored. Why do poorer people die younger than richer people? Why do those with the highest levels of need use services least? Do poorer people simply choose to engage in behaviours which put their health at risk? Should inequality be addressed at the individual or societal level? These questions and more will be addressed in this chapter.

An unequal society

Before focusing on inequality it is useful to think about what we mean by the term equality. Equality is central to modern politics and is the basis on which many of the revolutions of the world have been carried out. The French Revolution, the fight for the abolition of slavery in the United States, the Russian Revolution and the Black Civil Rights Movement were all about different issues and yet all were about equality (White 2007). What is confusing and complex about equality is that it is not a single concept but a collection of ideas, rights or duties:

> [T]he demand for equality is not a demand for a thing, but a demand for many things, and people can disagree about the relative worth of these different things. (White 2007: 4)

White suggests five forms of equality: legal, political, social, economic and moral equality, which may be weighted differently by different people or groups within society. Legal equality requires that all subjects are answerable to the laws of their society, whilst political equality relates to the ways that these laws are decided upon. Social equality refers to social standing and power, and economic equality relates to the ways in which resources are allocated within a society (incorporating ideas of meritocracy, land egalitarianism, ownership of the means of production and so forth). Whilst the first four forms of equality relate to specific forms of social relations, the fifth form, moral equality, can be seen as the motivation behind these demands, that each person is of equal moral worth. Inequality arises where one or more of the five types of equality are not met. For a more detailed explanation of the different forms of equality and the arguments for and against them, see White (2007: ch. 1).

Discussion Point

- Can the different forms of equality highlighted above be related to the experiences of people living on the Barringdon Estate? Can you identify any specific forms of inequality? How might these be addressed?

So how equal are we? Income and wealth can be used as ways of assessing equality and inequality. Income relates to the amount of money earned on a daily, weekly or monthly basis, whereas wealth relates to the assets that a person owns (in the form of houses, land, yachts, etc). Government figures on the distribution of real household disposable income from the 1970s to the 2000s show both that the top 10 per cent of the population earn significantly more than the bottom 10 per cent and also that the gap between the richest and the poorest is getting bigger as the income of the richest is going up at a considerably faster rate than the income of the poorest (http://www.statistics.gov.uk/cci). Further, in the UK children and older people, the two most vulnerable groups in society, are most likely to be living in households with an income below 60 per cent of the median. This is the official cut-off used to define those in poverty. Statistics and a full description of the data can be found on the UK government website (see http://www.statistics.gov.uk/cci/nugget.asp?id=1005).

When looking at wealth, the picture is even clearer. According to recent figures, the top 1 per cent of the population owns 21 per cent of the wealth.

The wealthiest 1 per cent owned approximately a fifth of the UK's marketable wealth in 2003. In contrast, half the population shared only 7 per cent of total wealth. The results are even more skewed if housing is excluded from the estimates, suggesting this form of wealth is more evenly distributed. Wealth is considerably less evenly distributed than income, and lifecycle effects mean that this will almost always be so. People build up assets during the course of their working lives and then draw them down during the years of retirement, with the residue passing to others at their death. (http://www.statistics.gov.uk/cci/nugget.asp?id=2, May 2006)

The evidence here shows clearly the inequality inherent in the UK. In addition, the level of inequality has grown over the past 20 years and the trend shows little sign of reversing as yet.

When looking at the global picture, inequalities within countries and inequalities between countries can be examined. There is little data on the former outside of the main developed countries, but there is clear data on inequalities between countries. What is clear from the statistics is that inequalities exist and are in many cases increasing rather than decreasing. What is also clear, and what we shall go on to explore in some detail in the following sections, is that these inequalities affect not only living standards and quality of life but also life expectancy, health and oral health. Figure 2.1 illustrates this point by comparing income per head and life expectancy in the richest and poorest countries (United Nations Development Programme 2006; cited in Wilkinson & Pickett 2009b).

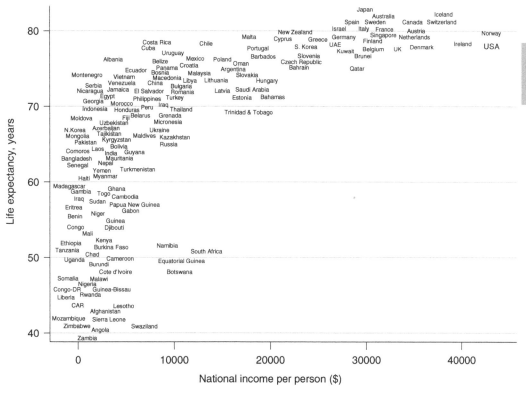

Figure 2.1 Income
per head and life
expectancy: rich and
poor countries
Source: United Nations
Development Programme
(2006); cited in Wilkinson
and Pickett (2009b)

In summary, we live in an unequal society within an unequal world. Not
only are income and wealth unequally distributed, but the gap between the
richest and the poorest is increasing and appears to correlate with higher
mortality and morbidity rates and lower life expectancy.

Social stratification

Inequalities can be found in all types of human societies and in all
regions of the world. These inequalities are not random events and nor
can they be reduced to differences between individuals. The evidence
(as we shall see) clearly shows that groups within society are in unequal
relationships with other groups. In addition, it is clear that these
unequal relationships are relatively stable and persist across time and
space with inequalities tending to continue through the generations.
This patterning of inequality is the basis of the concept of stratification.

Stratification is the differentiation of groups within a population
according to a specified criteria and resulting in a hierarchy, with
those at the lower end suffering in comparison with those at the top
of the system. Populations may be differentiated according to income
levels, wealth, educational achievement or length of education, housing

tenure, type of occupation, etc. Often these patterns will persist across groups, with those who are in a privileged position according to one measure being in a similar position when other measures are taken into account (and vice versa):

> Social stratification involves a hierarchy of social groups. Members of a particular stratum have a common identity, similar interests and a similar lifestyle. They enjoy or suffer the unequal distribution of rewards in society as members of different social groups. (Haralambos and Holborn 2000: 24)

Societies also vary in the severity of the gap between those at the top and the bottom of the hierarchy (in other words, some societies are more equal than others); in the explicitness of the stratification system in use; and the degree of mobility between strata within the system (how easy or difficult it is to move up or down).

Across time, four basic systems of stratification have been identified: slavery, caste system, estates and social class. The following explanations of the different systems of classification have been adapted from the work of Humphrey (1999).

- **Slavery.** This is the system by which some individuals are owned by others as property. The ways in which slaves have been used and the legal conditions under which they were kept and put to work have varied across time and place. In ancient Greece, for example, slaves were not permitted to take up political or military positions but could be found in most other occupations. In the Southern States of the United States, the positions available to slaves were far more restricted with slaves having virtually no legal rights or protection and working almost exclusively as plantation or menial domestic workers.
- **Caste systems.** Caste systems rank people in relation to 'social honour'. Historically, people were born into a particular caste and social mobility was not possible. The position that an individual was born into within the caste system would determine not only the type of occupation that they were able to undertake but also the people that they were able to associate with. In the Hindu caste system found in India, for example, those from the lowest caste were the only ones allowed to have direct contact with animals or substances regarded as unclean. They were therefore disproportionately found in related occupations. At the other end of the hierarchy, those in the highest caste were not permitted certain types of contact with those in the lowest caste. In more recent times, the caste system in India has been used as a framework for affirmative action (de Zwart 2000).
- **Estates.** In this system, the population is split into groups with different rights and duties towards one another, often determined by law. In Europe, a feudal estate system existed from the Middle

2

Ages and consisted of three divisions or strata. At the top were the aristocracy and gentry. The middle strata was composed of the clergy. Although they had less status than those at the top, they had certain privileges which set them above the lowest strata, that of commoners or serfs, free peasants, merchants and artisans. The feudal estate system is often depicted as a triangle with a broad base, signifying the fact that the vast majority of the population could be found in the bottom strata. Limited social mobility was possible within this system with intermarriage or the conferring or purchasing of titles.

- **Social class.** The final system of stratification is known as the class system. In this system socio-economic status is the key to determining people's positions within the hierarchy. Social class is not like the other systems in the sense that position within the system is not dictated or protected by law or religious provisions, and membership of a group is not automatically determined through inheritance. The boundaries between the classes are not rigid as they are determined by a combination of occupation type, social power and prestige and vary across time. Social mobility is relatively easy in this system, unlike the other three systems described, and it is more common for people to move up or down social class.

Power and advantage

Stratification is not simply a way of separating out people within a society. Members of different strata have different life chances, opportunities, quality of life and life expectancy and so it is important to examine different groups and explore why it is that people within those groups have different experiences. One possible explanation is that there are three different forms of power and those who are higher up within a stratification system experience more of all of these types of power. The three basic forms are:

- *Life chances.* Material advantages such as income, wealth, good standards of housing and job security all enhance a person's life chances. Those at the top of the hierarchy are more likely to experience all of these things.
- *Social status.* Status is a measure of characteristics by which one person is judged as superior to another. Although measures of status change over time and according to place, those at the top of the hierarchy are more likely to have high status (in no small part because they are likely to be the group who decides which characteristics convey status).
- *Political influence.* Political influence concerns power over decisions that are made and whose interest they serve. This power may be formal or informal.

Discussion Point

- How might ideas of power and advantage help us to think about the population of the Barringdon Estate? Use the case study presented at the start of the chapter to think about the life chances and social status of the average resident on the estate.

In summary, societies have been stratified in a number of ways across time and space, distinguished by the rigidity of the relationships between the groups and the ability to move between strata. Those at the top of the hierarchy are likely to benefit from more social and political power than those at the bottom.

Measuring socio-economic inequalities

It is clear, then, that there are many different forms of stratification and that human beings are grouped in a multitude of different ways across different countries and regions, using various systems, and across history. Similarly there are a range of measures that can be used when attempting to measure the relationship between socio-economic inequalities and factors such as educational chances or employment opportunities. The two main types of measure utilized in relation to health are deprivation measures and social class.

Defining and measuring deprivation

The term deprivation is one possible way of describing the situation of those groups and individuals who seem to have restricted access to a range of goods and services. Townsend and Whitehead (1988) distinguished between material and social deprivation.

- *Material deprivation*: A lack of goods, services, resources, amenities and a good physical environment.
- *Social deprivation*: Non-participation in roles, relationships, customs, rights and/or responsibilities implied by membership of society or a sub-group.

They went further to develop a measure of material deprivation, incorporating:

- Unemployment: percentage of economically active residents aged 19–59/64 who are unemployed.
- Car ownership: percentage of private households who do not own a car.
- Home ownership: percentage of households not owner occupied.

- Overcrowding: percentage of households with more than one person per inhabitable room (all rooms except the kitchen and bathroom)

The four combined parameters correlate well with area mortality levels.

Two other postcode-based measures of deprivation have been developed: the Jarman (1983) measure and the Carstairs measure (Carstairs & Morris 1991). Both use similar categories and are scored to show levels of deprivation in a given area. The scores are applied to geographical areas and correlated with health ratings for the area, such as levels of dental decay or mortality rates.

Defining and measuring social class

There is a wealth of evidence that social class and other forms of structural inequality in society have a significant effect on health and oral health. The concept of social class is contentious and is used in different ways by different social theorists. Whilst social scientists see all societies as stratified by some system, the most commonly used form of stratification in the UK is social class. When defining social class, there are two key concepts that need to be understood, those devised by Karl Marx and Max Weber.

Marx's concept of class

Karl Marx, the German political philosopher and sociologist, was writing about the concept of class in relation to early capitalist society at the end of the nineteenth century. Since this time his theories have been developed and modified many times by neo-Marxist theories to bring them up to date along with changes in capitalism. Marx's basic model of class is based on the construction of two classes in a relationship of perpetual conflict with one another, the bourgeoisie (capitalist class) and the proletariat (working class). The classes are in conflict but are dependent on one another. They have different interests: the bourgeoisie want higher profits whilst the proletariat want higher wages. Marx suggests that the bourgeoisie manipulate the proletariat via ideology and exploit their labour by making more profit than is given in wages. Because of the profit motive in capitalism, class conflict is inevitable, locally and globally.

Weber's concept of class

Max Weber, another key German philosopher and sociologist, proposed a different view of stratification. His model is multi-focal, highlighting class as a key element but also including status and power. Class relates to a person's occupation, status is the social standing that they have, and power relates to their social power – their ability to shape and have an active say in the running and organization of the society in which they live. These three facets interact with one another to form a model of social class. Weber's model is hierarchical – a model of stratified society where class relates to occupational standing. This includes a measure of occupation type but also social status and power. In Weber's model, occupations form a hierarchy in relation to scarcity of skill and demand in the marketplace, and conflict between classes is mainly between adjacent groups, constrained by forces of relative deprivation.

Weber's model of social class is hierarchical, whilst Marx's is relational, focusing on the interaction between classes. It is Weber's hierarchical model of social class which forms the basis for the measures of social class most often used within research into inequalities in the UK. The first measure (the Registrar General's Scale) was developed in 1911 and was initially introduced as a tool for analysing infant mortality rates. Occupations were allocated to classes according to the degree of skill involved and the social position implied by the occupation. Although the model was used consistently for over 80 years, there were a number of perceived flaws: a focus on status rather than economic class or living standards; a lack of homogeneity within classes; this was a male model of social class using the occupations of married men to classify their wives. In an attempt to address these flaws, the Registrar General Scale was superseded, in 1997, by the National Statistics Socioeconomic Classification.

National Statistics Socio-economic Classification (NS-SEC)

The Office for National Statistics NS-SEC is a model of social class consisting of eight classes or strata:

1 Senior professionals/senior managers
2 Associate professionals/junior managers
3 Other administrative and clerical workers
4 Own account non-professionals
5 Supervisors, technicians and related workers
6 Intermediate workers
7 Other workers
8 Never worked/other inactive

People are assigned to a social class according to a specific set of six criteria which lead to basic categorizations of employers, employees and the self-employed. These include the extent of job security in different occupations; the presence of a career structure with opportunities for promotion, autonomy to plan your own schedule of work and whether pay is monthly, weekly or hourly. Employers are categorized as those who are able to exercise control and authority, employees sell their labour and are under the control of the employees. A further division is categorized by the 'service relationship' between the employer and the employee and the type of 'labour contract' (Bartley & Blane 2008).

2

Discussion Point

• Looking at the different ways of measuring social class presented above, what might the social class profile of the Barringdon Estate look like?

In summary, socio-economic inequalities can be measure using the concept of deprivation or the theoretically derived models of social class. The most widely used measure in the UK is the ONS NS-SEC which is a hierarchical model based on the work of Max Weber.

Social class and health

There is a long history of studying health inequalities by social class in the UK. As far back as 1842, an influential report by Edwin Chadwick highlighted differences in death rates between the social classes with life expectancy ranging from 45 years for gentlemen and professionals to 26 years for tradesmen and 16 years for mechanics, servants and labourers (Chadwick 1842: cited in Bartley & Blane 2008).

One of the most significant studies of the twentieth century to look at inequalities in health was the Black Report (1980). The Black Report catalogued for the first time consistent gradients for mortality and morbidity between the social classes. Men, women and children from lower social classes were more likely to die from almost any cause of death, were more likely to be diagnosed with mental and/or physical illnesses and were more likely to self-rate their health as poor. In addition, the report found that those most in need of health services (those from lower social classes) used the health service least. This reflects work by Tudor-Hart (1971), who coined the phrase 'inverse care law' for this phenomenon. The Black Report was followed by other key reports such as the Acheson Report (1998), which again highlighted the growing gap between the richest and poorest in society in relation to health and life expectancy. The Acheson Report (1998) made public the results of an independent inquiry into inequalities which was the foundation of government strategy on reducing health inequalities (Department of Health 1999; 2000a, 2000b, 2003, 2010).

Regardless of whether you look at mortality, morbidity, life expectancy or self-rated health status, the gradients remain the same and the health of those at the bottom of the class system is worse than that of those at the top. Recent analysis on life expectancy suggests that men and women from social class 1 are likely to live 7 years longer than men and women in social class 5 (80.0 years at birth compared to 72.7 years at birth for men and 85.1 years at birth compared to 78.1 years at birth for women). In addition, they found that between 1972 and 2005 life expectancy increased for all groups but there was a larger increase for those from the non-manual (middle) classes than for those from the manual (working) classes (White et al. 2007). The data in relation to self-reported health status is also clear: those in social class 7 were over twice as likely to rate their health as 'not good' than those in social class 1. The highest rates of poor self-rated health (18.5 per cent rating their health as 'not good') could be found in the long-term unemployed and those who had never worked.

Discussion Point
- Describe what you would expect the broad patterns of ill-health to be in Barringdon and say why you think this is the case.

Mortality

Mortality rates for men (White et al. 2007) and women (Langford & Johnson 2009) were analysed separately using the NS-SEC. The data clearly show that the new NS-SEC model of social class shows the same gradients for mortality as the older Registrar General's Model of Social Class did. White et al. (2007) found statistically significant differences in mortality rates between all NS-SEC classes in a clear socio-economic gradient, with men in unskilled manual occupations (513 deaths per 100,000 in class 7) almost three times more likely to die than those in professional occupations (182 deaths per 100,000 in class 1). When the major causes of death were examined, the same patterns were found. In an analysis of specific causes of death using the NS-SEC, White et al. (2008) found that all major causes of death showed the same gradient, with those who were most deprived experiencing higher level of mortality from circulatory diseases, malignant neoplasma, respiratory diseases, digestive diseases, accidents, falls and suicide. The largest gaps between the most and least deprived were found in deaths from 'ischaemic heart disease, lung cancer, chronic lower respiratory diseases, suicide and all liver disease' (White et al. 2008: 30). In addition, death rates for the highest two classes were considerably lower than the average for all men and death rates for the bottom two classes were considerably higher than the average for all men.

Similar results were found when looking at the relationship between socio-economic status and mortality rates for women using the NS-SEC model. Women from lower social classes are more at risk of dying at all ages than women from higher social classes, whether categorized by their own or (for married women) their husband's occupation. Again women from the least advantaged social class were 2.6 times more likely to die than those in the most advantaged class (Langford & Johnson 2009). The mortality statistics have also been broken down

2

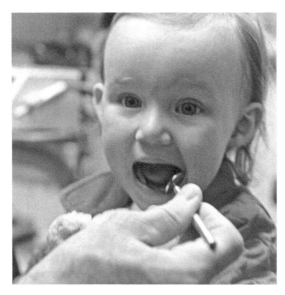

Image 2.1 Children from lower social classes are more likely to have decayed teeth
Source: 'First visit to the dentist', by Dave Buchwald. Own work. Licensed under CC BY-SA 3.0 via Wikimedia Commons.

by region to give figures across the UK. Although these figures are only available for men, they show that, wherever you go in the UK, there are inequalities and there is a clear gradient from social class 1 to social class 7 (Siegler et al. 2008).

> **In summary**, there is a strong and persistent link between inequality and health regardless of the measure of inequality or health used. Not only is there a gap between those at the top and those at the bottom, there is a clear and consistent gradient linking the two.

Child and adult oral health

There is clear evidence that social class affects health and that those with lower socio-economic status have poorer health. Although there are fewer studies available when looking at oral health, those that exist show the same gradients, with those from higher socio-economic groups experiencing better oral health and making more use of oral health services. Data from the 2009 Adult Dental Health (ADH) Survey showed that dental health is worse in the lower social classes than in the higher social classes and that there is a clear gradient. Taking the mean number and condition of teeth as an example (see table 2.1), adults from the highest social classes are more likely to have sound and undecayed teeth, and filled but otherwise sound teeth, than those from the lower social classes. This is likely to reflect both better oral health but also more frequent and active oral healthcare amongst those from the higher social classes.

Table 2.1 Mean number and condition of teeth by social class 1998–2009								
	Present	21 or More Functional %	Sound & Undecayed %		Decayed or Unsound %		Filled but otherwise Sound %	
	1998	2009	1998	2009	1998	2009	1998	2009
I, II, IIInm Managerial/ Professional	25.4	91	15.4	18.2	1.2	0.7	7.6	7.6
III m Intermediate	24.2	85	14.8	17.0	1.7	–	6.9	7.3
IV,V Routine/ Manual	23.6	79	15.3	17.5	1.9	1.3	5.7	5.7

Source: Adapted from Adult Dental Health Surveys 1998 and 2009

As with general health, considerable research is being undertaken to explore the relationship between socio-economic status and oral health in more detail in an attempt to understand the factors that create the relationship. A study by Sabbah et al. (2009), for example, used American data to explore the role of behaviours on inequalities. They found that there was a clear socio-economic gradient for all behaviours affecting oral health (including smoking, diet and frequency of dental visits). When adjusted for behaviour, however, they found that the relationship between socio-economic status and oral health attenuated but did not disappear, suggesting that inequalities in oral health are about more than simply behavioural differences between the socio-economic groups.

When looking at children's dental health, the same patterns can be found as in the adult population, although the picture is more mixed as many children across all social classes have dental decay and many do not. In general, children from lower social classes are more likely to have decayed teeth and older children from lower social classes are more likely to have unmet orthodontic need. Summarizing the key findings from the 2003 Children's Dental Health survey, Steele and Lader (2004) stated that:

> The prevalence of dental decay is associated with social factors, with children from more deprived backgrounds or from lower social status groups being substantially more likely to have decay in most age groups, with the differences most clear cut amongst younger children. At an individual level and when comparing just the children with decay, there is also a suggestion that more teeth are affected amongst children from less affluent backgrounds.

They also found that 15 year olds from routine manual backgrounds had twice as much unmet orthodontic treatment need (26 per cent) as those from professional backgrounds (13 per cent).

The same gradient can be found when using alternative measures of socio-economic inequality. The percentage of children with decayed

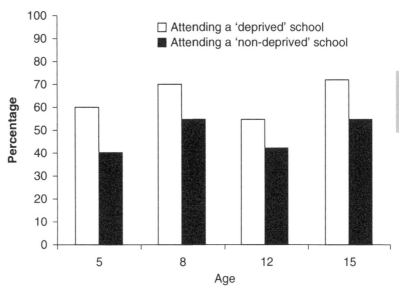

Figure 2.2 Percentage of children with decayed teeth attending schools in deprived and non-deprived areas

Source: http://www.statistics.gov.uk/cci/nugget_print.asp?ID=1000

teeth attending schools in deprived areas is consistently higher, across all age groups, than the percentage of children with decayed teeth in non-deprived schools, for example (see figure 2.2).

Overall, children from lower socio-economic groups were more likely to experience tooth decay, were more likely to have teeth extracted because of decay, and were twice as likely to have unmet orthodontic need than their wealthier peers.

Discussion Point

- If you were taking over the dental clinic in Barringdon, what interventions might you put in place to lower rates of decay amongst the children on the estate?

Access and service utilization

People from higher social classes are consistently more likely to attend the dentist regularly, whilst those from lower social classes are more likely to attend symptomatically and irregularly (Adult Dental Health Survey 2009). Whilst the number of people attending the dentist regularly has risen consistently since 1989, the gradient has remained the same (see table 2.2).

Unsurprisingly, working-class adults are also more likely to experience trouble meeting the costs of dental treatment and are more likely to attend irregularly. These issues are compounded by a perceived negative attitude towards working-class patients from dentists and a shortage of

Table 2.2 Dental attendance by social class				
Percentage who reported regular dental attendance				
	1989	1991	1993	2009
Managerial and professional	60	61	63	66
Intermediate	56	54	55	62
Routine and manual	39	39	43	55

Source: Figures for 1989, 1991 and 1993 adapted from Drever and Whitehead (1999); for 2009 from Adult Dental Health Survey (2009)

NHS dentists. Although dental contracts were changed in 2006 in an attempt to rectify this situation and make more NHS dentists available, a recent independent review (Steele 2009) suggests that the changes have not been successful and that further changes to the dental contract are needed to ensure that those who are most vulnerable and have the highest levels of unmet dental need receive the care that they need.

What the data presented here show is that there are clear socio-economic inequalities in oral health across the life-course and affecting both oral health status and access to and use of dental health services, just as there are when we look at general health. Some of the possible explanations for this are explored below.

Possible explanations for socio-economic inequalities in health and oral health

There is a pattern to the relationship between social class and health and between social class and oral health. This relationship is socially structured and not one of random distribution. This being the case, it is necessary not simply to chart the relationship between the two but to look for possible explanations as to why it is that social class affects health in the way it does. Moreover, an explanation is needed that covers the breadth and depth of the relationship, the fact that there is a gradient between social class and mortality, morbidity, life expectancy, self-reported health status and so forth. The fact that the pattern exists does not, in itself, imply causation, so further exploration is needed in order to understand the underlying factors which 'cause' this relation-ship. The seminal 'Black Report' suggested four possible explanations for the relationship. Two of these (the social selection explanation and the artefact explanation) have largely been discredited but the materi-alist and behavioural explanations are explored in more detail along with the two explanations that are in more popular contemporary use together with a further interesting thesis. The five proposed explana-tions or 'explanatory models' are:

- The Materialist Model
- The Behavioural Model
- The Psychosocial Model
- The Life-course Model
- The Wilkinson and Pickett Thesis

The Materialist Model

The materialist model is based on the premise that people from the lower social classes are systematically exposed to less material resources than those from the higher classes. They are materially deprived. At the same time they are also exposed to more hazards in the social and physical environment (people from lower social classes are more likely to live in areas of high pollution and overcrowding; live in damp housing; work with hazardous materials, etc.) and they do not have the material resources to protect themselves from, or mitigate the results of, such hazards. This model was the one favoured in the Black Report (1980). There is considerable evidence to show a link between material deprivation and poor health. Taking diet as an example, there is evidence that purchasing power affects the types of food that people are able to buy, and that those from lower social classes, with less disposable income, are more likely to buy foods high in sugar and refined carbohydrates (Barratt 1997; Turrell 1998). Diets consisting of large quantities of these types of food have been shown to be a risk factor for both oral and general health.

Further to this, in order to see the full impact of material deprivation on health, we need to take a life-course approach to exploring the relationship between social class and health. It takes considerably less money to buy enough food to survive in the short term than it does to buy the types of food needed to maintain health over a longer period. The results of persistent material deprivation need to be studied to get a true picture of its impact on health (Bartley & Blane 2008). In a review of health policy implemented to reduce health inequalities globally, Crombie et al. (2005) looked at policies in place in 13 countries. They found that policies on taxation and tax credits, old age pensions, sickness and rehabilitation benefits, maternity and child benefits, unemployment benefits and housing policies were the most important for reducing inequalities in health. All of these policies would fall under the remit of the materialist explanation.

The Behavioural Model

The behavioural model is built on the premise that material factors alone are not sufficient to explain the relationship between inequality and health and that we also need to look at elements of culture and behaviour. Behaviour can be either health-promoting or health-damaging and this model suggests that lower social class groups are more likely to engage in behaviour that is damaging and vice versa. This model is sometimes referred to as the cultural/behavioural model, as behaviour is shaped by the culture in which people live. Different types of behaviour are promoted or discouraged depending on the culture and this will affect the likelihood of individuals from within that culture engaging in that behaviour (Bartley & Blane 2008). This model posits the theory that health-related behaviours, such as smoking, excess alcohol consumption, poor diet and a lack of exercise, lead to inequalities in health. There is certainly considerable evidence to link these kinds of factors with health and oral health (see Elstad 1998; Watt & Sheiham 1999a,b; Bartley 2004). Other behaviour such as the uptake of immunizations, the use of contraception, or the use of preventive oral health measures such as flossing, have also been shown to vary with social class. This model has proved very popular, and policies and health promotion strategies developed by both the Conservative and Labour governments over the past 30 years have included behaviour change as a key element in reducing inequalities and/or improving health across the board.

Longitudinal studies focusing on behaviour have found, however, that behaviour accounts for only about a third of the differences in health between social classes (Bartley & Blane 2008). This suggests that the model is important but not sufficient in itself to explain the relationship. In addition, behaviour is shaped by the social and economic culture in which it occurs:

> Diet is influenced by both cultural preferences and disposable income. The ability of nicotine to maintain a constant mood in situations of stress and monotony might predispose towards cigarette smoking in repetitive and highly supervised occupations. (Bartley & Blane 2008: 126)

Following on from this, there is a danger that this model could lead to individualist or 'victim-blaming' attitudes towards ill-health and that responsibility could be unfairly apportioned to individuals. It is essential that we understand the social norms and values that act as constraints on people's behaviour and that the central value-system of society is a middle-class one. We need to avoid constructing norms and attendant behaviour from lower social classes as deviant (Scambler 2002).

The Behavioural Model has had a big impact on the way that we view inequalities and has been dominant within oral health research in the area (Towner 1993; Pearce 1996; Jarvis & Wardle 2006; Watt 2007). Davey Smith et al. (1990) suggested that the Behavioural and Materialist models cannot realistically be separated as explanations for the relationship between social class and health. For example, when looking back to the early 1900s, cigarette smoking used to be more prevalent amongst the middle classes and yet the social class gradients for mortality were similar to those we find today (Bartley & Blane 2008).

The Psychosocial Model

This model suggests that any understanding of inequalities in health needs to take into account the presence or absence of psychosocial risk factors such as social support, stress, levels of control and autonomy at work and the home/work balance (Bartley & Blane 2008). It is argued that lower socio-economic status directly affects psychosocial well-being and that this has a direct biological effect on health. People from lower socio-economic groups are more likely to experience multiple negative life events which impact on their psychosocial well-being and thus on their health. These include having occupations where they have little control or autonomy, having little job security and living in areas of high deprivation with 'lower levels of trust and higher levels of crime and anti-social behaviour' (Sisson 2007: 84). These negative life events can be posited to affect health directly through chemical changes to the body or indirectly through triggering damaging health or lifestyle choices or behaviours (Elstad 1998). This explanation is growing in popularity within oral health research, with links drawn between stress and periodontal disease (Aleksejuniene et al. 2002; Mengel et al. 2002), sense of coherence and poor oral health behaviours (Freire et al. 2001, 2002) and between work and/or marital stress and poor oral health behaviours (Marcenes & Sheiham 1992).

The Life-course Model

Until relatively recently, time aspects of the study of inequalities in health have largely been ignored. This means that traditional models for explaining social class inequalities in health have failed to adequately address the issue of the accumulation of disadvantage over time. In order to address this caveat, the Life-course Model was developed. The model is based on the premise that disadvantages experienced at any stage in the life-course cannot be understood outside the context of what has gone before and we need to study people from conception onwards to understand the causes of their deprivation (Krieger 2001). Health inequalities can thus be understood as a combination of materialist, behavioural and psychosocial factors and the ways in which these factors interact over time (Sisson 2007). Disadvantages may either be seen to have accumulated over time or to be the result of critical episodes which affect future development. Either way, this model suggests that we will not be able to tell the relative impact of the different key factors (material, behavioural or psychosocial) until we have studies which follow whole cohorts throughout their life-course, allowing us to see which factors impact at what point and their effect or effects. This model has been adopted both to look at the impact of children's circumstances on their oral health in adulthood (Poulton et al. 2002; Sanders & Spencer 2005) and specifically focusing on gingival status (Nicolau et al. 2003) and traumatic dental injury (Nicolau et al. 2003) in adolescence.

The major criticism of this model is that it is based on the flawed theoretical premise that changes in individual behaviour within a life-course are the key to improving health and reducing inequalities. As Sheiham and Watt (2000) argue, this ignores the fact that most determinants of oral health are far wider that simply behaviour. They further suggest that a wider approach is needed to deal with the social structures which shape our oral health. In his 2007 paper, Watt suggests the need within dentistry to move from 'victim blaming to upstream action' if the social determinants of oral health inequalities are to be tackled. He suggested that we need to move away from individual level interventions focusing on behaviour, or psychosocial factors, and look at upstream solutions more in line with the policies highlighted by Crombie et al. (2005).

Revisiting equality: the Wilkinson & Pickett thesis

A final approach that is worth exploring is posited by Wilkinson and Pickett and falls into the structural category of explanations for inequalities in health. Wilkinson and Pickett (2009a) use international research data to demonstrate that inequality is bad for almost all members of society and not just those at the bottom. They suggest that the extent of inequalities within societies, the gap between the richest and the poorest, radically affects not just health but a whole range of factors including violence, larger prison populations, drugs and obesity. They start their argument by using nationally collected statistics to demonstrate that health is related to income differences within countries but not across countries. Data previously presented show the gradient between poor health and inequality in the UK. If rich countries are compared to one another, however, it makes no difference how much richer the richest people in one country are than the richest in another. In other words:

> differences in average income or living standards between whole populations or countries don't matter at all, but income differences within those same populations matter very much. (Wilkinson & Pickett 2009a: 13)

To illustrate this, the richest countries in the world were ranked according to the gap between the richest 20 per cent and the poorest 20 per cent in each country. When ranked, it is clear that levels of inequality vary widely across countries, with the richest 20 per cent in Japan earning just over three times the income of the poorest 20 per cent and, at the other extreme, the richest 20 per cent in Singapore earning almost 10 times that of the poorest 20 per cent. It is also worth noting that the US and the UK are the second and fourth most unequal societies, respectively, whilst the Nordic countries are clustered at the top of the table as the most equal countries.

Wilkinson and Pickett then developed an index of health and social problems for which data are available across the 21 richest countries in

Health and Social Problems are Worse in More Unequal Countries

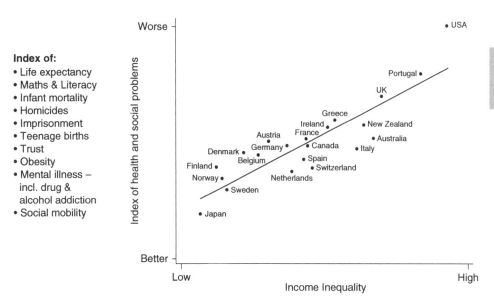

Index of:
- Life expectancy
- Maths & Literacy
- Infant mortality
- Homicides
- Imprisonment
- Teenage births
- Trust
- Obesity
- Mental illness –
  incl. drug &
  alcohol addiction
- Social mobility

Figure 2.3 Health and social problems are worse in more unequal countries
Source: Wilkinson and Pickett (2009b)

the world. The data were combined by country (with each item in the index having the same weight and positive measures such as life expectancy being reverse-scored to ensure that a higher score indicates poorer outcomes). What they found was that the most unequal countries had the highest levels of health and social problems (see figure 2.3). (Sources of data for the index can be found in box 2.2.) In addition, levels of health and social problems are not related to average incomes amongst the richest countries. The role of inequality thus seems obvious.

When looking at the data presented in this way, the resulting relationship is clear:

> there is a very strong tendency for ill-health and social problems to occur less frequently in the more equal countries. With increasing inequality (to the right on the horizontal axis), the higher is the score on our Index of Health and Social Problems. Health and social problems are indeed more common in countries with bigger income inequalities. The two are extraordinarily closely related – chance alone would almost never produce a scatter in which countries lined up like this. (Wilkinson & Pickett 2009a: 20)

The authors then document the same relationship when looking at: trust; child well-being; mental illness; drug use; life expectancy; infant mortality rates; levels of adult obesity; educational scores; teen pregnancy rates and teen birth rates; homicide rates; imprisonment rates; and environmental issues. It is not the level of wealth in a country but the level of inequality in the country which is key. They conclude with the following statement which both outlines their vision for the future and suggests a strategy for moving forward:

Box 2.2: Sources of Data for the Index of Health and Social Problems

Component	International data	US state data
Trust	Percent of people who respond positively to the statement "most people can be trusted" 1999–2001 World Values Survey Reverse-coded	Percent of people who respond positively to the statement "most people can be trusted" 1999 General Social Survey Reverse-coded
Life expectancy	Life expectancy at birth for men and women 2004 United Nations Human Development Report Reverse-coded	Life expectancy at birth for men and women 2000 US Census Bureau, Population Division Reverse-coded
Infant mortality	Deaths in the first year of life per 1000 live births 2000 International Obesity TaskForce	Percentage of the population with BMI >30, averaged for men and women, 1999–2002 Estimates from Prof Ezzati, Harvard University, based on NHANES and BRFSS surveys
Mental health	Prevalence of mental illness 2001–2003 WHO	Average number of days in past month when health was not good 1993_2001, BRFSS
Education	Combined average of maths literacy and reading literacy scores of 15 year olds 2000 OECD PISA Reverse-coded	Combined average of maths and reading scores for 8* graders 2003 US Department of Education, National Center for Education Statistics Reverse-coded
Teenage birth rate	Births per 1000 women aged 15–19 years 1998 UNICEF	Births per 1000 women aged 15–19 years 2000 US National Vital Statistics
Homicides	Homicide rate per 100,000 Period average for 1990–2000 United Nations	Homicide rate per 100,000 1999 FBI
Imprisonment	Log of prisoners per 100,000 United Nations	Prisoners per 100,000 1997–8, US Department of Justice
Social mobility	Correlation between father's and son's income 30-year period data from 8 cohort studies London School of Economics	N/A

Source: Wilkinson and Pickett (2009b)

The rich developed societies have reached a turning point in human history. Politics should now be about the quality of human relations and how we can develop harmonious and sustainable societies. (Wilkinson & Pickett 2009a)

This thesis presents a new and challenging way of looking at the relationship between socio-economic inequality and health and offers a different approach to reducing such inequalities. This work has created a huge amount of debate and polarized comments from the political left and right as to its validity. The consensus, however, seems to be that we need to look beyond individuals at the wider social structures shaping society if we want to address the range of issues correlated with inequality, not least that of general and oral health.

Conclusion

This chapter presents evidence for the relationship between social class, poverty and oral health. Data is used to demonstrate the clear gradient between social class and health, life expectancy, morbidity and use of health services. Furthermore, explanations presented suggest that whilst individual behaviour and psychosocial risk factors play a part in this relationship, much of the gradient can be accounted for by factors outside the control of individuals, requiring a structural approach to reducing inequalities. Furthermore, Wilkinson and Pickett's work suggests that this is the case globally and for a range of 'social problems' not restricted solely to issues of health. This has huge implications for public health, which focuses predominantly on targeted interventions and behaviour change and less on structural changes. Even upstream measures such as water fluoridation and policy initiatives on widening access for vulnerable groups do not come close to the kind of redistribution of wealth needed to reduce health and social inequalities if the materialist explanation proposed by Black (1980) is to be acted upon, or the individualist ideology of capitalism that is critiqued in the work of Wilkinson and Pickett (2009a) is to be challenged.

Gender and Oral Health

Sasha Scambler

IN THIS CHAPTER YOU WILL LEARN ABOUT:
- ▶ The profile of women in contemporary society
- ▶ The gender patterns of health
  - ▶ Mortality differences
  - ▶ Morbidity differences
  - ▶ Illness behaviour
- ▶ The relationship between gender and oral health
  - ▶ Dental health beliefs, attitudes and behaviours
  - ▶ Dental consulting
- ▶ Explanations for gender inequalities

Introduction

Gender is one of the key social divisions in all societies. In this chapter we consider the impact of gender on oral health from the wider perspective of the position of women in contemporary society. In this context it is important to understand the terminology and the distinctions between specific terms that we commonly see in use. The terms sex and gender are often used interchangeably, but in fact have distinct meanings. The term 'sex' relates to the biological differences that result in the male and female forms. Gender, however, is a term that is used to refer to the way in which society understands and has created a complex of meanings around the biological division of sex. As Scambler (2002) states, 'Gender encompasses a nexus of rules and values about the way the two main genders should behave, think, feel and dress, and what roles they should play in the public sphere of work and the private domestic sphere' (p. 44).

It is also worth bearing in mind that feminists focus our attention on the fact that the concept of gender itself is a social construction that

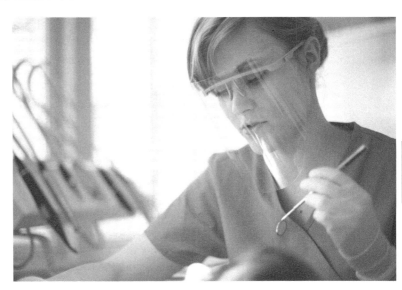

Image 3.1 The proportion of female dentists is rising
Source: Anna Jurkovska

has been created within a patriarchal system. This means that ideas about the roles of women in society, and the power, status, resources and expectations that they have access to are shaped by a society in which masculinity predominates and women have been subordinated as non-males. If we want to understand the relationship between gender and health or oral health we first need to have an understanding of the relative positions of men and women in contemporary society.

The following factfile illustrates the changing profile of dentistry across parts of the developed world and some of the debates sparked by the so-called 'feminization' of dentistry.

Box 3.1: Women in Dentistry – Facts and Figures

- In the US, women now make up almost half of all dental students and a quarter of practising dentists. Prior to the 1970s, fewer than 3 per cent of American dentists were female, the lowest percentage in the developed world (Sindecuse Museum, University of Michigan (2015) Women Dentists: Changing the face of dentistry. Available at: http://dent.umich.edu/about-school/sindecuse-museum/women-dentists-changing-face-dentistry).
- By the end of the 1970s approximately one-third of dentists in Norway, Sweden, Denmark and France, and half of dentists in Greece were female. Almost 80 per cent of dentists in Finland, Russia, Latvia and Lithuania were female (Carlisle 2015).
- Over half of UK dental students are female and over 50 per cent of dentists under the age of 35 are female. It is estimated that by 2020 half of all UK dentists will be female (Health and Social Care Information Centre 2012).
- Special Care Dentistry and Paediatrics are the only two dental specialities where women outnumber men, however, and men still dominate in the

> specialities which are perceived to have higher status. Over 70 per cent of dentists in oral surgery are male (General Dental Council 2013).
> - Male dentists contribute more working hours across their careers than female dentists. There are minimal differences in working hours prior to career breaks, but female dentists are more likely to take career breaks and more likely to reduce their hours once they return to work after taking a career break (Robinson et al. 2011).
> - Over 60 per cent of female and just over a quarter of male dentists take a career break (Newton et al. 2001).

This factfile illustrates the changing face of dentistry over the past few decades with increasing numbers of women entering the profession. This has led to a debate about the 'feminization' of dentistry as a profession and to some discussion about the implication of this on the future of the profession and the provision of dental care. A recent paper by McKay and Quinonez (2012) drew on Canadian data to suggest that the 'feminization' of dentistry could lead to dentists being less entrepreneurial, more focused on the work/life balance and could lead to the availability of fewer hours of clinical time for patients.

Gender impacts on both dental professionals and wider patterns of oral health within the population. Why is it that women live longer than men and yet experience more self-reported ill-health and use general and dental health services more? How can we explain differential use of oral health services amongst men and women? What is the link between gender and inequality? And how can this be explained? These are just some of the questions addressed in this chapter. The chapter starts with a brief overview of the gendered social context in which we live and work before moving on to look specifically at the relationship between gender and general and oral health. Potential explanations for gender patterns and inequalities are then presented and discussed.

Women in society

Women's and men's working lives are becoming increasingly similar. There are, however, clear demographic differences between them. Boys outnumber girls and in the latter years women outnumber men, with the population balancing out between 15 and 64 (see table 3.1).

When we look at the oldest old people, what becomes clear is that women make up the vast majority of this group. In the 85+ age group, women outnumbered men by 5 to 2. In addition, it is interesting to note that 72 per cent of men over the age of 65 were married in comparison with 44 per cent of women over the age of 65. This could be explained by a combination of the facts that men tend to marry younger women and that women live longer than men. Taking this into consideration, the average wife is younger than her husband

Table 3.1 Age Structure for Men and Women in 2011		
Age	Males	Females
0–14 years	51%	49%
15–64 years	50%	50%
65–79 years	44%	56%
80+ years	30%	70%

Source: Table 1, 2011 Census: Usual resident population by 5-year age group and sex, United Kingdom and constituent countries, ONS, 27 March 2011

3

and can expect to live longer. Gender distribution is one of the most important factors when looking at the older population, as we will see in chapter 4.

Women and power

The relative positions of men and women within society become evident when you look at power and some of the areas where power is exercised in society. Taking the central, or government, level of power in Britain as a starting point, it is interesting to look at the relationship between women and politics. British women gained the vote and the right to stand for election in 1918, but only women over the age of 30 and with additional qualifications were given the right to vote at this time. It was not until 1928 that women got the vote equally with men at the age of 21. If you look at the situation globally, what is clear is that, even with something as basic as voting, rights have only been extended to women gradually across the twentieth century (see table 3.2). In the United States of America, for example, although women were given the right to stand for election in 1788, it was not until 1920 that they were given the right to vote.

What is interesting about table 3.2 is that the reality of the equality in voting rights of women in different countries does not necessarily coincide with popular stereotypes. When the figures are broken down by individual countries, there are some surprising results. The USA, for example, ranks (at best) 68th out of 134 nations. In contrast, the most equal country is Rwanda with women making up 48.8 per cent of the lower house and 34.6 per cent of the upper house. In addition, out of the 186 states, only 13 have a female Head of Government and women only have limited rights to vote in Lebanon and United Arab Emirates and have no right to vote or even to appear before a judge without male representation in Saudi Arabia (International Women's Democracy Centre 2008b). Further details can be found on the 'Women's political participation factsheet' produced by the International Women's Democracy Centre, available at http://www.iwdc.org/resources/fact_sheet.htm.

The number of female Members of Parliament in the UK reflects the changing position of women in relation to power, but also

Table 3.2 A timeline of women's suffrage for selected countries	
Date	**Countries**
1900s	Australia (1902 with restrictions), Finland (1906),
1910s	Norway (1913), Denmark, Iceland (1915), Austria, Estonia, Georgia, Germany, Hungary, Kyrgyzstan, Latvia, Poland, Russian Federation (1918), Belarus, Luxembourg, Ukraine (1919)
1920s	Albania, Czech Republic, Slovakia, USA (1920), Armenia, Sweden (1921), Kazakhstan, Mongolia (1924), Turkmenistan (1927), Ireland, United Kingdom (1928)
1930s	South Africa (1930 Whites), Spain, Sri Lanka (1931), Maldives, Thailand (1932), Brazil, Cuba (1934), Philippines (1937), Uzbekistan (1938)
1940s	Dominican Rep (1942), Bulgaria, France, Jamaica (1944), Croatia, Italy, Japan (1945), Vietnam (1946), Pakistan, Singapore (1947), Belgium (1948), China (1949)
1950s	India (1950), Greece, Lebanon (1952), Syria (1953), Belize, Ghana (1954), Ethiopia, Peru (1955), Egypt, Somalia (1956), Malaysia (1957), Tunisia (1959)
1960s	Cyprus, Gambia, Tonga (1960), Sierra Leone, Paraguay (1961), Australia, Uganda (1962), Iran, Kenya (1963), Sudan (1964), Afghanistan, Botswana (1965),
1970s	Switzerland (1971), Bangladesh (1972), Jordan (1974), Angola, Mozambique (1975), Portugal (1976),
1980s	Iraq (1980), South Africa (1984 Coloureds and Indians), Namibia (1989)
1990s	Samoa (1990), Kazakhstan, Moldova (1993), South Africa (1994 Blacks)
2000s	Kuwait (2005), United Arab Emirates (2006 for advisors not those with power)

Source: International Women's Democracy Centre, 2008. http://www.iwdc.org/resources/suffrage.htm

demonstrates that the situation, whilst clearly improving, is by no means one of equality. Looking at the percentage of MPs who are female by year from 1945, it can be seen that up to 1997 only 9.2 per cent (n=60) of the 600+ MPs were women. The instigation of women-only shortlists by the Labour Party prior to the 1997 General Election led to a significant increase in the number of female MPs (up to 18.2 per cent, n=120), but such shortlists have since been judged illegal. A total of 101 female MPs represented the Labour Party after the 1997 election. By 2012, almost a quarter of MPs in the UK were female, and of the 145 women MPs elected, 49 were Conservative, seven were Liberal Democrat, 81 were Labour and five represented other parties (A. Scambler 2008; Cracknell & Gay 2013). This puts the UK parliament 11th out of the 27 EU Member States and 55th in the world, on a par with Malawi.

The same picture can be seen when you look at the representation of women in other positions of power both within Parliament and beyond. Figures from the UK Government Equalities Office 2012 show that women make up:

- 51 per cent of the population
- 5.6 per cent of the black and minority ethnic population
- 12.5 per cent of directors of FTSE 100 companies

- 26.7 per cent of the top 200 positions within the Civil Service
- 14.3 per cent of senior police officers

The picture is clear, even in what is considered one of the most equal societies in the world in relation to the position of women: women are enormously under-represented in every area when you look at the most powerful and highest status positions.

If you look at dentistry, what you see is that the number of women entering the profession has gone up dramatically in the last few years and there are now more female undergraduate dental students than males in the UK and many other developed countries. Whilst a majority of current qualified and practising dentists are male (61 per cent compared with 39 per cent female), when this is broken down by age, the changing gender demographics of the workforce can be seen. Fifty-four per cent of dentists currently practising in the UK and under the age of 30 are female (46 per cent male), whilst 86 per cent of dentists over the age of 60 are male (14 per cent female) (Office for National Statistics 2007).

3

Discussion Point

- The factfile at the start of the chapter illustrates the growth in the number of women entering the dental profession. How does this fit with patterns for other professions?

Income inequality

When you look at figures from 2007 in relation to the pay gap between men and women in different industries, what becomes clear is that the inequality does not relate only to positions of power but also to levels of pay. For example, figures from the Office for National Statistics (Self & Zealey 2007; Leaker 2008) show that whilst 79 per cent of those who work in health and social care are female, men in this sector earn 32 per cent more on average than their female counterparts. In education 73 per cent of the workforce is female and there is a 12 per cent pay gap, whilst in construction only 10 per cent of the workforce is female and there is a 12 per cent pay gap. If you divide the jobs according to private or public sector employers, what you find is that 41 per cent of those working in the private sector are female and the pay gap is 22 per cent, whilst 65 per cent of those working in the public sector are female and the pay gap is 13 per cent. Women are also disproportionately likely to be found in part-time positions that tend to be lower paid, with lower status and less additional benefits (sick pay, holiday entitlement, company car, private health insurance, gym membership, etc.).

Women are also more likely to be in receipt of benefits than men and still carry the bulk of caring and household tasks within the home as well as participating in increasing numbers in paid work outside of the home (Scambler 2002). In 1997 the Office for National Statistics calculated that:

- People in Britain spend 1.5 times as long doing unpaid jobs around the household than they do in paid work.
- Valued as paid employment, this equals £739 billion per annum.
- This would more than double the GDP of the country if it were added to it.
- AND women do twice as much of this work as men.

Clearly both inequalities in paid and in unpaid work lead to the levels of income inequality that have been identified.

The public and private spheres

One of the ways in which differences between the occupations (and related power, status and income) of men and women have traditionally been explained is through reference to division of society into two related spheres of activity. These have been termed the public and private spheres. These two sectors developed with the onset of capitalism and became entrenched in the latter part of the nineteenth century. The world of paid work became increasingly separated from the domestic sphere, both geographically and by gender. Initially this happened in the upper and middle classes, where it became a mark of status to have a non-working wife acting as a mother and home-maker and spiritual keeper of the family. This tied in neatly with work roles. The public sphere consisted of paid work, was predominantly male and was centred around production. Whilst the type of work that people do has changed, and the number of women working in the public sphere has increased dramatically, the distinction between the public and private spheres still remains. The institutions that create a functioning society are found in the public sphere.

'Real' work took place outside the home and what went on inside was differentially valued and called 'working for love'. Unpaid work in the private sphere was carried out predominantly by women and included reproduction and nurture of children, encompassing both their physical and moral well-being. Caring roles, whether for children or older parents, paid or unpaid, are still predominantly carried out by women and seen as low status.

Discussion Point

- The figures presented at the start of the chapter show that female dentists are more likely to take career breaks than their male counterparts. How might the public/private sphere roles be used to help explain this?

Another factor which plays a role in gender inequalities is the changes in family structure that have taken place over the last few decades.

The changing family

The size and shape of families has changed significantly over the past 40 years, reflecting not only the gender distribution in our ageing population but also reflecting changes in the constituent parts of families themselves. The rate of marriage has declined by 42 per cent since 1972. Alongside this, the age at first marriage has increased, with an average age of 29 for women and 32 for men by 2007, a rise of 6 years from 1971. Linked to a fall in the number of people getting married is a rise in the number who are choosing to cohabit. This figure has risen from 12 per cent in 1986 to 24 per cent by 2006. Not only are the number of people choosing to get married falling, but the number of marriages lasting the course is also falling. Divorce rates have risen by 50 per cent since 1972 and over 40 per cent of all marriages now end in divorce. This has had a knock-on effect on families, and now less than a quarter of all households in the UK comprise what would be recognized as a 'traditional' or nuclear family of two parents and dependent children. Seven per cent of households are single-parent families and, of these, 90 per cent consist of single mothers and their dependent children. If you look at this from the other side, it means that almost 25 per cent of dependent children live in lone-parent families and the vast majority of them live with their mothers (Self & Zealey 2007).

Explaining income inequalities

Attempts have been made to explain why it is that women earn less than men on average and that they are disproportionately likely to be found living in poverty. One suggestion is that female income is limited by the gender roles that we assume men and women do/can/should participate in. This is known as the 'Gendering of Poverty Thesis' (Scambler 2002), the main points of which are presented below:

- Unpaid work in the household limits the capacity for paid work.
- Lifetime earnings are substantially reduced.
- Unpaid work is more compatible with balancing paid and unpaid work, but is paid less and many workers get little or no holiday entitlement, sick pay or pensions.
- Women get less overtime and bonus pay because of their caring work obligations.
- Women get less access to company cars, shares, health screening and insurance, sports clubs and subsidized canteens.
- Pensions are lower because of gendered roles and low earnings. Women's weekly retirement income is on average 47 per cent less than men's.
- Women are disproportionately dependent on social security benefits.

In addition, evidence is emerging that austerity and cuts to welfare in the UK in 2012 are disproportionately affecting women. What is clear from this is that a combination of factors around our conception of male and female roles, both within the private sphere of the family and the public sphere of paid work, conspire to reduce the amount of income available to women in comparison to their male counterparts.

> **In summary**, despite significant improvements in the position of women globally in recent years, they are still under-represented in positions of power, get paid less, are more likely to be in receipt of benefits and living in poverty and are more likely to juggle public and private sphere roles than their male counterparts.

Explaining gender inequality

A range of suggestions have been made as to why women are consistently disadvantaged and suffer inequality when compared to men. The main explanations given are the biological determinist explanations, Lukes' power explanation, and a range of feminist explanations. These are explored in more detail below.

Biological determinist explanations

These explanations suggests that it is the fundamental biological differences between men and women that are the foundation for gender inequalities in society. The focus is on four different levels of biological differences, which are all seen to impact on the differential roles, experiences and life chances of men and women. These are:

- physical differences: men are bigger and stronger and therefore better at certain types of jobs;
- reproductive differences: men and women have different biological functions, and women are constrained by their mothering role;
- physiological differences: men and women are emotionally different – women are too emotional for certain roles;
- genetic differences: men's and women's social roles are controlled by the genetic imperative – women need a husband and men need to spread their seed (Scambler 2002).

These foundations are based on traditional gender stereotypes to the extent that they incorporate both the biological differences between men and women and the assumed social differences that tie in with these biological differences. Whilst it is clearly the case that women carry and give birth to children, it is no longer the case that women need to take sole or even the main role in raising children. It can be argued that this is a social decision rather than a biological one. Even where a mother chooses to breast feed her baby, technology has made it relatively easy to express milk, which can be frozen and stored, and so there is still no need for the mother to take the main caring role. Decisions that are made will depend, amongst other things, on the presence of the father, finances, preferences, family and/or societal pressures and so forth.

Lukes' Three Levels of Power (1974)

Another possible way to explore the subordination of women is to look at the arrangement and exercising of power within society. Lukes suggests three faces of power:

3

- *Visible or overt power by force or public decisions*: Power is easy to see at this level, women may be excluded by rules, or laws or quotas. This type of power includes domestic violence and rape, and also the legal systems that affect the ways in which these crimes are dealt with.
- *Distorted or agenda-setting power*: This type of power is less easy to see. Eighty to ninety per cent of the workers that gained from the introduction of the minimum wage in the UK were women, and yet the minimum wage was not defined as a gender issue; it was defined economically. It has been suggested that issues that are important for women often fail to make the political agenda. For example, childcare was, and to an extent still is, defined as a private matter, and rape in marriage was not made illegal in the UK until 1991.
- *Hidden or ideological power*: This is the most insidious level of power. Ideology controls our perceptions and we have defined the male as the norm. Language is gendered, citizenship is a masculine attribute and ideologies create images of the ideal wife or mother. These hidden powers can be seen in the images of the ideal women portrayed in adverts and arguments over size zero models or airbrushing. Within health it has been argued that women accept the male norm for mental health and see themselves as lacking.

All of these types of power can be seen to promote the subordination of women to men, or the continuation of gender inequality.

Discussion Point

- How might the patterns of power presented here help to explain the figures presented at the start of this chapter? Why are women underrepresented in higher status specialisms within dentistry? Is this changing and if so, why?

Feminist explanations

Four key feminist schools of thought have provided alternative explanations for the inequalities faced by women in contemporary society.

Liberal feminism

Liberal feminism forms the backbone of the feminist movement. They contend that gender inequalities have developed from a traditional focus on overt biological differences between men and women that have led to stereotypes emerging about the proper roles for men and women and false ideas about lack of intelligence, emotionality and so on. Liberal feminists campaign for education, legal and civil rights' changes. These are the feminists who campaigned for the vote, for the Sex Discrimination Acts and so forth. Despite this legislation, we still see a great deal of inequality in society today, however, and other theories emerged in the 1960s to explain the perceived lack of success of liberal feminism.

Marxist feminism

This form of feminism developed from the work of the social and political theorist Karl Marx and focused on capitalism. Marxist feminists suggested that women, in their traditional roles, were useful to capitalism because they maintained the household, including the male workers, and reproduced the next generation of labour force workers at low cost to the capitalist system. They were also able to act as a reserve army of labour when the economy needed extra workers.

Whilst this strand of feminism is a useful critique of capitalism, it does not explain where the traditional view of the role of women came from. It also needs amending or updating to take account of changes in work, such as the laying off of men from full-time, relatively secure work to be replaced by women doing part-time, low-paid contract work.

Radical feminism

This theory asserts that the other forms of feminist theory have failed to explain the persistence of discrimination against women. Pay was not increasing, there was a glass ceiling at work and men were still not doing an equal share of unpaid work within the household despite the emergence of equality laws and the increasing numbers of women working in paid employment outside the home. Radical feminism focused on the concept of patriarchy. They suggested that the implementation of new laws would not be successful on its own because the power structure of the whole social system was controlled by men and in the interests of men. They highlight disparities such as the lack of women in the most influential positions at the top of all of the main institutions in society, such as Parliament, the law, industry and the City, science and so forth.

Radical feminists also point to the gendered language that we use (mankind, chairman, the fellowship of man, etc.) and they focus on the family as the lynchpin of women's subordination. They suggest that women, in their domestic role, reproduce their own inferiority by socializing children and maintaining the institution of patriarchy.

Socialist or dual-systems feminism

This theory states that the forces of capitalism and patriarchy act separately and not together and that they both work in concert to suppress and oppress women. Thus it is suggested that socialism is needed to break this pattern and promote equality.

> **Discussion Point**
>
> • How might the different schools of feminism address the issue of the feminization of the dental workforce? How would they explain current trends?

The fracturing of feminism

Recently there has been a backlash against these feminist theories of gender inequalities. Male studies have developed and the focus has been on boys doing badly at school and on 'girl power' (think of the Spice Girls!). Whilst there have undoubtedly been changes, there is little doubt that fundamental inequalities remain, and yet feminism as a force has been severely weakened.

Sub-groups have appeared, focused on groups such as black and gay women. The postmodern perspective, which suggests that all grand social theories are merely social constructions that can never explain the ever-changing complexities of the social world, has also contributed to the demise of feminism. Postmodern feminism has denounced the notion of a widespread patriarchy, focusing on the local empowerment of women and thus encouraging separatism and weakening the wider cause. Following on from this, post-structuralist feminism emphasizes the ambiguity of gender and sexuality and rejects the gender binary. The fluidity of personal identity is emphasized, allowing women to define feminism for themselves, incorporating personal identities.

As can be seen from the picture presented here, there are wide social and economic differences between men and women and their relative positions, influence and power in society. Although a number of improvements have been made to boost the position of women in society, inequalities remain, particularly in relation to income and power. In the next two sections the position of women in relation to health and to oral health will also be considered.

> **In summary,** a range of theories have been put forward to explain why women are consistently disadvantaged and suffer inequality when compared to men. All but one of these explanations focus on the norms, expectations and power relations that shape the social roles adopted by men and women.

Women and health

The evidence shown above illustrates inequalities between the men and women in society in a whole variety of ways, including power and income. Given these overarching inequalities it could be expected that there are also inequalities between men and women in relation to health. What is interesting about health inequalities in relation to gender is that, in spite of the widespread subordination of women to men that we looked at in the previous section, women live longer than men. Not only do women live longer, the difference is so great that even with the social class gradient, women from the lowest social class live longer than men from the highest social class.

The differences do not end here, however. The evidence suggests that not only do women live longer than men, they also suffer from more ill-health throughout their lives. Thus the saying, 'women sicken, but men die' (Scambler 2002). Table 3.3 shows the relative differences in life expectancy and healthy life expectancy between men and women. What is interesting about these figures is that whilst women live on average 3.6 years longer than men, they spend 1.8 more years in poor health than men and 2.5 more years with disability. So, whilst women experience more ill-health than men overall, they still, on average, spend more years in good health than men.

Table 3.3 Life expectancy, healthy life expectancy and disability-free life expectancy at birth by sex in the UK, 2002

	Males	Females
Life expectancy[a]	77.7	81.9
Healthy life expectancy[a]	63.0	65.0
Years spent in poor health[a]	14.7	16.9
Disability-free life expectancy[b]	62.3	63.9
Years spent with disability[b]	14.6	17.4

Sources: [a] Office for National Statistics (2011a); [b] Office for National Statistics (2009b)

As already mentioned, women live longer than men and to such an extent that women from the lowest social class live longer than men from the highest social class. Thus gender has a greater protective effect than social class. It is also worth noting that these figures reflect a picture that is found across Western, developed countries. In many developing countries the gap in life expectancy between men and women is much closer and in some Asian and African countries the gap is reversed with men living longer than women. This being said, women outlive men in the majority of countries across the world. In the UK, life expectancy rates are still rising and the gap in life expectancy between men and women is falling, slowly.

The main gender differences in mortality

The statistics consistently show that mortality is greater in males of all ages. Acheson (1998) illustrated the mortality differences between the genders. He suggested that the gap between men and women would be even greater if it were not for the high mortality rates associated with cancers which hit only (or overwhelmingly) women, such as cancers of the uterus, cervix or breast. Acheson found that between the ages of 1 and 15 the excess in male mortality is mainly due to accidents, injury or poisoning. By the age of 15, boys have a 65 per cent higher mortality rate than girls. This gap remains throughout adulthood, with men aged 20–24 having a mortality rate 2.8 times higher than women, again mainly due to motor accidents, other accidents and suicide.

The most common causes of death for both men and women in the UK between 1971 and 2005 were circulatory diseases, including the cardiovascular diseases, coronary heart disease and stroke. The rate of deaths from circulatory diseases has come down dramatically in both men and women during this time, and by 2006 cancers had overtaken circulatory diseases as the largest cause of death for women (Office for National Statistics 2009b). Interestingly, a relationship between decreased income and increased rates of cardiovascular disease has been found in men over the age of 35, but the same relationship has not been found in women. In fact, for women, rates of cardiovascular disease were highest for women in the highest income group. Mortality rates for men and women by leading causes of death are shown in figure 3.1.

The second most common cause of death for men and women between 1971 and 2005 was cancer, which became the most common cause of death for women from 2006 as death rates from cardiovascular disease fell. Death rates from cancer tend to be lower in females than males, which tends to reflect the types of cancers that men and women get, the risk factors associated with these different types of cancers and their survival rates (Office for National Statistics 2009b).

Rates per million population

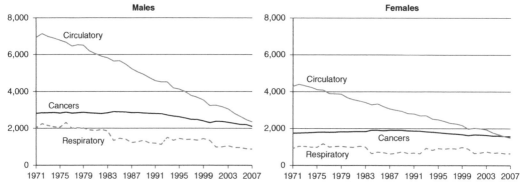

1 Data are for all ages and have been age-standardized using the European standard population.

2 Data for 2000 are for England and Wales only.

Figure 3.1 Mortality[1] by sex and leading cause groups, United Kingdom[2]

Sources: Office for National Statistics (2009b, 2011a)

Explaining gender differences in mortality

When it comes to explaining mortality differences, both biological and social/gender roles are implicated. It has been suggested that men are more likely to take part in dangerous or hazardous activities both at work and as part of their leisure time and that these activities are more likely to result in death. Hazardous working conditions or environments have been linked to mortality through accidents, dangerous machinery, hazardous environmental conditions and so forth. Men are more likely to work in fields associated with these kinds of risks such as the construction or mining industries, fishing or oil rig work. In addition, men working in these kinds of industries are more likely to come into contact with toxic chemicals or other substances which carry long-term risks related to cancers and respiratory diseases (A. Scambler 2008).

It is not just in employment that men encounter situations which are hazardous to their health. Men are also more likely to participate in dangerous leisure activities than women and they consume more alcohol than women, with 24 per cent of men and 13 per cent of women drinking over the recommended weekly limit (Office for National Statistics 2006). Men are also more likely to smoke than women, although this trend is reversed in the younger age groups: in 16–19 year olds 23 per cent of men and 26 per cent of women smoke. Men drive more, drive faster and account for 60 per cent of road casualties (Office for National Statistics 2006). They are more prone to accidents generally than women, have higher suicide rates, are more likely to be the victims of violent crime and murder and take less good care of their health (Office for National Statistics 2009a, 2009b). All of these factors impact on the differences in mortality rates between men and women. It is worth bearing in mind, however, that these 'gender role based' explanations are not static and change across time and place. Women are increasingly participating in more dangerous leisure activities and the number of women who smoke has also increased. The mortality rate for women from lung cancer is rising, whilst that for men is dropping.

Gender differences in morbidity

The morbidity differences reported between men and women are small but nonetheless consistent. Women are more likely to report long-standing illness and limiting long-standing illness than men, and men are more likely to rate their health as 'very good' or 'good' than women in studies measuring self-reported health status. Conversely women are consistently more likely to rate their health as 'not good', although again the difference between men and women is small (Office for National Statistics 2004). Further to this, women are also 2–3 per cent more likely to suffer from long-standing illness than men and 4 per cent more likely to suffer limiting long-standing illness than men over the lifespan. However, there is a clear male excess up to the age of 14, and a clear female excess throughout the childbearing years (15–44) and then up to the age of 74, when men catch up (Self & Zealey 2007). Thus, whilst women experience relatively more long-term and limiting long-standing illness across the life-course, there are fluctuations at different (and specific) points in time.

Approximately 1–3 per cent more women consistently report problems with pain, with mobility and with self-care and in performing 'normal' daily activities such as getting up, washing, dressing, bathing, etc. (Office of Populations Censuses and Surveys (OPCS) 2002). Alongside higher rates of physical morbidity, women also report more mental health problems with 7 per cent more women reporting anxiety and depression over the life-course (OPCS 2002), and women over the age of 16 being more likely to use out-patient or community mental health services than men (Office for National Statistics 2009b). Overall, the consensus is that there are gender differences in morbidity but that these may actually be smaller than the research implies and may be an artefact of the way in which women are viewed by society and the medical profession.

Gender differences in illness behaviour

So far we have seen that women live longer than men but suffer more ill-health over the life-course. In addition to this, women also exhibit different illness behaviour to men. Women are more likely to consult a health professional than men, they consult more for each condition that they have, and they take more prescribed drugs. In a survey carried out in 2005, 16 per cent of females and 11 per cent of males had seen a General Practitioner (GP) in the 14 days prior to the data collection and women averaged five GP consultations a year while men averaged only three (Office for National Statistics 2005a). Women consult more for mental health problems, particularly anxiety and depression, and are over twice as likely as men to have treatment for depression. They also consult more for preventive care (after controlling for reproduction), self-examine more and take more health supplements (General Household Survey 2005).

The above data demonstrate gender differences in general health across all measures: mortality, morbidity and health behaviour. Now we move on to consider the evidence on gender differences in oral health.

> **In summary**, women live longer than men, and are less likely to die than men at all ages, but are more likely to suffer from long-term and long-standing limiting illnesses than men. Men are also less likely to access healthcare services, take prescription drugs or engage in self-care practices.

Women and oral health

For more than a decade dental studies have shown that gender has a significant effect on subjective dental health experiences, although there is still a dearth of good data on differences in clinical dental health by gender. Studies suggest that women experience more communication problems with their dentists and report higher levels of worry, pain and other symptoms. This is very similar to the findings on general health. Overall, it is suggested that women suffer a greater impact from oral disorders than men. It has been suggested (Covington 1996) that the genders have different oral health needs but that the use of a male norm has decreed that teeth are gender-neutral. Covington suggests that it is, in fact, unlikely that teeth are gender-neutral given the depth of gendering around body image and experience more generally. She illustrates gender differences by pointing out that the main gender differences highlighted by dentists relate to pregnancy gingivitis. She further suggests that women's medical problems are often misdiagnosed, ignored or trivialized by medical practitioners and asks whether this also happens in dentistry. She notes that it is difficult to find research specifically on women's experience of dentists and that often, in multi-factorial studies, gender is sidelined.

Gender differences in oral health

A number of differences can be identified when comparing the dental health of men and women in the UK. Women in the UK have poorer dental health than men (although the reverse was found to be the case in Scandinavian countries). Women also suffer more coronal caries and less surface root caries than men (Redford 1993) and have more fillings than men across the age ranges. Women have less periodontal disease than men and suffer lower levels of gingivitis, except during pregnancy. They also suffer less from oral cancer than men but are more likely to be edentulous. The most recent Adult Dental Health Survey (2009) shows that gender was not found to be a significant predictor of the number of sound and untreated teeth in young adults. Men were more likely to have teeth that were unrestorable and more women (7 per cent) than men (5 per cent) were found to be edentulous, although age would have to be taken into account here, as we have already established that women live longer than men and the older you are the more likely it is that your teeth will fall out. The 2009 Adult Dental Health Survey also found that men are more likely to smoke and more likely to have high sugar intake and have more calculus than women, and women are marginally more likely to have excellent oral health (9 per cent of men and 11 per cent of women).

Studies from America (Nowjack-Raymer & Gift 1990) seem to show that women, irrespective of ethnicity, have worse access to dental care, more dental disease and worse diets than men. Similar studies by Todd and Lader (1991) and Downer (1994) in the UK also indicate that women's dental health may be poorer than men's. In contrast, studies from various Scandinavian countries indicate that women have better dental health than men (Scambler 2002). Kent and Croucher (1998) indicate that edentulism seems to be a greater problem in women than in men, but it is unclear whether this is a social class effect (women are poorer than men), or purely to do with age, or could it be due to women's relative lack of status in relation to health professionals? It is clear that more data is needed if we are to draw definitive conclusions about the link between gender and dental health status.

Dental health beliefs, attitudes and behaviour

Differences between men and women have been found in studies exploring a range of factors related to dental health, from prevalence of dental anxiety to dental health and illness behaviours. Some of the key differences with related studies are presented below.

Dental anxiety

One of the reported differences between men and women relates to the incidence of dental anxiety. Various studies have found a correlation between women and higher levels of dental anxiety. Liddell and Locker (1997), for example, found that dental anxiety relating to the fear of a future experience of dental pain had a higher incidence amongst women than men. A study in Germany similarly found that women are more likely to be dental-anxious than men but that it is previous painful experiences that are most likely to trigger the anxiety (Enkling et al. 2006).

Aesthetics and eating disorders

It has also been suggested that gendered concerns with body image may lead women towards the adoption of better oral hygiene practices than their male counterparts. It can, however, also lead to higher rates of eating disorders such as bulimia or anorexia nervosa, which have been associated with oral health problems. Both Nunn (2007) and Studen-Pavlovich and Elliott (2001) highlight the particular challenges posed to oral health by these disorders and also the fact that eating disorders of this kind are disproportionately found amongst women.

Atypical facial pain

Atypical facial pain is an interesting condition (or group of conditions) which appears to affect significantly more women than men. Studies in the United States such as that by Zakrzewska (1996) suggest that between 25 and 45 per cent of the adult population is affected by this condition at some point in their lives and that the female to male ratio amongst 30–59 year olds is 4:1. Agostoni et al. (2005) also suggest that atypical facial pain is much more common amongst women and older people, due to the impact of oestrogen levels. Atypical facial pain is thought to be stress-related and manifests itself as non-muscular and non-joint-related aches and pains in the face, head and neck, which can spread to other parts of the body.

Temporomandibular joint (TMJ) disorders

This is a diffuse syndrome of pain of a variety of different types, which affects the craniofacial muscles, causes the jaw to 'stick' and can cause limitation of function in this area. As with atypical facial pain, this condition is diagnosed disproportionately amongst women and has been related to stress and depression (Scambler 2002). In a study of female dental patients in the United States, Zakrzewska (1996) found that the number of women diagnosed with TMJ disorders is three times the male rate, with a ratio of 5:1 found in those requiring hospital treatment. This raises the question of whether the diagnosis or reporting of conditions such as atypical facial pain or TMJ disorders could be related to the stereotyping of female patients. Thus this would be an interesting area for future research.

Hormonal, menstrual and childbirth oral health effects

In addition to the conditions outlined above, there are some oral conditions found in women that seem to be related to the reproductive system. Menstrual gingivitis and progressive periodontitis are often problems found in younger women. Some oral contraceptives also cause gingival changes in women of childbearing age. Pregnancy is also related to the problem of gingivitis, with bleeding gums recognized as a common side-effect of pregnancy (Christensen et al. 2003). In the UK this has led to the provision of free dental care for women whilst they are pregnant and for the first year postpartum.

Dental hygiene

3

Research evidence suggests that oral hygiene levels amongst women are higher than those amongst men. Sakki et al. (1998), for example, found that women brushed their teeth more often than men and were less likely to take sugar in coffee and tea. In addition, Davidson et al. (1997) found that women are more likely than men to use a range of oral hygiene aids within the home and on a regular basis. In this North American study, women were also found to clean their teeth more often than men and to floss and use mouthwash more frequently. These earlier studies reflect the findings of the most recent UK Adult Dental Health Survey (2009), which also found that women are more likely to clean their teeth regularly, and are more likely to use additional oral hygiene aids, whilst men are more likely to have high sugar intake levels.

Gender and dental consulting

The evidence outlined above suggests both that there are various conditions that are more common amongst women than amongst men, and also that women make better use of oral hygiene measures and practices within the home. In addition to this, evidence from a variety of countries suggests that women also consult dental professionals more than men, are more likely to seek preventive care and are more likely to have teeth restored. A report by the Department of Health, Social Services and Public Safety (2004) raised concerns that men were less likely to be registered with dentists than women, with almost one in five men failing to register with a dentist. They suggested further that this mirrors reluctant use of a range of other health services by men. The difficulty of accessing appointments during the working day, cultural norms making it difficult for men to admit to feeling pain and a lack of confidence in discussing health issues were all suggested as potential reasons for the lower rates of dental consulting by men.

Earlier studies produced similar results. Steele et al. (1996) found that there is a north/south divide in England with the most significant differences between men and women in the north of the country. They found that men were less likely to opt for restoration, were less worried about edentulism and visited dental professionals less frequently than women, and that these differences were more pronounced in the north than in the south. A similar study in Finland (Sakki et al. 1998) found that men consulted less than women. This finding was also replicated in Canada (MacEntee et al. 1993), where they found that men were more likely to attend symptomatically, particularly when in pain, whilst women attended for preventive care.

There are very few studies that focus fully on gender differences in oral health and oral health behaviour. Women tend to be included more in samples of ethnic minority groups or older people rather than as a group in their own right. Of the studies that have specifically looked at women, the majority focus on pregnant women and new mothers. In 1991, Rogers carried out a study of dental attendance amongst pregnant women in Birmingham. Five hundred women were interviewed postpartum to look at dental care during pregnancy, the justification being that dental care is seen as a way to promote better maternal health but also to instruct on the dental health of the new baby. The results showed that only 61 per cent of the women interviewed had visited the dentist during pregnancy in spite of the fact that 96 per cent of the sample were aware that their dental care at the time was free. This suggests that free care is not enough, on its own, to encourage dental attendance. Previous patterns of dental attendance were strongly influential and the study found that non-attenders were most likely to be previous irregular attenders, Muslim mothers, first-time mothers or those from lower socio-economic groups.

A Danish study carried out in 2004 similarly found that, whilst the majority of pregnant women in their survey had good oral hygiene and attended the dentist regularly, there was a lack of awareness of the increased likelihood of gingivitis during pregnancy and the need for increased oral care (Petersen et al. 2004). Similarly, a study of Kuwaiti pregnant women found that a large proportion of the pregnant women sampled had oral health problems during their pregnancy but only half sought dental care at this time (Honkala & Al-Ansari 2005). In a similar study in Manchester in 1992, Crawford and Lennon focused on dental attendance amongst mothers in an area of deprivation. Only 44 per cent of the mothers in the sample had attended the dentist in the previous 12 months, but 61 per cent of their children had seen a dentist during this time. This suggests, interestingly, that mothers may make some attempt to obtain dental care for their children even whilst avoiding it themselves, although attendance of mothers tends to correlate well with attendance of their children. A study in Japan found that women were more likely to engage in good oral health behaviours (tooth brushing, flossing) than men (Tada & Hanada 2004).

Scambler (2002) summarized seven main gender differences in relation to dental attendance and consulting behavior. Women attend the dentist more often than men and make more visits for preventive care or to see the hygienist, whilst men are more likely to attend for symptoms. Women brush their teeth more frequently and use other methods of cleaning such as dental floss or mouth wash. Women eat less sugar, drink less alcohol and smoke less.

A range of possible explanations has been suggested as to why women consult with dental professionals differently from men. It could be that women are more frequent attenders at dental surgeries because they are more anxious about their health in general and they report higher levels of worry, pain and symptoms relating to their oral health. It has also been suggested that women attend dental appointments more frequently because they make appointments for, and take their children to visit, the dentist. Case studies also suggest that men of all ages are less concerned with their oral health than women. The explanations presented here are possible explanations for gender differences but it is important to read these in the context of a very limited body of research specifically exploring gender differences in oral health and oral health behaviour. More research is needed in this area before the explanations given above can be substantiated or discredited.

In summary, there are few studies which focus on the relationship between gender and oral health. There is, however, some evidence that women are more likely to suffer from a range of oral diseases but are also more likely to engage in positive oral health behaviours.

Conclusion

This chapter provides some insight into the impact of gender on health and oral health within the context of an unequal society. The chapter started with an illustration of the fact that we do not live in an equal society (locally or globally) despite gender discrimination legislation. Women are under-represented in positions of power and are more likely to be found in lower status poorly paid work. The health statistics demonstrate that women live longer than men, but experience relatively more general and dental health problems over the life-course. Women also consult doctors and dentists more than men, are more concerned and informed about health issues and also engage in more preventive action. Whilst there is a considerable amount of research exploring the relationship between gender and health, there is a dearth of literature focusing specifically on gender differences in oral health and most of the studies that do exist focus on pregnant women and mothers rather than on gender more generally. The aim of this chapter, therefore, has been to set out the context within which more research is needed, particularly in light of recent changes in smoking and alcohol consumption amongst women and the potential impact of this on oral health.

Ethnicity and Oral Health

Sasha Scambler

> **IN THIS CHAPTER YOU WILL LEARN ABOUT:**
> ▶ What the terms race and ethnicity mean and how they are used
> ▶ The profile of black and minority ethnic groups in the UK
> ▶ The relationship between ethnicity and health
> ▶ The relationship between ethnicity, oral health and oral health care
> ▶ Explanations for ethnic inequalities in oral health

Introduction

In previous chapters we have started to unpick some of the ways in which society is stratified and the social groups into which people are either placed or place themselves. We have looked at social class, socio-economic status and gender so far and now we turn our attention to ethnicity. Ethnicity is another way in which we group people within society and is used as a tool for looking at the impact of various social factors such as culture, religion, language and immigrant status on health and oral health. When we talk about ethnicity, however, a number of different groups are often taken together, and in the UK the phrase 'black and other minority ethnic groups' (BME) is used as a shorthand to refer to the many different sub-groups represented.

The term minority is used in a specific way in sociology to refer to a group of people who share distinct characteristics and are exposed to inequality because of these characteristics. They occupy low social status because of prejudice and/or discrimination and this can be seen in all areas of social life, from education to employment levels to health. The BME population in the UK is one group that can be classified as a minority in the sociological sense along with groups characterized by social class, sexual preference, age and disability. It is important to note that the term 'minority', when used sociologically, is not a numerical measure and a minority group is one that holds low status in relation to other groups regardless of size. In this chapter we explore the implications of ethnicity and BME status on health and oral health with a specific focus on inequality.

The following case study highlights the importance of social contextual knowledge in thinking about the health and oral health of people from BME groups, focusing on the description of an encounter in a dental clinic.

Box 4.1: A Clinical Encounter

Mrs S, a 53-year-old woman of Bangladeshi descent, makes an appointment to visit her local dental clinic as she is experiencing pain in her mouth and one of her teeth feels loose. Mrs S is accompanied to her appointment by her daughter Amolika.

On entering the clinic for her appointment, Amolika explains that her mother is in some discomfort and is concerned that one of her teeth is going to fall out. The dentist asks when Mrs S last visited for a check-up, but neither Mrs S nor her daughter can remember.

An initial examination shows signs of gingivitis. The dentist raises his eyebrows, looks Mrs S straight in the eye and asks how well she is caring for her teeth as the evidence clearly shows that she is not flossing her teeth regularly as she should. The dentist asks Mrs S why she does not look after her teeth properly and asks whether she owns a toothbrush. He further tells Mrs S that her plaque and gingival scores are very worrying and that not looking after her oral health may lead to chronic periodontitis. Amolika translates what the dentist says to her mother and then translates Mrs S's answer back to the dentist. Amolika explains that her mother brushes her teeth every day and that she showed her mother how to do it after a dentist visited her school.

Further examination shows signs of a worrying patch of sore skin in Mrs S's mouth. The dentist asks her how long she has had it and whether she smokes or drinks alcohol. Amolika discusses this with her mother and explains that her mouth has been sore for several months and that she does not drink alcohol or smoke. The dentist asks Amolika whether her mother chews betel nut and she says yes. The dentist explains to Mrs S that he is concerned about the sore in her mouth and will refer her to the local dental hospital for further investigations. He tells her she will receive a letter with an appointment date and time from the hospital. Amolika explains this to her mother who looks worried as she leaves the surgery.

This case study highlights some of the social, clinical and practical considerations that need to be taken into account when providing care for people from different ethnic minority groups in a clinical setting. The UK, like many other countries, is becoming increasingly multicultural as people move more freely and easily across the world in search of new opportunities. This raises specific issues for people providing healthcare in an ethnically and culturally diverse community. This chapter starts with a brief overview of key terms and their meanings before providing an overview of ethnicity in the UK as an example of the potential implications of minority status in this context. Issues relating specifically to health and oral health are then explored.

Defining terms

The terms 'race' and 'ethnicity' are often used interchangeably along with other confusing terms such as 'cultural diversity' and 'minority status'. It is worth being clear what is meant by these terms from the outset to avoid confusion.

Race

The term 'race' has been used in an attempt to categorize and define groups according to their genetic homogeneity. Racial categories can only be used, however, to make broad statements about general racial characteristics, referring to loose categories such as 'caucasian'. Biological differences between the groups are restricted to features that do not affect the basic nature of the 'human being' such as skin colour, bone structure or hair type (Scambler 2002).

Ethnicity

In contrast to race, 'ethnicity' is a social concept which is applied to social groups. Members of these social groups are seen to share common characteristics associated with 'race' or physical appearance but also include the unique *culture* of the group. Ethnicity can be seen to relate to groups of people who share:

- cultural heritage
- common language
- religion and values
- customs
- common history including a homeland outside of the UK
- they may also be aware of a sense of 'difference'

In this context culture is taken to incorporate the organization of the family, group traditions, styles, musical and literary preferences, religious practices and so forth. An ethnic group may be defined in terms of a dominant cultural characteristic, for example religion or language. Thus the Jewish community might be defined by the former and the Gaelic speakers of the Scottish Islands by the latter.

The complexity of the concept of ethnicity was captured in a definition offered by Yinger (1986):

> ... a segment of a larger society is seen to be different in some combination of the following characteristics – language, religion, race and ancestral homeland with its related culture; the members also perceive themselves in that way; and they participate in shared activities built around their (real or mythical) common origin or culture.

It can be seen from the above that ethnicity is a far more useful concept than race when trying to explore inequalities, as it contains within it both obvious physical differences and the social context. There are, however, difficulties experienced when operationalizing the concept of ethnicity in a research context, as ethnicity is a self-defined and determined category. Thus the following limitations need to be considered:

- Ethnicity cannot be predefined by researchers looking at the relationship between ethnicity and health.
- Ethnicity is about how people define themselves and to which groups they belong.
- It is, thus, difficult to compare studies over time as identities can change and adapt over time.
- Sampling is also difficult as self-classified sampling is needed – which may result in a biased and unrepresentative sample.

It is in this context that any research on ethnic groups needs to be understood.

Discussion Point

- Drawing on the definition of ethnicity given above, how might the ethnicity of Mrs S have impacted on her consultation?
- It is clear that Mrs S is using her daughter as an interpreter during the consultation. What are the implications of this for the consultation? How might the dental team handle consultations with patients who do not speak English?

Valued attitudes

In the context of ethnicity, it is also worth noting that some characteristics, whether physical or cultural, are valued more highly than others. This varies both geographically and historically but there is evidence that some physical attributes (e.g. lighter skin and an aquiline nose; taller rather than shorter people; slim rather than a stocky build) tend to be valued more than their opposites in British society. These preferences, again, change across time.

All members of society carry many of their physical attributes overtly, but their impact varies significantly. Negatively valued attributes carry a stigma, and the depth and scope of the stigma of dark skin in a predominantly white society is profound and can be seen in the raft of academic papers, media coverage and legal guidlelines related to the issue of the systematic devaluing of physical and cultural differences, or *racism*. In Britain there is now an acknowledgement of the presence of widespread institutionalized racism.

The very issue of race has come to be seen as a political statement, referring to the negative and discriminatory aspects of cultural and ethnic differences. In this context the word 'ethnicity' has come to be seen as a neutral term which de-politicizes the issue.

Minority status

As outlined in the introduction, in sociological terms 'minority status' does not simply refer to the small size of the population or groups who are being studied. Members of minority groups tend to be socially distanced from the rest of the population. This means that they are socially isolated and that barriers are set up between them and everyone else. This is manifest in the denial of access to accommodation or jobs or equality and was seen in its most extreme form in South Africa under apartheid where the *majority population* had *minority status*.

In summary, the terms 'race' and 'ethnicity' are often used interchangeably but are quite specific in their meaning. Ethnicity is the term which is most commonly used in relation to research on health and oral health. It is a self-defined category and relates to a range of social and cultural characteristics.

Ethnicity in the UK

Figures from the 2011 Census in England and Wales (Office for National Statistics 2011a) show that in 2011 19.5 per cent of the population were from minority ethnic groups. White was the majority ethnic group accounting for 86 per cent of the population, with White British people making up 80.5 per cent and the remaining 5.5 per cent (3.1 million people) consisting predominantly of White Irish and White Europeans. The White majority population has decreased by 8.1 per cent in the past two decades whilst the remaining ethnic groups have increased in number. The breakdown of the ethnic minority population can be seen in figure 4.1.

The figures show that England and Wales have become more ethnically diverse over the past two decades with the broad white ethnic group decreasing in size and the minority groups expanding in number. The largest increases were found in the Asian and Asian British groups. General factors affecting the changes over the past two decades include births, deaths, migration and country of birth. Specific factors include the addition of White non-British categories since 1991, Poland joining the EU in 2004 giving residents rights to free movement and to seek employment in the UK, and the movement of the Chinese tick box

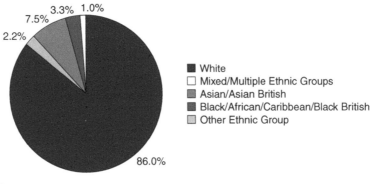

Figure 4.1 Breakdown of the ethnic minority population in England and Wales according to the 2011 Census

Source: Office for National Statistics (2011a)

from 'Other' to 'Asian/Asian British' for the 2011 census. There has also been a change in language from cultural to ethnic background, which may have changed how people categorize themselves (Office for National Statistics 2012a).

Figures from 2011 show London as the most diverse area of the country, whilst Wales is the least diverse. Less than half of those living in London are White British (44.9 per cent), but London also has the highest level of non-British White people (12.6 per cent) and above average numbers of African (7.0 per cent), Indian (6.6 per cent) and Caribbean (4.2 per cent) people. Ethnically diverse areas, such as the West Midlands and London, have seen the greatest changes in the past decade, whilst the least diverse areas, such as Wales, have seen

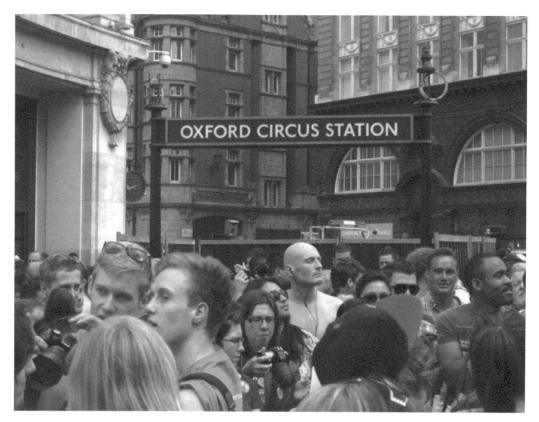

Image 4.1 London is the most diverse area of the country

Source: By Roger (Flickr: IMG_1191). Licensed under CC BY 2.0 via Wikimedia Commons.

the least change. If you look at ethnic groups by age, it is clear that the White groups have a significantly older population with the White Irish Group having the largest proportion of its population (1 in 4) over the age of 65. The youngest groups, conversely, are those from mixed ethnic background, where half were under the age of 16 (Office for National Statistics 2004).

Inequality and ethnicity

The inequality faced by many from the minority ethnic population in the UK can be seen when key aspects of society are presented. Educational achievement, rates of poverty and unemployment can all be used as examples of inequalities.

Education

The highest achieving minority groups in respect of education in 2004 were Chinese and Indian pupils with Black Caribbean pupils getting the poorest GCSE results. It is also worth noting that for all ethnic groups the girls in each group outperformed the boys at GCSE level. Similar results can be found when looking at the rate of exclusions only in reverse with Black Caribbean, Other Black and Mixed White and Black Caribbean pupils among the most likely to be permanently excluded from schools in England (Office for National Statistics 2005b). Again, in all groups boys were more likely to be excluded than girls. This clearly has implications for employment and income levels, but, as we will see, education does not necessarily override discrimination even where high levels of education are achieved.

Poverty

Figures published by the Department for Work and Pensions (2011) show that people from ethnic minority groups are significantly more at risk of poverty than the majority population, with those from Bangladeshi and Pakistani groups at most risk. Figure 4.2 shows the proportion of the households below 60 per cent of median income by ethnic group. Whilst proportions have fallen in the past decade, 70 per cent of the Bangladeshi population and over 60 per cent of the Pakistani population live in low income households.

Platt (2011) conducted a study on poverty amongst ethnic minority groups and found that there were differences between the groups in terms of the types of poverty being experienced (income, material deprivation) and the sectors of the population most affected (older people, children). She highlighted the fact that over half of Bangladeshi, Pakistani and Black African children are growing up in poverty. In addition, she found that Muslims are more likely to live in poverty

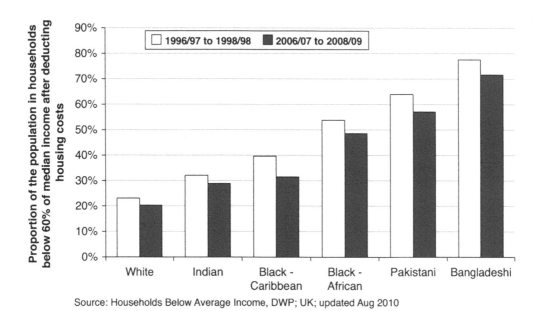

Source: Households Below Average Income, DWP; UK; updated Aug 2010

Figure 4.2 Proportion of Bangladeshi and Pakistani population living in low-income households. Whilst rates have been falling for all ethnic groups, more than half of people from Bangladeshi and Pakistani ethnic backgrounds still live in low-income households

Source: DWP (2011), reproduced from poverty.org.uk

than other religious groups and discrimination and 'ethnic penalties' can counter the effect of factors such as education. Black Africans, for example, have high rates of higher education but also high rates of unemployment and poor occupational outcomes.

Unemployment

As with poverty, rates of unemployment among most ethnic minority groups were higher than those found in the majority population, with the exception of Chinese and Indian men who had similar rates to the majority White population. Figures from the 2011 UK census also show that while Pakistani and Bangladeshi men have seen large falls in levels of unemployment over the past two decades, employment rates for these groups remain much lower than for White men (Office for National Statistics 2011a). A similar picture can be seen for women, with White women being significantly more likely to be in employment than any other ethnic group except Black Caribbean women. Pakistan and Bangladeshi women remain least likely to be in the labour market (ESRC Centre on Dynamics of Ethnicity 2013a). These trends are important as unemployment is associated with poverty and is also directly linked to higher risks of poor physical and mental health, both for the unemployed person and their family.

In addition to the inequalities highlighted above between ethnic groups, a recent report by the Joseph Rowntree Foundation (Barnard & Turner 2011), drawing on work by Hills et al. (2010), highlighted the importance of acknowledging inequality within groups as well as between them. By focusing on inequality and poverty as distinct concepts, the report shows how some sectors of the populations, particularly women and older people, are disproportionately affected and may fall well below average levels for the ethnic group that they fall into.

In summary, clear inequalities can be seen when ethnic minority and majority groups are compared. It is important to distinguish between groups, however, as the minority ethnic population is not a homogeneous group and some groups are consistently more likely to live in poverty, have higher levels of unemployment and have lower levels of educational achievement than others.

Ethnicity and health

When looking at the relationship between ethnicity and health we are mainly limited to statistics on morbidity (with the exception of infant mortality), as ethnicity is not recorded at death registration. This means that we only have accurate mortality statistics by country of birth, which rules out second- and third-generation, British-born, ethnic minority groups. There are, however, accurate figures for infant mortality which show that ethnic minority groups have higher rates of infant mortality than the White British population. Recent figures show that infant mortality rates for Caribbean and Pakistani babies were twice that of the majority White population at 9.8 and 9.6 deaths per 1,000 respectively, compared with 4.5 deaths per 1,000 live births in the White British group (Office for National Statistics 2008).

Mortality aside, there are a range of studies that have looked at the relationship between ethnicity and health. A summary document produced by the ESRC Centre on Dynamics of Ethnicity (2013b) based on the 2011 census data suggested that poor health is caused by a range of social (education, income, discrimination) and biological (age, sex, hereditary factors) determinants that are unequally distributed across social groups. Studies in the US have found similar patterns (Nazroo 2003). A summary of inequalities in health according to ethnicity can be found in the parliamentary paper 'Postnote' (Parliamentary Office of Science and Technology 2007) which outlines key inequalities, possible causes of those inequalities and the impact on and reaction of health services. The report suggests that:

> Black and minority ethnic (BME) groups generally have worse health than the overall population, although some BME groups fare much worse than others, and patterns vary from one health condition to the next. Evidence suggests that the poorer socio-economic position of BME groups is the main factor driving ethnic health inequalities.

In addition to the above, it is worth noting that health inequalities also vary by gender and age. Self-reported health status, levels of long-standing limiting illness and health-related behaviours such as smoking are presented here to give an example of the relationship between ethnicity and different aspects of health.

Self-reported health status

Self-reported health status data from the 2011 census suggest that the White Gypsy or Irish Traveller ethnic group has the worst self-reported general health status with 29.8 per cent reporting their health as 'not good', followed by 27.8 per cent of the Irish population (Office for National Statistics 2013a). The only other group with poorer self-reported general health than the White British people (20 per cent) were the Black Caribbean group at 22.9 per cent. In all other ethnic groups, less than 20 per cent of people rated their health as 'not good', with the lowest percentage amongst the Black African population. It is also worth noting, however, that self-reported poor health ratings go up with age and the White British and Irish populations had the highest median ages at 42 and 53 respectively (Office for National Statistics 2013a).

Long-standing limiting illness

The picture with regard to long-standing limiting illnesses is complex, with men from White Irish, Black Caribbean, Mixed White-Black Carribean, White Gypsy or Irish Traveller groups experiencing more long-standing limiting illness than White British men, and Pakistani, Bangladeshi and Arab men experiencing less. Interestingly, though, this second group still reported poorer self-reported health than White British men (ESRC Centre on Dynamics of Ethnicity 2013b). A similar picture can be seen when looking at women, with some groups experiencing higher rates of illness (Pakistani, Bangladeshi and White Gypsy or Irish Traveller) and others experiencing lower levels of illness (Chinese, Other White and Black African) than White British women. The Chinese group have consistently reported the best health out of all ethnic groups over the past two decades, with half or under half White illness rates for both men and women.

Amongst older people, inequalities in health by ethnicity are significantly greater. Fifty per cent of White British men over the age of 65 report limiting long-term illness, whilst this figure rises to 69 per cent of White Gypsy or Irish Traveller men, 69 per cent of Bangladeshi men and 64 per cent of Pakistani men. Amongst older women, three quarters of women aged 65+ in the Pakistani, Bangladeshi and White Gypsy or Irish Traveller communities reported limiting long-term illness, with Arab women (66 per cent) and Indian women (68 per cent) also experiencing substantially more limiting long-term illness than the total female population aged 65+ in England and Wales (56 per cent). The lowest rates were to be found amongst Chinese women at 46 per cent.

Risk behaviours

The statistics on smoking and drinking suggest that Bangladeshi, White Irish and Black Caribbean men were most likely to smoke and more likely to smoke than the majority White population, which had similar rates to the Pakistani and Indian male populations. Again, Chinese men were less likely to smoke than any other group. The results for women are much clearer with White Irish women being the only group to smoke more than the majority White population, and the rest of the minority groups have significantly lower rates. The statistics relating to the consumption of alcohol are marked, with men and women from the White Irish group drinking more than any other group. All of the other ethnic minority groups consumed less alcohol than the majority population (Office for National Statistics 2001).

Religion and health

The Office for National Statistics breaks down data by religion as well as by ethnic minority group and, whilst religion is only one aspect of ethnic status, it is nevertheless interesting to look at the impact of religion on health. The statistics show that Muslims and Sikhs were most likely to rate their health as 'not good', whilst Christians and Jews were least likely to do so. Disability rates also varied markedly by religion with Christians and Jews experiencing the highest rates of disability. When age was taken into account, however, Jews and Christians were found to have the lowest age standardized rates, whilst Muslim women had the highest rate (24 per cent), followed by Muslim men (21 per cent) (Office for National Statistics 2001).

The picture presented here is one of inequality in relation to health with men and women from ethnic minority groups exhibiting a different, and largely a poorer, relationship with health than the majority White population. In many cases the health of the minority groups is poorer than that of the majority population, although there are some notable exceptions relating to health-damaging behaviours and also to the superior health profile of the Chinese population.

4

In summary, as with other measures, the ethnic minority population are heterogeneous in relation to health. White Gypsy or Irish Traveller, Bangladeshi and Pakistani men are disproportionately likely to experience poor health, whilst Chinese men and women have better health, regardless of which measure is used, than the majority population.

Ethnicity and oral health

This leads us on to consideration of the relationship between ethnicity and oral health. There is a dearth of quality information on the oral health of people from ethnic minority groups in the UK. Dhawan and Bedi (2001) suggest that the heterogeneity of the various groups makes it difficult both to draw conclusions and to design and implement health promotion strategies that would be effective and meet the needs of all groups. The limited data available in relation to caries, periodontal disease and oral hygiene, oral cancer and oral health-related knowledge are presented here.

Dental caries

Studies by Anantharaman et al. (2011) and Gray et al. (2000) showed high rates of caries amongst pre-school children from ethnic minority groups in different parts of the UK. A further study carried out by Marcenes et al. in 2013 focused on a highly deprived part of North London and found that pre-school children from White Eastern European, Pakistani and Bangladeshi backgrounds had significantly higher caries rates than those with Black, Asian, Indian and White British parents. Levels of untreated decay were found to follow a similar pattern. This demonstrates the heterogeneity of ethnic groups and the difficulty of making broad assertions based on a general category of ethnic minority status.

The evidence on dental caries shows that the levels of caries has reduced across all developed countries but there are still significant differences in caries experiences in pre-school children (Watt & Sheiham 1999a; Ahmed et al. 2008). In this age group the caries rates of ethnic minority children are higher than those of the White British population.

There is some debate about whether this is an 'ethnicity' issue or a 'deprivation' issue, however, as the samples with the highest levels of caries are also from the most deprived areas. Interestingly, when older children and adult's teeth are examined, there is less caries found in the minority ethnic groups than in the majority population. Robinson et al. (2000), for example, found that ethnic minority adults in the South Thames region had less caries and more sound teeth than adults across Southern England as a whole. They also found that levels of caries were related to how long people had lived in the UK, with caries rates going up as the length of time people are in the country increases. Ahmed et al. (2008) suggests that four factors need to be considered when assessing caries levels amongst ethnic minority groups. These are: religion of the family; the mother's ability to speak English; the age of the child (younger children have higher caries rates); a lack of evidence on dental service useage (Ahmed et al. 2008: 1). These factors influence how we look at caries and the programmes that will be developed and implemented to address the problem (Bedi et al. 2000; Dhawan & Bedi 2001).

Oral cancer

There is a lack of data on the incidence of oral cancer across the UK and, in particular, data related to ethnic minority groups. This being said, there is some evidence that there are higher rates of cancers in some ethnic minority groups, which have been related to tobacco and alcohol use (Moles et al. 2007). It is suggested that dietary factors and genetic predispositions may also play a role in making some groups more susceptible than others (Ahmed et al. 2008). Moles et al. (2007) suggest that ethnic minority groups may also use cancer services less and so it remains very difficult to build an accurate picture of the situation in the UK. In addition, poor data collection in relation to ethnicity within the cancer databases also hampers understanding and research in this area. This said, there are some risk factors that are common to a relatively small sector of the population (chewing tobacco in the South Asian community, for example), which means that targeted interventions should be relatively straightforward in these cases.

Discussion Point

- Thinking back to the case study at the start of the chapter, is Mrs S at a higher risk of oral cancer because of her ethnicity? What, if any, risk factors does Mrs S show?

Oral health-related knowledge and dental attendance

There is limited oral health knowledge in some ethnic minority groups, particularly in relation to caries and oral cancer (Babu et al. 1996). There is also some evidence to suggest that, even though oral health-related knowledge levels increase amongst British-born ethnic minority parents, caries rates are actually higher in these groups than in immigrant ethnic minority parents (Godson & Williams 1996). This seems to suggest that factors other than knowledge are important here, and the authors suggest that diet is of particular importance. There is also evidence that attendance at dental clinics remains low despite relatively high levels of dental need (Nazroo et al. 2009).

The picture is further complicated by the fact that different cultures have their own health beliefs which result in specific forms of illness behaviour. They may also have different lay and formal healthcare structures. As we saw in chapter 1, Western societies predominantly follow a biomedical model of illness causation. There may, however, be gaps between the beliefs of ethnic minority groups in relation to healthcare and the biomedical model. Although this may have wider implications for general healthcare, it may also impact on dentistry.

Various studies have suggested that differences in consulting behaviour exist between the various ethnic groups. Some commentators have even suggested that ethnic minority groups are overusing the National Health Service. This accusation is not borne out by the evidence, however. Mattin and Smith (1991) found that less than 15 per cent of Asians over the age of 55 in their sample attended the dentist regularly and then attended only for pain or dentures. Waplington et al. (1998) further found that South Asian children in Birmingham were disproportionately likely to use community dental services (54 per cent) rather than be registered to a General Dental Practitioner (10 per cent). They suggested that the extension of community dental services could be a good way of increasing attendance amongst these hard-to-reach groups. In a more recent study exploring ethnic inequalities in access to and outcomes of healthcare using data from the Health Survey for England, Nazroo et al. (2009) found that, whilst ethnic minority groups made good use of Primary Care services, reflecting the findings of other studies (Rudat 1994; Nazroo 1997), they were less likely to use hospital services and there were 'marked inequalities in the use of dental care'. They suggest that this may be due to ethnic differences in the use of private healthcare, with ethnic minority groups less likely to use private healthcare services (Nazroo 1997) or difficulties finding NHS dental services or paying the fees associated with dental care (Nazroo et al. 2009).

Discussion Point

- Read through the case study at the start of the chapter again. How might Mrs S's consultation have been better managed to ensure that her needs were met?
- What assumptions does the dentist make about Mrs S in the case study at the start of the chapter? How might these assumptions affect the quality of care she receives?

Reducing inequalities in oral health for ethnic minority groups

The picture we are putting together here is one of ethnic minority groups in the UK who are at risk of poorer health and oral health than the majority White population and yet use hospital and dental services less often that the White British population. Attempts are being made to address this, and Wagner et al. (2008) report on the implementation of a cross-cultural patient-instructor programme to improve dental students' understanding of, and attitudes towards, ethnically diverse patients. This demonstrates the increased importance placed on this and programmes like this could go some way towards improving the experiences of those patients from ethnic minority groups who utilize dental services. It will not, however, address the underlying issues of widespread social inequality and the financial constraints that make it difficult for people to pay for NHS dental care or access private care. In a paper published in 1999, Watt and Sheiham stress this very point, suggesting that, whilst oral health has improved substantially over the past two decades, inequalities in oral health have widened with the most substantial oral health inequalities found in pre-school-aged children. They suggest that these inequalities will only be addressed if the wider social determinants of disease are addressed, a point Watt returns to in later work (2007, 2012). Scambler (2014) suggests that we need to go further still if we want to tackle the social determinants of oral health and look at the inequalities that are at the heart of the global capitalist system.

Conclusion

Previous chapters have explored the relationship between poverty, social class and oral health. In addressing ethnic inequalities in oral health, Watt and Sheiham (1999a) take this idea further to suggest that socio-economic status is the confounding factor which influences all others:

> . . . being a member of an ethnic minority group in the UK does not necessarily correspond to having poorer oral health. Caries experience in the primary dentition is higher in children of Asian origin than in White children but when matched for social class and mother's ability to speak English there

were no differences. In the permanent dentition children of Asian origin had less caries than Whites. Children of Asian and Afro-Caribbean origin had similar permanent teeth decay scores as Whites. There are no differences in oral health among minority ethnic groups of the same socio-economic status. The inclusion of ethnicity as a variable for dental caries may no longer be relevant as it could divert attention from more important variables such as income and social class.

This suggests that oral health differences are just one of the inequalities faced by ethnic minority groups in the UK. In this chapter we have reviewed data on the wider social inequalities in relation to poverty and employment levels. It is also worth noting that people from ethnic minority groups are disproportionately found in the lower socio-economic groups and living in the most deprived inner city areas. This being the case, it would seem that the social class-related inequalities outlined in chapter 2 would be equally relevant to these groups and that any inequalities experienced through ethnic minority status would be experienced alongside and compounded by socio-economic inequality. As Watt and Sheiham (1999a) state, any solutions to the oral health problems experienced by these groups would need to tackle the underlying socio-economic inequalities and not just focus on ethnicity per se.

4

Oral Health in Later Life

Sasha Scambler

> **IN THIS CHAPTER YOU WILL LEARN ABOUT:**
> ▶ The different ways in which older people are socially positioned
> ▶ Sociological theories of ageing
> > ▶ Disengagement Theory
> > ▶ Structured Dependency Theory
> > ▶ The Theory of the Third Age
> ▶ The relationship between health and ageing
> ▶ The relationship between ageing and oral health
> > ▶ Age-specific oral health problems
> > ▶ Oral healthcare and older people
> ▶ Explanations for age differences in oral health

Introduction

We are living in a world with an ageing population. The World Health Organization estimates that between 2000 and 2050 the proportion of people aged over 60 in the world will double from 11 per cent to 22 per cent (World Health Organization 2011a), resulting in approximately 2 billion older people globally. It is further suggested that low- and middle-income countries are ageing most rapidly, and that by 2050 four in five older people will live in low- and middle-income countries. There will be a fourfold increase in the number of people over 80 in the population and a corresponding increase in the need for improved primary and long-term care provision, with non-communicable diseases being the largest cause of illness and death amongst this sector of the population. Furthermore, older people are particularly vulnerable to neglect, discrimination and abuse (World Health Organization 2011a). For the sake of clarity, in this chapter the term older people is taken to refer to those over the age of 65, with the 'oldest old' referring to those over the age of 80 years.

Whilst not a homogeneous social group in relation to background, socio-economic status, gender or ethnic group, there are certain experiences which are more common amongst older people and which need to be considered in relation to their impact on health and oral health.

The following case study highlights the importance of a social contextual knowledge in thinking about the health and oral health of older people.

Box 5.1: Perceptions of Health and Illness

Enid Anderson is a 78-year-old retired shop worker who lives with her husband Victor in a flat in a small industrial town in the Midlands. She has limited mobility due to rheumatoid arthritis and hip pain, and is currently on the waiting list for a hip replacement operation. Enid finds it difficult to move about outside the flat and her husband does the food shopping and the heavy housework, whilst Enid does the cooking and lighter jobs. Enid and Victor both have full dentures and attend the dentist irregularly. Both experience some discomfort when chewing and they avoid foods that they find difficult to eat and have adapted their diet to contain softer foods that require less chewing. On a Tuesday Enid and Victor visit a local drop-in centre to have lunch with friends and they see one or other of their children most weekends.

At a recent visit to the GP surgery Enid and Victor were asked to fill out a self-assessment form. Enid rated her health as fair and Victor rated his as good, and both Enid and Victor rated their quality of life as good. Health and oral health problems were dismissed as a natural part of ageing.

This case study highlights some of the social factors that need to be taken into consideration when thinking about the relationship between ageing and oral health and the provision of oral healthcare for an ageing population.

Discussion Point

- How do Enid and Victor's assessments of their health relate to the details provided in the case study? What kind of questions would you need to ask in a clinical history to pick up the contextual details needed to build a picture of Enid and Victor's oral health needs?

In order to better understand the oral health needs of an ageing population, we need to think about ageing more widely. How do we see older people within society? How is the ageing process viewed? Is old age seen as a positive or negative stage of life? And why? What are the implications of the social positioning of older people on the provision of oral healthcare for this growing sector of the population?

To this end, this chapter starts with an outline of the main sociological theories that have developed in an attempt to explain ageing from a social perspective. An overview of the position of older people in contemporary society is then provided before the chapter focuses on the relationship between old age and health and oral health.

Understanding ageing

The study of ageing (gerontology) is multi-disciplinary, with different disciplines focusing on different aspects of the ageing process. The way in which ageing is understood varies from discipline to discipline and this means that a range of different theories of the ageing process are used to frame the study of older people. There are biological, psychological and sociological theories that aim to explore what ageing is and how it affects people.

Why theorize ageing

Theory is a set of conjectures or tentative explanations of reality which helps us to orientate our reaction to situations. We all use theory constantly and have our own theories or models that represent the way in which we see the world around us. There are many different theories about concepts that we use in everyday life (such as ageing, culture, ethnicity), and we use these to make sense of what is going on around us. This is why we do not all see the world in the same way. Facts do not speak for themselves and we interpret facts according to our own particular theoretical framework. It is because of different ideas about the nature of illness, old age and the role of women that we have different views about the way that society should care for sick older people. A good example of this is the case of depression. Recent figures suggest that one in four older people have symptoms of depression (Craig & Mindell 2007) and the figure is thought to rise to approximately 40 per cent of people over the age of 85 (Reynolds et al. 1999).

There are a number of different theories as to why this might be. Clinical work suggests that depression is due to changes in the ageing brain, whilst psychological explanations focus on changes in the way in which older people see themselves. Sociological theories, on the other hand, suggest changes in the social roles that older people are involved in and in their levels of participation. These theories have led to a range of vastly different interventions:

- Pharmacological interventions have been used to combat changes in the brain.
- Psychological therapy has been used to address the self-concepts older people use.
- And the promotion of day centres, luncheon clubs and befriending schemes have been used to try and maximize participation.

The evidence suggests that none of the separate theories offers the whole answer to the question of depression in older people. It seems much more likely that it is a combination of all three approaches that would explain why it is that older people are more likely to experience depression than younger people. The example of depression demonstrates how our understanding and approaches to issues are dictated to a greater or lesser extent by the ways in which we theorize concepts. We cannot ignore theory; we can only choose which of the alternatives we feel best explain a concept or experience.

Theories of ageing

We are so familiar with the human and social effects of ageing that there is a tendency to dismiss the biological implications of the ageing process. Most living organisms show an age-related decline in functional capacity. This can be studied at various levels, from the intact organism (be it plant or animal), through its component organs and their cellular constituents, to the molecular structure. The terms 'ageing' or 'senescence' are used interchangeably and imply decline and deterioration. Therefore the growth of children is thought of as development rather than ageing because it is beneficial rather than detrimental. The culmination of senescent decline (cell death) is the death of the individual. Not all cell death is damaging to the organism, however, and it may be a natural part of the organism's biological economy. Ageing is seen, therefore, as the process through which the organism becomes more vulnerable to extrinsic or intrinsic factors which will result in cell death. So death may result from an organism's inability to maintain its intrinsic function or from an extrinsic source such as illness or an accident.

Comfort (1960) defined ageing as:

> an increased liability to die, or an increasing loss of vigour, with increasing chronological age, or with the passage of the life cycle.

Another biologist, Strehler (1962) went further, suggesting that there are four distinct criteria of ageing:

1 Ageing is universal – it occurs in all members of the population – and therefore is unlike disease.
2 Ageing is progressive – it is a continuous process throughout the life-course.
3 Ageing is intrinsic to the organism – all organisms are designed to age, they necessarily age – they have no choice about it.
4 Ageing is degenerative – as opposed to developmental or maturational changes – ageing necessarily involves decline.

The biologist is concerned, therefore, with measuring the nature and extent of ageing changes and understanding how these changes are caused and controlled and how and whether the effects of ageing can be manipulated or mitigated.

Sociological theories of ageing

Sociologists are interested in the social implications of ageing and the ways in which society might impact on or shape the ageing process. There are a number of different perspectives on ageing within the sociological literature. Social gerontologists suggest that theories of ageing move through phases, with theories developing to mirror the predominant trends of the time. Thus sociological theories of ageing have moved from individualist theories to social structural theories, through to identity and cultural theories. Examples of three of the most widely used of these theoretical approaches to ageing are outlined below. These are: Disengagement Theory, Structured Dependency Theory and the Theory of the Third Age.

Disengagement Theory

Disengagement Theory was one of the first generalized sociological accounts of old age. In the US, social gerontology very much centred around the approach of Disengagement Theory which was first proposed by Cummings and Henry (1961). Disengagement was seen as the process by which older people in industrial societies disengaged from the roles that they had been performing in wider society. They did this to enable the younger generation to develop and to take society forward. Disengagement was suggested to occur in relation to work roles and also in relation to families, where retired generations became less central to their children's lives. Old age thus presented the individual with many problems. In pre-industrial society, inheritance of skills and property accorded older people a function within society. In industrial societies, however, the lack of skills and property to hand on meant that older people did not have scripts with which to negotiate their new roles. This led many researchers to stress the importance of finding ways to facilitate successful ageing – with the priority being psychological adjustment. Much research was carried out in the 1950s and 1960s in the US to prove that this theory was accurate.

Neugarten (1984) carried out a longitudinal study in Kansas City that showed that older people did indeed disengage. She suggested that for women this process started in widowhood and for men it started on retirement. The process was seen as to do with the different roles that people would play as they got older, and therefore the answers to the problems encountered would come from psychological adaptation to these new roles. This approach was dominant for a long time in social gerontology. The way in which ageing occurs in modern societies was seen as inevitable rather than as a process.

There are a number of criticisms of Disengagement Theory, however, which led to its downfall in gerontology. Firstly, questions about whether people wanted to disengage or not and whether they were forced to do it were never asked – it was assumed that they actively chose to disengage. The emphasis on psychological adjustment was also challenged as it avoided looking at the very real social structures and processes that can be seen to structure old age. In addition, men and women are now much more likely to both work and retire, and this affects the time at which they supposedly 'disengage'. Retirement ages have gone down and so the rigidity is no longer there, and there is increasing evidence of different, very active roles – e.g. in the research around grandparents (Wilson 2000). All of these criticisms led to the discrediting of Disengagement Theory and the promotion of alternative theories of ageing.

Structured Dependency Theory

5

Disengagement Theory focused on the perspectives of individual older people. Structured Dependency Theory conversely stresses the importance of social policy in creating the circumstances in which older people find themselves. This theory predominantly developed in the UK through the work of Townsend (1981), Walker (1981) and Phillipson (1982), and hinges on the existence of the notion of retirement. In most industrialized societies the age at which this occurs has been set by the state and it is from this point that people are entitled to claim a state pension. Retirement therefore marks formal withdrawal from the labour market and the shift from making a living to being dependent on the state. Up until the 1990s in the UK it was actually a requirement that in order to receive a state pension the recipient was not allowed to do any paid work. In this way the state pensioner was treated in the same way as unemployed people on state benefit. As a consequence, decisions of governments have a huge impact on the ways in which older people live their lives.

A large proportion of older people live in poverty and proponents of the Structured Dependency Theory see this as a direct consequence of the way of life imposed on retired older people. They suggest that state retirement pensions are kept at a deliberately low level, even falling in relation to average living standards. Figures from the Department for Work and Pensions (Kotecha et al. 2013) suggest that as many as 20 per cent of pensioners are living in relative poverty. The Government Work and Pensions Committee further suggest that the benefits system is too complex with as many as 1.7 million people failing to claim the pension credit to which they are entitled to top up low state and private pensions (Kotecha et al. 2013). Structured Dependency Theory suggests that the disengaged status of many older people is due to low pensions and not as a result of an active decision to disengage brought about by the ageing process. This theory is not limited solely to the economic sphere, however, and covers all aspects of society seeking to explain the inferior status that many older people have. The cultural emphasis on youth sees ageing as purely bad and can lead to ageism, where discrimination against older people is accepted as part of the ageing process. This can manifest itself in policies that seek to limit the medical or healthcare resources available for older people or to discriminatory employment practices or to the poor treatment of physically frail or mentally confused older people. If the dependency of older people is structural, then the obvious response is to change the policies that most disadvantage older people. The most obvious answer is to raise pensions.

The main criticism of Structured Dependency Theory is that it sees older people as a homogeneous group. With retirement ages changing and becoming both later in statutory terms and earlier and more flexible for those able to take an early retirement option, there is no longer a fixed cut-off date and the differences between older people are becoming more apparent. In addition, Structured Dependency sees all older people as in poverty and in need of care and services. It has been argued that this is no longer the case and with increased longevity we not only have more people living longer but we also have people living longer as active participatory citizens without health problems. In addition, it is argued that there are many older people who do not have financial problems and are comfortably off, particularly amongst early old ages now, as the baby boomers of the 1960s move into their 50s and 60s (Wilson 2000). Interestingly, as we shall see later in the chapter, media attention has recently focused on the 'baby boom' generation as the lucky generation who had the best of the National Health Service, the grammar school system, grants to study at university and benefited most from the dramatic increase in house prices over the last 30–40 years.

The Theory of the Third Age

The 'Theory of the Third Age' was developed by Laslett (1989), partly in response to the changes perceived in the ageing population in the late 1980s and partly as a challenge to Structured Dependency Theory. He argues that modern society presents opportunities for a fulfilling third age of relatively good health and affluence and that there are actually four ages:

- 1st age – from birth to the end of full-time education
- 2nd age – the period when people are economically and family active
- 3rd age – where people are no longer economically and family active
- 4th age – where health declines into death

Laslett argues that increasing time is being spent in the third age after retirement but with no or few health worries. In addition, the idea of fixed retirement is being challenged all the time with many people taking early retirement or redundancy. For many, this offers a period of opportunity for self-enrichment activities, which they had no time for in the second age when they were busy working and bringing up children. This idea meshes well with the sociology of culture, which argues that there has been a blurring of the distinctions between middle and old age, and more cultivation of lifestyles and consumerism by an increasing number of people. In this theory, old age is seen as a mask detracting from the person underneath. This has led to a denial of some of the negative effects of ageing in favour of youth-orientated activism. 'Third agers' are more able to enjoy the pleasures previously deemed inappropriate to their age.

The most obvious criticism of the Theory of the Third Age is that, in contrast to Structured Dependency Theory, it fails to acknowledge the large number of older people who are living in poverty, with health problems, or who are forced to work on beyond retirement age and who are not able to partake in consumerism, travel and so forth (Wilson 2000).

Discussion Point

• Why might older people assume that tooth loss is a natural part of the ageing process? How might theories of ageing perpetuate this idea? What are the implications of this for the provision and use of oral health services?

In summary, old age can be seen in a variety of ways both by, and within, different disciplines. Biological theories on ageing focus on when and why ageing occurs, whilst sociological theories on ageing focus on the extent to which society is shaped by or shapes the experiences of older people. The way in which we classify and understand old age depends on the theory or theories we adopt.

Older people in contemporary Britain

Data from the 2001 census in the UK (Office for National Statistics 2001) showed that, for the first time, in 2001 people over the age of 60 years (21 per cent) outnumbered those under the age of 16 years (20 per cent). When we talk about older people in Britain and across the developed world we are talking about a significant, and growing section of the population. Just over 16 per cent of the population in England and Wales in 2011 were aged 65 or over (growing from 8.3 million people in 2001 to 9.2 million in 2011). This is slightly below the EU average of 18 per cent, with Italy and Germany topping the table at 20 per cent and 21 per cent, respectively (Office for National Statistics 2013b). Over a third of the UK population are now aged over 50 and the Office for National Statistics predicts that the number of people over 75 will double in the next 30 years whilst the number of people over 85 will double in the next 20 years and treble in the next 30 years (Office for National Statistics 2009a). In 2012 just under 1 per cent of the population were aged 90 and over in England and Wales and there has been a 33 per cent increase in the number of people in this age bracket over the past 10 years (Office for National Statistics 2013c). These figures suggest that it is not just the proportion of young older people that is growing but that significant numbers of people are living into their 80s and beyond. The census data thus show that we have an ageing population and it has been suggested (Wilson 2000; Bond et al. 2007) that there are two socio-demographic factors underlying this process: a fall in fertility rates across the developed world and increased longevity. At the turn of the twentieth century, 4.7 per cent of the population in Britain were aged 65 or over and just 0.13 per cent were aged 80 or over. By 2001, as we have seen, these figures were 21 per cent and circa 7 per cent, respectively.

These figures suggest not only that we have an ageing population, but that the population is going to continue ageing for the foreseeable future. When we look at the oldest old people, what becomes clear is that women make up the vast majority of this group. In the 90+ age group there are estimated to be 2.6 women per man and there are almost six women for every man in the 100+ age group (Office for National Statistics 2012a). In addition, it is interesting to note that 72 per cent of men over the age of 65 were married in comparison with 44 per cent of women over the age of 65. This could be explained by a combination of the facts that men tend to marry younger women and that women live longer than men. Taking this into consideration, the average wife is younger than her husband and can expect to live longer. Gender distribution is one of the most important factors when looking at the older population, as can be seen from these Census (2001) figures:

- 0–19 years: 49 per cent of the British population female
- 20–64 years: 50 per cent of the British population female
- 65–79 years: 56 per cent of the British population female
- 80+ years: 70 per cent of the British population female

When these figures are put into the context of the inequalities faced by women that we explored in chapter 3, some of the potential problems to be faced by an ageing, predominantly female, population can be guessed at.

Inequality in old age

In the context of the demonstrable link between socio-economic circumstances and poor health and oral health, it is worth noting that older people are more likely to be living in poverty than any other sector of the population. Some 14.4 per cent of all households in the UK are made up of single people over pensionable age, and of these 75 per cent are women. Data from the Department for Work and Pensions (Kotecha et al. 2013) show that 14 per cent of pensioners in the UK live below the poverty threshold and of these, 1 million (8 per cent) live in severe poverty. DWP figures also showed that in 2008–9 46 per cent of pensioner couples and 73 per cent of single pensioners depended on state benefits for at least 50 per cent of their income. To put this into context, the basic state pension in 2012–13 was £102.15 per week for a single pensioner and £163.35 per week for a couple. The most severe deprivation is experienced by pensioners living alone, who are mainly dependent on state pensions; for this group, 49 per cent of expenditure goes on housing, food and fuel.

Social inequality is harder to measure in the 65+ age group as it is usually measured through occupational status. Poor pensioners are, however, more likely to become sick or disabled than rich pensioners and, if they become ill, poorer pensioners are more likely to die and to die younger (Arber & Ginn 1993). In addition to this, premature death in those under 65 leaves many more people as widows or widowers in the more deprived areas with the worst health records than in the richer and healthier areas. Mortality rates of people aged 60–74 living in council housing, for example, are 16 per cent higher than the national average for that age group.

Taking a social model of ageing approach to the study of the relationship between ageing and health allows us to incorporate the social context in which older people live into our understanding of their health. Such a model implies the importance of social factors in shaping the experiences of growing old. Ageing can be seen as shaped by socio-economic conditions and cultural values throughout the life-course and each cohort of older people experiences social, cultural and economic conditions specific to their time. Therefore older people are not a homogeneous group. Health and illness in later life is also influenced by the social roles of older people as the theories presented above suggest. It is in this context and through adopting a social model approach that we move on to look at the relationship between ageing and health and oral health.

Ageing and health

The number of older people in the population is increasing. One of the factors that has already been suggested as a partial explanation for this is the increasing life expectancy. Current estimates for life expectancy in the UK are 82.3 years for women and 78.2 years for men (Office for National Statistics 2012a). This is compared with a life expectancy of 43 years for women and 41 years for men in 1841. It is clear from this that life expectancy has almost doubled in the last 150 years.

If we want to judge the health of our ageing population, we need to know not just how long people can be expected to live but how long they are likely to live free from illness and disability. Thus we also need to look at healthy life expectancy. This tells us how healthy people are likely to be in the future. When we look at healthy life expectancy, we look not just at how long people will live but at how many of those years will be free of limiting long-term illness. There are two views on healthy life expectancy: the optimistic view and the pessimistic view.

The optimistic view

This is the idea put forward by Fries (1980) that an ageing population with increased life expectancy can be expected to live both a longer and a healthier life. A number of studies support this viewpoint. Victor (1991), for example, found lower levels of chronic illness in later cohorts of older people within a study on ageing and health. Similarly, Doblhammer and Kytir (2001) conducted a longitudinal study over a period of 20 years in Austria and found that both life expectancy and healthy life expectancy increased over the period of the study. This supports Sutherland's (1999) assertion that social and environmental improvements have led to a longer and healthier life expectancy.

The pessimistic view

This view was put forward by Taylor and Field (2003), who suggest that there are four reasons to be cautious and not to assume that an increase in life expectancy will automatically result in an increase in healthy life expectancy:

1 Evidence about the nature of chronic illness and disability amongst older people does not provide any conclusive evidence that illness is becoming markedly less common in older age groups.
2 The socio-economic inequalities in health continue and are not ameliorated in old age.
3 There is no guarantee that succeeding generations of people will continue the trend of continuous health improvement.
4 Illness is subjective in nature.

Thus people are living longer, but this does not necessarily mean that there are not health problems within the population. Indeed, an ageing population could potentially bring with it a surge in health problems and put pressure on an already stretched healthcare system. Data from the Office for National Statistics (2012) suggests that when they reach the age of 65, men can expect to live in good health for another 10.1 years on average, whilst women can expect a further 11.6 years of good health. This constitutes just over half of their predicted remaining life expectancy. These figures also suggest that a considerable amount of time is likely to be spent in ill-health at the end of life.

> **Discussion Point**
> • How might the different views of ageing be used to make sense of Enid and Victor's experiences of old age?

Disability and long-term illness amongst older people

In the context of exploring healthy life expectancy, it is interesting to look at rates of disability and long-term limiting illness amongst older people. These are illnesses which last over an extended period of time and affect multiple areas of daily life. Data from the General Lifestyle Survey (Office for National Statistics 2010) reported that 40 per cent of people over 65 have a limiting long-standing illness. When broken down by age, there is a very clear relationship between long-standing limiting illness and ageing, as 36 per cent of people aged 65–74 have a limiting long-standing illness and the rate goes up to 47 per cent of those aged 75 and over and up to 69 per cent of those aged 85+.

The most common disability reported was locomotor disability which, again, was particularly prevalent in those over the age of 80 years. It is important to note when looking at these figures that, whilst disability is clearly a significant issue for older people, 80 per cent of

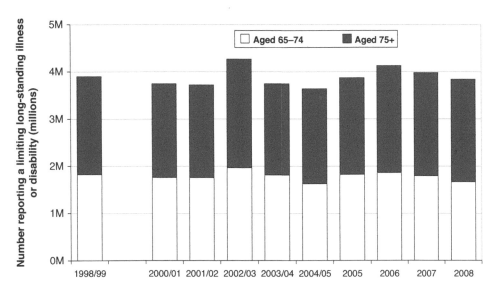

Figure 5.1 Number of adults over the age of 65 with a limiting long-standing illness or disability, 1998–2008. Four million adults aged 65 and over report a long-standing sickness or disability. This is a similar number to a decade ago

Source: General Lifestyle Survey, ONS, Great Britain, 2010. Accessed through poverty.org.uk

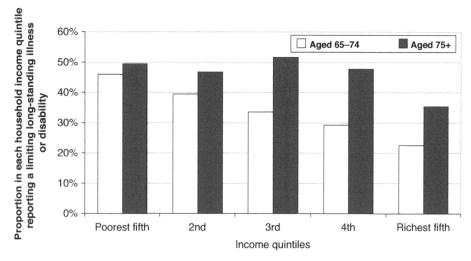

Figure 5.2 Proportion of adults over the age of 65 with a limiting long-standing illness or disability, by income group. For those aged 65–74, the proportion with a limiting long-standing illness or disability increases as income decreases. The differences by income are less for those aged 75 and over

Source: General Lifestyle Survey, ONS, Great Britain, 2010. Data is the average for the three years to 2008. Accessed through poverty.org.uk

men and women over the age of 85 are able to perform the tasks classified as the main 'activities of daily living' (i.e., they are able to feed themselves, bathe themselves, get in and out of bed and use the toilet) without help.

The proportion of people aged 65+ with a long-standing illness or disability has remained relatively stable over the past decade as can be seen in figure 5.1, but there is a relationship with income, particularly for those age 65–74, where rates of long-term illness or disability increase as income decreases (Office for National Statistics 2010). Furthermore, those who had previously worked in manual or routine jobs are more likely to experience long-standing illness than those who had previously had non-manual occupations (see figure 5.2). These figures show not only that rates of limiting long-standing illness increase substantially with age, but also that there are both gender and social class differences when we look at the figures for those aged 65+.

Multiple pathology

An important factor to consider when looking at the results of 'activities of daily living' tests, and the presence of limiting long-standing illness amongst older people, is the prevalence of multiple pathology. In addition to higher rates of disability and limiting long-standing illness, it is also worth noting that older people are likely to have more than one medical condition and that these will often be of a disabling nature. This leads to a situation where older people may find themselves on multiple different drugs to treat a variety of different conditions. It is also worth noting, however, that although the average number of multiple pathologies increases with age, nearly two-fifths of older people are not subject to any disabling conditions.

Discussion Point

- In the case study at the start of the chapter, it is clear that Enid's locomotor disability means that she is unable to move easily outside the home and experiences pain and discomfort when travelling around. This is the most common form of disability reported by older people. How might this information be used to develop targeted dental services for older people?

Use of healthcare services

A final factor to consider when looking at the relationship between ageing and health is health and illness behaviour in relation to health service use. Figures suggest that the use of healthcare services also increases between the middle and later years of life, and people over the age of 75 are particularly likely to make use of these (Higgs 2008b). There are significant differences in the frequency of health service usage amongst older and younger people. Older people are the largest users of hospital services and make use not just of specialisms such as geriatrics but of most major specialisms. The admission rate also increases with age. Interestingly, however, whilst two-thirds of those utilizing the National Health Service (NHS) are aged 65 or over, figures from the Department of Health (2008) show that they account for only 40 per cent of total expenditure. Furthermore, data from the NHS (Robinson 2010) show that emergency hospital readmission rose by 88 per cent for those aged 75+ between 1999–2000 and 2009–10. This ties in with findings from two recent surveys which found that approximately one-third of the general public do not feel that older people are treated with dignity in hospital (AgeUK 2013; ICM Research 2008).

Rates for primary care usage also increase with age, and older people are more likely to consult their General Practitioner, and to consult them repeatedly. This being said, the number of GP consultations made is similar for children under the age of 4 and people over the age of 65, so older people are not the only group to make substantial use of primary care services. In addition, whilst the number of home visits by GPs fell from 22 per cent in 1971 to 4 per cent in 2006, older people are still more likely to receive home visits than any other age group (Age Concern Policy Unit 2008). In 2006, 15 per cent of GP consultations amongst people aged 75 and over were undertaken as home visits.

In summary, the picture presented here in relation to the health of older people suggests that whilst life expectancy is increasing, this does not necessarily mean that people are living longer in good health, and there is some debate about the idea of 'health life expectancy'. The figures suggest that older people are more likely to experience limiting long-standing illness and disability than any other section of the population and use health services more than any other group except very young children. This being said, it is worth stressing that the majority of older people do not have limiting long-standing conditions, do not have disabilities and are able to care for themselves within their own homes and without assistance.

Ageing and oral health

In the previous section we explored the relationship between age and health. A similar relationship exists between age and oral health. Oral health has been identified as a particular area for concern by the World Health Organization, which suggests that the rise in the prevalence and importance of chronic conditions globally can be seen in the rates of 'tooth loss, dental caries experience, and the prevalence rates of peri-odontal disease, xerostomia and oral precancer/cancer' amongst older people (Petersen & Yamamoto 2005: 81). The negative impact of poor oral health also adversely affects quality of life. Multiple regression analysis on data from the 1998 Adult Dental Health Survey showed that, in Britain, age accounted for the biggest predicted difference in sound and untreated teeth. Age is the single biggest reason for the decrease in sound and untreated teeth across the population as a whole, with the next most important factor being region of the UK. Unsurprisingly, the least deprived regions are the ones with the highest levels of sound and untreated teeth and vice versa. Again this ties in with the link between socio-economic status and oral health and to the previous section, where we looked at the relationship between poverty and old age.

There is very little published work on oral health in later life and particularly in relation to the social implications of poor oral health for this age group. MacEntee et al. (1997), however, carried out a qualitative study looking at 'the significance of the mouth in old age' and focusing specifically on older people's experiences of poor oral health and their relationship with their mouth. They found that 'comfort, hygiene and health' were identified as the most salient factors, and that respondents in their study focused on the need to manage their oral health in order to function on a daily basis. For the full WHO report, see Petersen and Yamamoto (2005) and see also MacEntee et al. (1997), both of which are recommended reading.

Oral health problems specific to older people

A range of oral health problems have been identified as more common amongst older people than any other group. There is still a relatively high rate of edentulism amongst older people and, although the rates have improved since the 1960s, a significant number of people over the age of 65 are still losing their teeth and almost half of those aged 85 and over are edentate (Adult Dental Health Survey 2009, see figure 5.3). People from lower socio-economic groups are more likely to lose their teeth than those in higher groups, as we saw in the previous chapter,

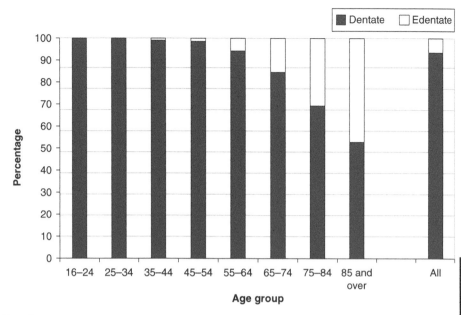

Figure 5.3 Dental status by age group

Source: Adult Dental Health Survey 2009.

and women are also more likely to lose their teeth than men, although as rates of edentulism increase with age and women live longer than men, this is perhaps unsurprising. The data also suggest that older people suffer from poor quality prosthesis as they have higher rates of denture-related mucosal disorders than other denture-wearing groups (Adult Dental Health Survey 2009).

The Adult Dental Health Survey (2009) also found that levels of functional dentition decrease with age. The percentage of people with fewer than 21 functional teeth rose dramatically after the age of 55, with fewer than 10 per cent of those under the age of 55 with less than 21 functional teeth. This figure rose to 26 per cent of those aged 55–64 years, 39 per cent of those aged 65–74, 60 per cent of those aged 75–84 and to 74 per cent of the 85+ age group. The proportion of adults with visible coronal caries varied between age groups but with no obvious pattern, although it was highest amongst adults aged 25–34 years (36 per cent) and lowest in adults aged 65–74 (22 per cent). The number of sound and untreated teeth also varied significantly by age, and adults aged up to 44 had over 20 sound and untreated teeth on average. However, this declined steeply in those aged 45+. Adults aged 55–64 had the highest number of restored, otherwise sound, teeth (10.1) whilst the youngest adults (16–24 years) had the lowest number of restored but otherwise sound teeth at 1.8 teeth on average. The average number of restored but otherwise sound teeth rose steadily up to age 64 and then began to fall again, reflecting a reduction in the total number of retained teeth amongst older adults. Interestingly, those aged 65–84 report significantly less extreme dental anxiety than any other age group, and even those aged 85+ experience less extreme dental anxiety than those aged 16–64 (Adult Dental Health Survey 2009).

Image 5.1 Older patients suffer disproportionately from certain conditions like edentulism
Source: leezsnow/iStock

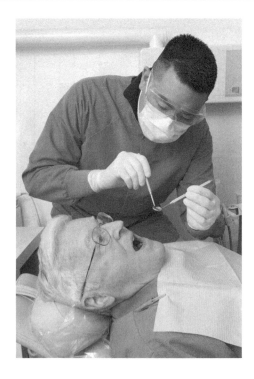

- Looking back at the case study presented at the start of this chapter, what are the social implications of poorly fitting dentures and the limitations that this may place on food choices? What are the wider implications of this for the health of older people?

Oral healthcare for older people

Research suggests that alongside specific oral health problems associated with ageing, there are treatment issues for older people. Strayer et al. (1986), for example, conducted a study of dentists' attitudes towards older patients and found that dentists saw older people as less satisfying to treat than younger people. The respondents used stereotypes in their assessment, saw older people as less competent and were likely to offer simplistic explanations of treatments given. The authors suggested that this increased the negative response to dentists amongst patients.

A similar study by Pyle et al. (1999) in the US looked at dental students' perceptions of older patients. The results indicated that, while patient age did not affect the treatment given, a high level of negativity existed towards older patients generally. Interestingly the level of negativity increased with increased edentulousness in patients.

Recent work by Borreani et al. (2008, 2010b) looked at barriers to dental service usage amongst older people and found that the research participants were aware of the benefits of attending the dentist regularly but many did not do so. Reasons given included fear (often

Table 5.1 Regular dental attendance by age and percentage				
Age	Regular check-up	Occasional check-up	Only when having trouble	Never been to the dentist
All	16	10	27	2
16–24	51	14	33	2
25–34	44	14	38	3
35–44	60	11	27	2
45–54	67	7	25	1
55–64	72	6	21	1
65–74	77	5	17	1
75–114	70	6	22	2
85+	65	5	26	4

Source: Adult Dental Health Survey 2009. Copyright © 2015, Reused with the permission of the Health and Social Care Information Centre. All rights reserved.

5

stemming from traumatic childhood experiences of dentistry), cost and the fear of cost, practical issues such as the need for a companion when attending for treatment under sedation, and very distinct ideas about the right to 'free' dental care, including the vilification of private dentists and strong ideas of citizenship. It was suggested that dentists need to be aware of the foundations of patient attitudes towards dentistry if they are to successfully counter them and promote regular, preventive treatment amongst this group.

Statistics from the 2009 Adult Dental Health Survey show that those aged 45+ are more likely to access dental services for regular check-ups than their younger counterparts, and are less likely to access care occasionally or symptomatically. This can be seen in table 5.1.

The quarterly NHS dental statistics do not routinely report on the number of older people requiring dental care, but a study undertaken by Age Concern Policy Unit (2008) found that just over 50 per cent of respondents were registered with an NHS dentist, although the numbers declined with age and there were variations across the country. Care Quality Commission statistics on accessing primary care (2009) show that 7.4 million people across England and Wales would like to access NHS dentistry but are unable to do so, and a further 2.7 million stated that they were unable to access a dentist at all. This was across all age groups.

Explanations for age differences in oral health

There is some evidence that, amongst older old people, tooth loss is seen as an inevitable part of the ageing process and, therefore, older people are less likely to look for preventive treatments and expect to lose their teeth. This is changing as rates of edentulousness fall and it is becoming widely accepted that most older people will keep their teeth into old age. It is also worth considering, in line with the evidence presented on poverty amongst older people, that the costs of dental treatments and dentures may be prohibitive for older people who are more likely to live in poverty than other age groups. With the increased focus on the maintenance of youth and of young-looking teeth and the growth of cosmetic dentistry (as evidenced by the inclusion of dentists on programmes such as *10 Years Younger*), it seems unlikely that older patients are going to be seen as a priority until sufficient numbers are demanding restorative and cosmetic treatments themselves, when they will become both attractive and lucrative patients.

In summary, older people experience higher levels of poor oral health than other groups and overall they make use of dental services less and receive poorer care than other groups. There is also evidence, however, that the newer old people are increasingly likely to make regular use of dental services and make increasing use of restorative and cosmetic treatments. This, along with the decrease in the number of older people losing their teeth and the overall increase in the older population, suggests that provision of dental care for older people is going to change dramatically over the next few decades.

Conclusion

This chapter provides some insight into the impact of ageing on health and oral health within the context of an unequal society. The chapter started with an outline of the position of older people in society, taking the example of contemporary Britain and in the context of an ageing society. The health statistics demonstrate that people are living longer but not necessarily in good health, with significant numbers of older people living with limiting long-term conditions. Older people make more use of general and dental health services than their younger peers, are more likely to use dental services preventively, and experience significantly less dental anxiety than those under the age of 65. There has been little research looking at older people's experiences of the mouth, however, and of the impact of living with a less functional mouth over time. This is an area highlighted for future work. The aim of this chapter, therefore, has been to set out the context within which more research is needed, particularly in light of the ageing population, the retirement of the baby boomer generation, and the potential impact of this on oral health and future oral health services.

Disability and Oral Health

Sasha Scambler

> **IN THIS CHAPTER YOU WILL LEARN ABOUT:**
> ▶ The profile of disability and disabled people in the UK
> ▶ The importance of definitions of disability and disabled people
> ▶ The three main models of disability
>   ▷ The Medical Model of Disability
>   ▷ The Social Model of Disability
>   ▷ The International Classification of Functioning, Disability and Health
> ▶ Approaches to disability in dentistry
> ▶ Access to and use of oral health services

Introduction

In 2011 the World Health Organization published the first *World Report on Disability*. They estimated that more than 1 billion people across the world, approximately 15 per cent of the population, live with a disability. A rise in numbers from the 1970s is accounted for by the ageing population and the increasing number of people living with long-term disabling conditions. Considering the UK, one in ten people live with a disability – which equates to over 11 million disabled people and/or people with long-term disabling conditions in the UK (Department for Work and Pensions 2012). The prevalence of disability increases with age, rising from 6 per cent of children to 16 per cent of working age adults and 45 per cent of those over state pension age reporting a disability, and mobility problems are the most commonly reported impairments in the UK. The evidence from the WHO suggests that disabled people experience poorer health outcomes, lower educational achievement, increased levels of dependency and restricted

Box 6.1: Use of Health Services – Facts and Figures

- Disabled people make up a significant proportion of NHS users. 30% of people report they have a chronic condition. This 30% accounts for 52% of all GP visits, 65% of all out-patient visits and 72% of all hospital stays. [Ham 2009, *Health Policy in Britain*, Palgrave Macmillan, London, p. 107]
- Difficulty in accessing the NHS is widespread. In 2010, 33% of disabled people reported difficulties accessing local services, including local health services. [Office for Disability Issues 2011, Disability Facts and Figures, http://odi.dwp.gov.uk/disability-statistics-and-research/disability-facts-and-figures.php#gd]
- 20% of disabled people found it difficult or impossible to get the healthcare they needed as a result of inaccessible transport. [Leonard Cheshire Disability 2010, Rights and reality: disabled people's experiences of accessing goods and services. http://www.lcdisability.org/?lid=12274s]
- 16% of disabled people reported that due to impairment, a healthcare professional has demonstrated a negative attitude towards them in the past 12 months. [Leonard Cheshire Disability 2009, Disability Review, http://www.lcdisability.org/?lid=11009]
- 30% of disabled people reported that for reasons relating to their impairment, healthcare professionals have made negative assumptions about their quality of life. [Leonard Cheshire Disability 2009, Disability Review, http://www.lcdisability.org/?lid=11009]
- 71% of disabled people reported they have never heard of the Disability Discrimination Act, or knew little or nothing about it. [Leonard Cheshire Disability 2010, Rights and reality: disabled people's experiences of accessing goods and services. http://www.lcdisability.org/?lid=12274s]

participation in society, have lower employment rates and are more likely to live in poverty than their non-disabled peers.

The factfile above illustrates the impact of disability on just one aspect of life, health service usage. This is an issue not just for disabled people but for service providers and society as a whole.

This factfile illustrates a number of issues that will be explored in this chapter; significant numbers of disabled people are still unable to access the healthcare that they require and feel that they have been discriminated against or viewed negatively and the vast majority are unaware of the legal protection that they have against discrimination. Disability activists say disabled people are consistently discriminated against, oppressed and stopped from achieving their potential in a world designed for non-impaired bodies. There is much debate about what disability is and how it should be defined, but underlying this is the undisputed and global fact that the vast majority of disabled people (or people with impairments) experience exclusion, poverty and dependence on a daily basis (WHO 2011b; Oliver & Barnes 2012).

The chapter starts with a brief overview of the social context of disabled people before debates around what we mean when we talk about disability are presented in the context of the profile offered above. How is disability defined? And does it matter? The chapter then focuses on the relationship between disability and oral health, outlining key trends before examining access to and use of oral health services, policy initiatives and the emergence of special care dentistry as a specialism.

The social context of disabled people in the UK

The position of disabled people in the UK has improved over the past decade and disabled people are more likely to be in employment now than they were in 2002 (Office for National Statistics 2012b). This said, however, disabled people are still significantly less likely to be employed than their non-disabled peers, with 46.3 per cent of working age disabled people in employment compared to 76.4 per cent of non-disabled working age people. Disabled people are also more likely to live in poverty, to struggle in school and further or higher education, to face discrimination and to face barriers accessing leisure facilities or being active in the community than their non-disabled peers. They are more likely to live in inappropriate (not up to standard) accommodation, significantly less likely to live in households with internet access, and significantly more likely to be victims of crime than their non-disabled peers.

By 2010–11 almost 90 per cent of 16 year olds in the UK achieved five or more GCSEs at grades A*–C. This compares with almost 60 per cent of children with special educational needs and 25 per cent of students with a statement (statutory support provided by schools with additional resources provided by the local authority) of special educational needs (Department of Education 2011). This trend goes through to further and higher education, with disabled people about three times less likely to hold professional qualifications and half as likely to hold a degree than their non-disabled peers (Office for National Statistics 2012b). In addition, disabled people are more likely to experience discrimination both in the workplace (Department for Business, Enterprise and Regulatory Reform 2010) and in the community (Office for National Statistics 2011b). And almost two in five disabled 16–34 year olds report being victims of crime in comparison with just over a quarter of non-disabled people (Home Office 2011). As we have already seen, disabled people are also less likely to be able to access the healthcare services that they need and face discrimination and negative treatment when they do.

Moreover, it is not just disabled people themselves who are affected. Families with a disabled member are also disproportionately more likely to live in poverty than those without. Almost one in five individuals living in families with at least one disabled family member live in relative income poverty and the situation is slightly worse for children, 21 per cent of whom are living in poverty when living in a family with at least one disabled member (Department for Work and Pensions 2012). This compares to 16 per cent of children in families with no disabled members.

Against this backdrop, there has been the emergence over the last four decades of the disability rights movement, which has raised the profile of disability and disabled people. There has been a campaign for inclusive education and the introduction of the Disability Discrimination Act (DDA) in the UK which requires businesses and services to make 'reasonable adjustments' to ensure that disabled people can access services. There is still no universal understanding of the concept of 'disability'. The nature, meaning and impact of disability depend on the geographical, historical, social, cultural and economic environment in which the person with the disability is located. In addition to being culturally specific, the concept of disability is also historically specific and the treatment of people with disabilities has changed over time.

> **Discussion Point**
>
> - Figures suggest that accessibility of services is a big problem for disabled people in all realms of life. What kind of 'reasonable adjustments' could dental surgeries make to address issues of accessibility?

Defining disability

The central debate concerning definitions of disability has been ongoing since the late 1970s, with the major arguments surrounding the medical and social models of disability and their corresponding advantages and disadvantages as ways of understanding exactly what disability is and what it means to people living with disabilities. The importance of developing an adequate definition of disability was seminally highlighted by Mike Oliver (1990). Human beings give meaning to the objects that they encounter within the social world and orientate their behaviour accordingly. Thus, if disability is given a strongly negative meaning, then its onset will be experienced and treated as a tragedy and disabled people will be treated as tragic victims. Oliver suggests that official or bureaucratic definitions attached to disability define who is and is not able to work, offering quasi-legitimate social status to people who are not able to work as opposed to people who choose not to work. This is particularly salient in light of current changes to benefits for disabled people and media representations of disabled people in the UK as 'scroungers' who are too lazy to work.

In order to reclaim disability as a positive state, the terms surrounding disabilities and their meanings need to be redefined in a positive way. Oliver likens this to the fundamental redefinition work that has been undertaken by women's movements, black movements and gay and lesbian movements since the 1960s, which have systematically challenged public perceptions, language use and overt and covert discrimination. The Disability Discrimination Act in the UK (1995) and the more recent Equalities Act (2010) and equivalent legislation in the US and Europe are part of this process. Alongside this, a growing body of theoretical work has explored how disability and disabled people are (and should be) understood in relation to bodies, impairments and wider society. The main theories are presented below.

Disability theory

There is ongoing debate about how disability should be defined and the impact of definitions on the provision of care. The debate sees disability defined either as functional limitations based on an impaired body or oppression caused by a social world which is not made accessible to everyone regardless of impairment (Scambler et al. 2010). The argument hinges on the extent to which disabled people are seen as tragic victims to be 'helped' (the medical model approach) or individuals who happen to have an impairment but have the same rights and needs as their non-disabled peers (the social model approach). Whilst much dental training adopts, often unconsciously, a medical model approach, there is a growing awareness of the need for a social, patient-centred approach, which is reflected in the World Health Organization's International Classification of Functioning, Disability and Health (ICF) which was ratified in 2001. The main facets of each of these models, along with critiques, are presented below. The definitions presented are now over 30 years old; however, the debates that rage around them continue unabated.

6

The medical model of disability

The polarity of the two main definitions or positions, the 'International Classification of Impairment, Disability and Handicap' (ICIDH) (WHO 1980) and the 'Social Model of Disability' (UPIAS 1976) is clear when looking at the emphasis placed on the role of the body. In 1981 the World Health Organization adopted the ICIDH, which became the most commonly used definition of disability amongst medical practitioners and other professionals, including medical sociologists. The definitions provided in ICIDH state the following:

> **Impairment** – an impairment is any loss or abnormality of psychological, physiological or anatomical structure or function.
> **Disability** – a disability is a restriction or lack (resulting from an impairment) of ability to perform an activity in a manner or within the range considered normal for a human being.
> **Handicap** – a handicap is a disadvantage for a given individual, resulting from an impairment or a disability, that limits or prevents the fulfilment of a role that is normal (depending on age, sex and social and cultural factors) for that individual. (WHO 1980)

The ICIDH has been widely criticized for placing the emphasis on the individual and not on society. It has also been pointed out that the ICIDH places the emphasis on the impairment as the cause of disability and handicap. The environment is seen as neutral and the onus is placed on the individual to fit into the environment with the use of medical aids (Oliver & Barnes 2012). Rather than being viewed as the result of an inadequate social environment, as may originally have been intended, a number of researchers have suggested that the 'handicap' category gives the impression that handicaps are 'merely complex disabilities' (Bickenbach et al. 1999), a view echoed by Grimsby et al. (1988) and Orgogozo (1994). Bickenbach et al. go on to suggest that:

> Although identified as a classification 'of circumstances in which disabled people are likely to find themselves', there is never any reference in the handicap classification to features of the social world that create those circumstances. It is a classification of limitations of people's abilities. (1999: 1175)

Furthermore, underlying this is the assumption that disabled people should be willing to adjust themselves to become more normal (e.g. through the use of medical aids, artificial limbs or cochlear implants) and adjust their expectations to make the best of their 'diminished circumstances' (Finkelstein 1993).

It is important to note, however, as Williams (1999) points out, that despite the many criticisms that have been levelled at it, the ICIDH definition of disability has been adopted, if unconsciously, by the majority of sociologists working in this field to date as well as by most of those working in the health and allied fields. The danger here is that health professionals see disabled people as having something wrong with them, as either needing to be willing to adapt and be 'normalized' or risk becoming a 'social problem' (Oliver & Barnes 2012).

The social model of disability

The social model of disability developed alongside the medical model, providing an alternative definitional framework for understanding disability. The clearest version of this definition of disability is as follows:

- **Impairment** – lacking part or all of a limb, or having a defective limb, organ or mechanism of the body.
- **Disability** – the disadvantage or restriction of activity caused by a contemporary social organization which takes no or little account of people who have an impairment (whether it is physical, sensory or intellectual) and thus excludes them from participation in the mainstream of social activities (adapted from UPIAS 1976).

This definition rejects the idea that the body, and any impairment it may have, has anything to do with an individual's experience of disablement. It was designed to politicize the disability movement's struggle (Albert 2006; Bickenbach 2009). Writers such as Oliver (1990) and Swain et al. (1993) suggested that it is social oppression which prevents individuals from participating fully in society and, thus, that the body is immaterial. In addition, it has been suggested that medical sociologists are implicitly or explicitly adding to this social oppression through their conscious or unconscious acceptance of the medical model approach. It has further been suggested that the whole area of disability can only be understood and conceptualized fully by disabled people themselves, thus rendering much work done in the area as fundamentally lacking.

A number of criticisms have been levelled at the social model of disability and its disassociation of the body from disablement. It has been suggested that by removing the body from the debate around disablement, the social model of disability is moving in the opposite direction to the sociology of the body which claims to look at the same issues (Williams 1999). It has also been suggested that removing the body from the realm of sociology gifts it to medicine unchallenged (Hughes & Patersen 1997). Further criticism surrounds the issue of bringing impairment back into the debate about disablement, with the idea that this allows the social, as well as the biomedical to have some command over the body. This has led to the development of an area of disability studies concerned primarily with the disabled body and the impairment debate.

The International Classification of Functioning

Problems with the existing definitions of disability led the WHO in 1993 to begin the process of developing a new definitional framework for understanding disability, based on a revised ICIDH. The 'International Classification of Functioning, Disability and Health' (ICF) was released by the World Health Organization in 2001 as an international standard to measure health and disability (World Health Organization 2014). It was incorporated into the United Nations Convention on the Rights of Persons with Disabilities in 2006 (United Nations 2006). The ICF is a scale composed of measures of body functions and structures, activity, participation and contextual factors, which has been designed to incorporate aspects of the social model of disability, and to include environmental factors. It has also been designed with the aim of utilizing neutral terminology and avoiding past stereotypes and negative connotations. The ICF is described by the WHO Information office as follows:

1   The <u>Body</u> dimension comprises two classifications, one for functions of body systems, and one for the body structure.
2   The <u>Activities</u> dimension covers the complete range of activities performed by an individual.
3   The <u>Participation</u> dimension classifies areas of life in which an individual is involved, has access to, and/or for which there are societal opportunities or barriers. (WHO 2001)

The three elements of ICF are designed to be co-participants in a new definition of the aspects which, when combined, create this concept of disablement. It is important to note that they are designed to be seen as equal participants. Equally important is the assertion that ICF was designed as a health classification and cannot be seen as more than a way of classifying the consequences of health conditions. Bickenbach et al. (1999) suggest that the ICF embodied a biopsychosocial approach to disablement, with each dimension conceptualized as interaction between the individual and their social and physical environment. A fourth 'environment' dimension lists environmental factors which are recognized as determinants of disablement. The ICF model is presented in figure 6.1.

The ICF is in wide use as a standard epidemiological tool in research across medicine and many allied fields (Bickenbach 2012). It is no secret that the disability movement and many people within the disability field were unhappy from the outset at the idea of revising the ICIDH, which they see as fatally flawed. The definitional frameworks and their critiques are complex, hinging on the role of biomedicine in defining and 'treating' disability and the role of society in shaping the experience of disability. It is this interface between the biomedical and the social that is at the heart of the most recent debates around the introduction of a sociology of impairment. Whilst the impact of society and the environment on disability are acknowledged in ICF, advocates of the social model say that the latest changes do not go far enough, and that disability has nothing to do with impairment and everything to do with the social environment and the ways in which it discriminates against non-able-bodied people.

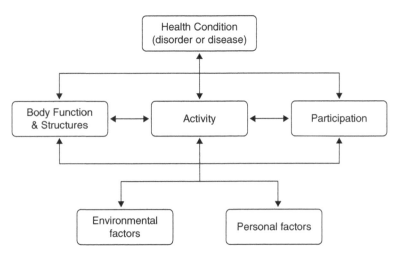

Figure 6.1 The International Classification of Functioning, Disability and Health (ICF) Model

Source: Reprinted from 'Towards a Common Language for Functioning, Disability and Health'. World Health Organization, 'The Model of ICF', p. 9. Copyright 2002

Scenario

To help you think about the differences between the medical and social models of disability, consider the following scenario.

There is a woman sitting outside the doors to a dental surgery. She has an appointment to see the dentist but is unable to access the building because of the steps up to the door. The woman is in a wheelchair and has arthritis.

Discussion Point

- How would each model describe the problem faced by the woman? What would each model say was the solution to the problem? Which model do you think gives the most useful explanation of the scenario?

Explanation

Once you have thought about these questions, read through this explanation. The medical model would identify arthritis as the root cause of the problem faced by the woman. The only solution would be to depend on someone helping the woman negotiate the steps if this was possible given the woman's condition and the nature of the steps. If this was not possible, then needing to find an alternative dental surgery would be seen as part of the personal tragedy of disability.

By contrast, the social model approach would say that the woman's medical condition is irrelevant. Rather, it would identify the stairs as a barrier. These could be removed through, for example, the provision of a ramp or of an alternative accessible entrance.

In summary, the way in which we understand disability and disabled people depends on the theory or theories we adopt. Disability is often presented as a binary, either caused by an impaired body or by an oppressive social environment. These definitions are important as our understanding of disability shapes the way that we respond to and treat disabled people both on an individual level and as a society.

Disability and oral health

Research suggests that disabled people and people living with long-term disabling conditions (such as a mental illness or a learning difficulty) have poorer oral health than their non-disabled peers (Melville et al. 1981; Scott et al. 1998; Cumella et al. 2000). This can cause physical problems but may also have a wider impact. For example, it has been found that good oral health can have a positive effect on self-esteem, quality of life and general health (Dahl et al. 2012). Improving the levels of oral health for disabled people and those living with long-term disabling conditions is, consequently, a major issue for the dental care services.

There is relatively little research available on the oral health needs of disabled people. Broadly speaking, disabled children and adults suffer from the same common oral diseases and conditions as the rest of society. There is evidence, however, that they experience poorer outcomes and the impact of oral disease on quality of life can be profound as it impairs eating, speaking, socializing and comfort. Caries rates amongst people with learning disabilities, for example, are comparable, but the decay is significantly less likely to be treated (Cumella et al. 2000; Owens et al. 2011), resulting in a poorer oral health outcome. In one Australian survey where the levels of disease were not significantly different across settings, higher odds of missing teeth were associated with type of impairment, whether general anaesthetic was required for dental treatment, and low and high levels of carer contact. Higher odds of filled teeth were associated with age, no oral hygiene assistance and high carer contact. Higher odds of caries experience were associated with age and a lack of oral hygiene assistance (Pradhan et al. 2009). The evidence suggests that whilst there are a small number of disabilities that incorporate direct oral symptoms (Plauth et al. 1991; Bell et al. 1999; Chandra & Bathia 2011), the oral diseases experienced by disabled people are similar to those experienced by the non-disabled population. And yet the oral health of disabled people is poorer than that of their non-disabled counterparts. This suggests that the problem, and potentially the solution, lies in dentistry and access to and use of dental care services.

Discussion Point

- The figures presented at the start of the chapter suggest that societal barriers such as stereotyping and negative attitudes are encountered by many disabled people when accessing healthcare. Can you think of any examples of this kind of barrier in a dental setting and how these kind of barriers might be addressed?

Approaches to disability within dentistry

The approach of dentistry towards disability and the provision of care for disabled people has been shaped, at least in part, by the conceptual framework for measuring oral health status developed by Locker in 1988. This emerged from the medical model of disability (WHO 1980).

Locker's model made the link between impairment and a range of psychosocial and functional outcomes of oral disease (Locker 1988a) and has been 'pivotal' in the development of dental research on the impact of oral disease and disorders on daily life (Allen 2003). Locker moved beyond the impaired body as the cause of disability, however, to suggest that disability is both a product of society and is dynamic in nature:

The extent to which functional limitations and activity restrictions cause a problem, or are otherwise handicapping, is not only variable historically and culturally but is also somewhat dependent on more immediate contexts: their meaning is not the same across different social and environmental settings. (Locker 1983: 5)

This acknowledged the socially contextual nature of functional limitations whilst stopping short of questioning the nature of disability itself. More recently, studies have looked to utilize the ICF (WHO 2001) as a way to calculate the number of people in need of special care dental services, acknowledging the role of the environment in the creation and perpetuation of disability (Allison et al. 2001). Again, however, the assumption that disability hinges on an impaired individual is not questioned.

The growing awareness of the limitations of the medical model of disability (ICIDH) led to calls for the dental profession to challenge negative attitudes towards disability within dentistry. In 2007 an editorial in the journal *Disability and Oral Health* called for dentistry to adopt the social model approach as a means of focusing on the environmental barriers, including attitudinal and awareness issues, which prevent disabled people from accessing dental services or promote dependency and powerlessness.

6

These are, by no means, always explicit or deliberate but can, sometimes, be borne out of low levels of disability awareness, which can result in anxiety and, at worst, a lack of enthusiasm and/or willingness to treat disabled people. (Goss 2007)

This call to action tied in with the publication, in 2007, of *Valuing Oral Health: A Good Practice Guide for Improving the Oral Health of Disabled Children and Adults* (Department of Health 2007). The report recommended that the majority of dental provision for disabled people should take place within primary care; that accessible health information should be available to promote choice and inclusion; that quality healthcare is a right for disabled people as it is for all other groups; that this healthcare should be responsive to their specific needs; and that oral healthcare should be part of holistic packages of care for disabled people.

Following the publication of the Department of Health report, Scambler et al. (2010) conducted a study to explore dental and allied professionals' attitudes towards disability within a special care dental context. Retroductive analysis of a series of focus groups and interviews with dental and allied professionals (n=30) was conducted using a theoretical framework modelled on the key tenets of the social model approach to disability. This incorporated the social cause of disability (Oliver 1990; Swain et al. 1993); a patient-centred approach (Charlton 1998); disability as secondary to dental care needs; and equality of care (Galipeault 2003). They found evidence that community special care dentistry staff held attitudes in support of the social model of disability with an underlying ethos of equality and awareness of the environmental, social and organizational barriers facing people with impairments, but demonstrated no explicit knowledge of the social model itself.

Access to oral healthcare

Special care dentistry (SCD) has evolved from the former community and salaried dental service (General Dental Council 2008) in response to identified need for a specialty (JACSCD 2003; Gallagher & Fiske 2007). SCD aims to cater for those with 'a physical, sensory, intellectual, mental, medical, emotional or social impairment or disability or, more often, a combination of a number of these factors' (Fiske 2006: 61). The majority of disabled people are cared for within general dental services and special care dentistry was established to support primary care practitioners in providing the majority of routine care and provide care for people with complex special needs (Gallagher & Fiske 2007). Despite the establishment of special care dentistry, there is some evidence that not all those who should be able to, or want to, access dental services can do so (Oliver & Nunn 1995).

Whilst some of these issues stem from difficulties experienced in accessing existing services, others stem from the adoption of the medical model approach to disability and disabled people prevalent across dentistry (Locker 1988a). A study by Scully et al. (2007) suggests that there are four categories of barriers which prevent people with learning disabilities from accessing oral healthcare. These are: barriers with reference to the individual; barriers with reference to the dental profession; barriers with reference to society; and barriers with reference to government. These categories are relevant to the experiences of people with a wide range of disabilities and are not simply limited to those with learning disabilities.

Individual barriers include a lack of perception of need by individuals (Hallberg & Klingberg 2005) or their carers (Cumella el al. 2000); difficulty following instructions with relation to oral self-care (Bollard 2002); and access problems, including those related to travel to and from the dental surgery (Dougall & Fiske 2008). Barriers relating to the dental profession include a lack of training specific to the requirements of the job (Gallagher & Fiske 2007; Scambler et al. 2010); poor communication skills (Sentell et al. 2007); high staff turnover, which results in a lack of trust and continuity of care (Pratelli & Gelbier 1998; Scambler et al. 2010); and a lack of time and resources (Scambler et al. 2010). In addition, cramped and inappropriate clinical environments and a lack of funding were identified (Edwards & Merry 2002; Scambler et al. 2010), as well as poor communication skills (Sentell et al. 2007).

Societal barriers include a general lack of awareness of the importance of oral healthcare, and a lack of positive attitudes towards oral health promotion (Owens et al. 2011). They also include a lack of appropriate service planning and provision (Rouleau et al. 2009) and a lack of research into the oral health needs of disabled people (Daly et al. 2002). Finally, governmental barriers include a lack of resources for oral health services and the resulting inability to put planning and policy into practice and ensure good quality oral healthcare for everyone (Dougall & Fiske 2008). This suggests that whilst the oral health needs of people with learning disabilities are broadly similar to their non-disabled peers, there are significantly more barriers to ensuring that their needs are met and that they receive good quality care.

By categorizing research on the barriers to accessible oral healthcare for disabled people using Scully et al.'s categories, it is possible to discern the micro-, meso- and macro-level responses to the problem of poor oral health outcomes amongst disabled people. What is clear from this is that the majority of research that has been undertaken in this area focuses on disabled people and their 'inability' to use general dental services. As Owens et al. (2011) argue, 'the literature displays a tendency to represent people with learning difficulties as a problem and pay[s] less attention to adjusting their environment to reduce the barriers that they encounter' (Owens et al. 2011: 18). This demonstrates the prevalence of the medical model approach focusing on the impaired individual rather than the disabling society in which they find themselves.

6

> **In summary**, the rhetoric around disability is moving from a medical towards a social model approach, but there is a lag between the theory and practice within dentistry. Relatively little research has been conducted looking at the oral health needs of disabled people, but studies that have been conducted suggest that the oral diseases encountered are similar to those within the non-disabled population, but that oral health outcomes are significantly worse. A range of individual and societal barriers have been identified in an attempt to explain this trend.

Conclusion

This chapter has not outlined the structure of dental service provision for disabled people, nor the practicalities of providing dental care for people with a range of different impairments. The aim of this chapter, rather, is to set the oral health of disabled people and dental care provision for this group into a wider context, exploring attitudes towards disability and disabled people and how these manifest themselves in the discrimination and social disadvantages that disabled people are forced to deal with on a day-to-day basis. The move towards a social model approach to disability within medicine and dentistry is welcomed, but it is worth noting that the poor oral health outcomes currently experienced by this group when compared with their non-disabled peers can be explained through the individual, professional, societal and policy-level barriers that they face in accessing dental care.

Symptoms and Help-Seeking

Suzanne E. Scott

Introduction

Think about the last patient you treated. Think about their journey into healthcare. What symptoms did they notice? What made them visit a dentist? Did they come to the dentist as soon as they developed symptoms? Why do people sometimes put off seeking help?

On first consideration, it may appear that a patient's treatment journey begins at the point at which they enter the healthcare system. However, there are a number of decisions, processes and actions that occur *before* healthcare use. For example, a person may or may not notice symptoms. After noticing a symptom, a person may choose to ignore it and will not seek healthcare. Alternatively, they may initially attempt self-medication and consult friends or family. Sometimes people decide the symptom requires attention from a healthcare professional and then need to negotiate access to healthcare. Help-seeking behaviour has been defined as a process involving 'symptom perception, interpretation, appraisal and decision-making, in addition to having the ability and motivation to enforce the decision by visiting a healthcare professional' (Scott & Walter 2010).

Help-seeking behaviour does not just involve whether or not someone decides to seek care, but also the timing or speed of healthcare use. This is crucial, because for many diseases, the timeliness of treatment is important. Morbidity and mortality rates are often improved when diseases are identified and treated at an early stage. For instance, if oral cancer is identified and treated when it is small and localized, 5-year survival rates can be as high as 90 per cent, yet if it is identified at an advanced stage (when large and metastatic), 5-year survival rates can be as low as 20 per cent (Cancer Research UK 2011). Consider the following case study. It is cases like this that underpin the investigation into help-seeking behaviour. If we can better understand the decisions behind healthcare use, we can use this knowledge to develop ways to encourage prompt presentation of disease.

Box 7.1: Case Study

Mr McNally is a 53-year-old gentleman. He works for the local council as a planning officer. He is unmarried, smokes 10–15 cigarettes a day and drinks about 18 units a week. He is a fairly regular attender at the dentist, usually visiting once every 12–18 months.

Today Mr McNally has come to visit you for his annual dental check-up, but he also tells you he has a sore patch on his tongue – he thinks it may be 'an ulcer that might have got infected'. It has been sore for about 5 months. He said that initially it ached but sometimes it becomes very painful, particularly when eating, so he has been avoiding hard foods such as crusty bread and has been trying to eat on one side of his mouth to stop aggravating it. Mr McNally tells you he has tried a few different mouthwashes, which seemed to provide some temporary relief and asks you if you can prescribe him something stronger to clear it up.

On clinical examination you can see a very tender, solitary ulcer with rolled borders on the lateral border of his tongue. You believe it requires an urgent referral to the local oral medicine unit to determine whether this suspicious lesion is a sign of oral cancer.

A few weeks later you hear back from the Oral Medicine Consultant. Your suspicions have been confirmed. Mr McNally has been diagnosed with advanced stage oral cancer. He is due to have an operation to remove the tumour and some lymph nodes, but the prognosis is not good. You are saddened to hear this news. If only Mr McNally had sought help sooner, maybe the lesion could have been diagnosed at an earlier stage. You wonder why he waited so long.

This chapter discusses research and theory on help-seeking behaviour, including the detection and interpretation of symptoms. The chapter will begin by outlining how people become aware of signs and symptoms (symptom perception) and how they are appraised. It will distinguish between biomedical and psychological models of symptom perception and highlight the relative inaccuracy of symptom perception and interpretation, and the possible reasons for this. The role of symptoms in help-seeking behaviour will be discussed and the concept of the clinical iceberg will be introduced. The chapter will then outline theoretical approaches used to understand help-seeking behaviour, factors which contribute to the decision to seek help, the topic of access to healthcare, and interventions to encourage early presentation. Wherever relevant, this chapter will use examples from oral diseases, but it will also draw on research about other symptoms and diseases to help understand and exemplify the general processes of symptom perception and help-seeking behaviour.

Symptom perception

Biomedical models of symptom perception state that the presence of illness (i.e. pathology, injury) will directly cause bodily changes and these will be detected by the individual as symptoms, and these symptoms will be perceived as indicators of illness. Biomedical models also assume that as pathology intensifies, symptoms will be increasingly obvious or distressing to the patient. For example, a life-threatening disease will lead to more severe and debilitating symptoms than those caused by a minor condition. However, there is mounting evidence that contradicts and challenges biomedical models of symptom perception. For example, there are a multitude of changes that occur within our body every day and across our lifetime, and there are a number of reasons why these bodily changes occur (Kolk et al. 2003). Whilst bodily changes can arise from disease (e.g. a lump due to cancer), these bodily changes can also arise from emotions (e.g. increased heart rate due to anxiety) or from environmental conditions (e.g. change in hand temperature due to cold air) as well as from fluctuations in normal bodily processes (e.g. bloating due to indigestion). Throughout the rest of this chapter, the terms 'signs and symptoms' are used to refer to bodily changes (either objective bodily events which can be measured and verified by others, or subjective experiences such as nausea that are 'felt' by individuals and are therefore only apparent to the affected person unless communicated; Pennebaker & Brittingham 1982). The term 'symptom perception' is used to refer to *awareness* of the signs and symptoms. This distinction is important because it appears that, contrary to the assumptions of the biomedical model, the presence of signs or symptoms does not necessarily mean we are aware of them. For example, reconsidering the case study in box 7.1, initially, before a painful ulcer developed, Mr McNally may have had oral erythroplakia (a cellular change leading to a raised red area on his tongue). However, he may not have been aware of the red lesion unless he (or someone else) had looked in his mouth and realized it looked different from normal. Thus a person may have signs or symptoms (a red lesion on the tongue) but symptom perception has not occurred. Indeed, this scenario has been reported in studies of oral cancer where up to 13 per cent of cases are picked up as an incidental finding during routine dental appointments (Allison et al. 1998). This example also contradicts the assumption of the biomedical model that 'serious' disease will have obvious symptoms.

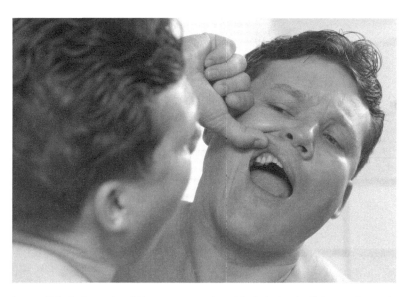

Image 7.1 Patients should be encouraged to visit their dentist if they notice oral symptoms such as a red patch, white patch, ulcer or lump that last more than three weeks
Source: schankz

Further, the occurrence of symptom perception does not necessarily mean that disease is present. Many people have 'false alarms' whereby they notice and become preoccupied with symptoms, concerned they may be a sign of serious disease. In fact, the symptoms turn out to be due to emotions, environmental conditions or fluctuations in normal bodily processes. It has been estimated that in 25–50 per cent of all primary care visits, there is no somatic disease that could explain the patient's presenting symptoms (Barsky & Borus 1995; olde Hartman et al. 2009). Of course, this is not to say those symptoms should be dismissed – they may be just as debilitating as those arising from disease. However, it does indicate that people may be relatively inaccurate at perceiving symptoms (Broadbent & Petrie 2007). Indeed, using experimental tests of symptom perception, Pennebaker and Brittingham (1982) found that there is only a low correlation between physiological states (e.g. skin temperature) and reported symptoms (e.g. self-reported warm hands).

With regard to oral symptoms, Patton (2001) assessed the accuracy of self-reports of oral infections by patients with HIV/AIDS. Comparison of these self-reports with results of an examination by an oral medicine practitioner indicated the sensitivity (agreement between the practitioner and patient) was generally low, ranging from 11 per cent for changes in the colour or texture of the tongue, to 56 per cent presence for ulcers. In a study of the accuracy of mouth self-examination for potentially malignant oral lesions, Scott et al. (2010) asked 53 adults to look in their mouth to check for any ulcers, white or red patches, or lumps/swellings. On comparing the findings

Table 7.1 Findings of mouth self-examination compared to findings of dental examination for potentially malignant oral lesions

		Findings from examination by dentist	
		Lesion present	Lesion absent
Findings from mouth self-examination	Lesion present	4 (4 adults correctly identified lesions that were present)	19 (19 adults had false positives: they thought a lesion was present when there was no lesion)
	Lesion absent	8 (8 adults had false negatives: they thought there was no lesion, when there was one)	22 (22 adults correctly noted there were no lesions)

Source: Adapted from Scott et al. (2010)

from the adults to those from an examination by a dentist (see table 7.1), the sensitivity and specificity of mouth self-examination were found to be low. The participants often missed oral lesions that were there (as seen by the dentist) and believed oral lesions were present when they were not (presumably by interpreting normal anatomic structures as pathological changes).

Psychological models of symptom perception

Psychological models of symptom perception (e.g. Pennebaker 1982; Cioffi 1991; Gijsbers Van Wijk & Kolk 1997) encompass cognitive (e.g. our thoughts and those of others), emotional and contextual/environmental processes involved in the awareness of symptoms. In contrast to biomedical models, they allow for the variability and inaccuracy in symptom perception and the psychosocial aspects that influence awareness of signs and symptoms. The impact of the environment and cognitive influences on symptom perception are now considered in turn.

How does the environment influence symptom perception?

Our external environment produces a constant stream of sensory information. For instance, think about the shapes, sounds, light, smells, movement and temperature of your current surroundings. At the same time, our brains are constantly receiving and processing masses of internal sensory information from our organs (e.g. indicators of hunger, thirst, arousal) and other body parts (e.g. physical comfort, aches or pains) (Rief & Broadbent 2007). It would be impossible to consciously process all of this external and internal information at once, as our brains have a limit in their capacity (Pennebaker 1982). As such, it has been proposed that there is a 'competition of cues' between the external and internal sensory information – if there is a mass of internal information, we will notice less about our environment. Conversely, if there is a lot of sensory information from our environment, we may not notice internal, bodily information. An example of this is the sports player who is so 'involved' in the game that they fail to notice they have an injury.

Further, it is thought that we also filter the incoming information. 'Selective attention' is the term used to describe this filter. Selective attention determines the type and extent of information that we consciously process (and thus are aware of). If we selectively attend to the body, we focus on bodily changes and therefore increase the likelihood of symptom perception (at the cost of missing aspects of our environment). If we selectively attend to external information, we focus on what is going on in our environment (at the cost of missing changes within our body). The 'competition of cues' theory and the concept of selective attention have been supported by a number of experimental and observational studies. For example, those who live alone or have boring, undemanding jobs (and thus have fewer environmental cues) report more physical symptoms than those who cohabit or have demanding jobs (Gijsbers van Wijk & Kolk 1997).

The influence of the environment on symptom perception can also be observed within the dental setting. For instance, many practitioners use the technique of 'distraction' when treating anxious patients. Distraction in the dental setting may be achieved by asking patients to focus on interesting wall displays, playing music or a radio or film in the clinic, asking patients to perform some kind of mental task (e.g. puzzles, guided imagery) or use of virtual reality technology (Frere et al. 2001). Distraction directs the patient's focus onto something unconnected to themselves or the dental work. In line with psychological models of symptom perception, distraction encourages selective attention to environmental cues, and so shifts a patient's focus away from the procedure, thus increasing the competition of cues from the environment. In turn, the potential for being aware of pain or discomfort (internal information) is reduced.

How does cognition influence symptom perception?

Symptom perception is not solely determined by the balance between internal and external information. Our cognition (e.g. thoughts, beliefs, expectations) and emotions can direct our attention towards or away from our body, and thus influence the likelihood of noticing symptoms. Expectation or anticipation of a symptom can influence symptom perception. We are more likely to become aware of a symptom that we are expecting, as opposed to something we did not anticipate (Cioffi 1996; Janssens et al. 2009). This is because expectations lead to selective attention, which in turn creates bias in our awareness of bodily changes. For example, Pennebaker and Skelton (1981) told some participants in their study that an ultrasonic noise (actually fictitious) would make their hands warm. They told others the noise would make their hands cold, and others were told the noise would have no effect. Participants' subsequent symptom reports (perceived hand temperature) were consistent with the suggestions they were given.

Within dentistry, use of phrases such as 'this might hurt' or 'you may feel some pain', implying the experience will be unpleasant, may create an expectation that pain will occur and thus direct patients' attention to their body, resulting in an increased likelihood of detecting and experiencing pain. Another example of the influence of expectations on symptom detection is the placebo effect, whereby patients report a reduction in symptoms after taking medication even though the medication is actually inert.

Symptom perception can also be influenced by our beliefs about diseases. If we have, or think we have, a disease, we will search for signs and symptoms that we believe occur as part of that disease, and this results in an increased likelihood of noticing these symptoms (Leventhal & Diefenbach 1991). For example, participants who were told they had a condition related to a particular enzyme deficiency (which was actually fictitious) were more likely to report symptoms consistent with their knowledge of that condition than individuals who were told they did not have the enzyme deficiency (Croyle & Sande 1988).

Although less extensively studied, it appears that emotions also influence symptom perception. For instance, Costa and McCrae (1980) found individuals with low mood report two to three times as many symptoms as those in a positive mood. Experimental studies indicate that people made to feel sad report more physical symptoms than those made to feel happy (see Salovey et al. 2000). This is particularly relevant to dentistry, as anxiety can be a contributing factor to pain. This may result from anxiety increasing our sensitivity to pain or by increasing our expectations of pain, resulting in selective attention to internal sensations. Therefore a reduction in anxiety should lead to a reduction in pain (Kent & Croucher 1998). See chapter 11 for further discussion.

7

Discussion Points

- What are the differences between biomedical and psychological models of symptom perception?
- Why may a patient fail to notice a change in their oral health?

In summary, symptoms arise for a number of reasons, including, but not limited to, the occurrence of disease. Awareness of symptoms or 'symptom perception' is not as straightforward as it first seems – some bodily changes are not detected, others are dismissed and sometimes disease does not seem to trigger symptoms. As psychological processes play a crucial role, symptom perception is subject to inaccuracies. Our environment, emotions and thoughts influence the symptoms we experience.

Symptoms and healthcare use

So far, this chapter has focused on how people may become aware of symptoms. What happens once someone is aware of a symptom? Does the experience of symptoms lead to healthcare use? To answer these questions, data on the occurrence of symptoms, disease and corresponding consultations with healthcare providers will be considered.

Perception of signs and symptoms is common. In fact, diary studies indicate that we notice symptoms almost daily (Gijsbers van Wijk et al. 1999). In a prospective study, Scambler et al. (1981) asked women to complete a symptom diary over 6 weeks and also note their healthcare use for those symptoms. In support of previous studies, experience of symptoms was found to be common (e.g. among the 79 women there were 180 episodes of headache, 71 episodes of aches or pains in joints, muscles, legs or arms and 45 episodes of stomach pains over the 6 weeks). Corresponding healthcare use was relatively rare, with one medical consultation for every 18 symptom episodes. So for most 'illness episodes', people do not seek help for symptoms. This phenomenon, whereby health professions are only consulted about a small proportion (the tip) of the sum total of ill-health, is referred to as the 'clinical iceberg' (see figure 7.1). There is evidence of this clinical iceberg for oral symptoms and disease and the use of dental services (Locker 1988b; Department of Health 2000).

It is noted that some healthcare use is not dependent on symptoms at all (e.g. preventive healthcare programmes such as those for screening and vaccination). This is particularly relevant to dentistry, where patients are asked to attend regular check-ups in the absence of symptoms. However, the best predictors of dental service utilization have been reported to be perceived need, dentate status and recent symptom experience (Holtzman et al. 1990).

The presence of the clinical iceberg highlights that even though consultation with healthcare professionals is often stimulated by the experience of signs and symptoms, symptom perception will not necessarily result in healthcare use. This is because presence of symptoms (even debilitating symptoms) does not necessarily mean a person will consider themselves ill or in need of healthcare (Komaroff 2001). Further, the number and severity of symptoms does not appear to have a major role in determining the timeliness of healthcare use: some people attend a healthcare professional fairly quickly with seemingly trivial symptoms, whereas others do not seek care or delay seeking care, despite having symptoms that are bothersome or grave (Prochaska et al. 1990).

Reflection Point

Consider the last 10 patients you have seen who had similar symptoms. It is likely that some will have sought help sooner than others. This suggests that it is something other than the nature of the symptoms that drives the speed of healthcare use.

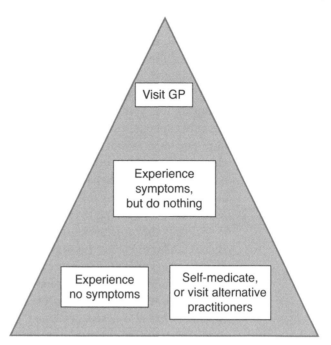

Figure 7.1 The 'clinical iceberg': the proportion of ill-health referred to health professionals
Source: Adapted from Alder et al. (2004)

7

Are some people in denial about their symptoms? Simply doing nothing in response to symptoms? This is not usually the case: there are a whole host of alternative responses. For instance, dismissing symptoms as 'normal', monitoring symptoms for change, hoping symptoms will resolve naturally, self-medication, adaptations to life-style, use of complementary or alternative medicines, or seeking lay (non-professional) advice. This occurred in the case study: Mr McNally did not consult a healthcare professional about his sore tongue for 5 months. However, he did not ignore his symptoms. Instead, he tried to manage them himself. In order to relieve the discomfort, he changed what he ate, the way he ate and he also used mouthwash.

Theoretical approaches to help-seeking behaviour

A number of theoretical approaches have been proposed to understand how people make the decision to seek help and barriers to healthcare use. Examples of these approaches are discussed in this section.

Ronald Andersen's 'Behavioural Model of Health Services Use' (Aday & Andersen 1974) describes people's use of healthcare services as a product of their predisposition to use services, factors that enable or impede healthcare use and their need for care. Predisposing factors involve demographics such as age and gender, position within the social structure and general health beliefs. Enabling factors involve structural or organizational barriers and triggers to seeking care (e.g.

income, accessible services, health insurance cover, having a regular source of healthcare) and need factors involve health status and the severity of the illness. Research using this model has demonstrated that evaluated need (professional judgement about people's health status and their need for medical care) is a common predictor of healthcare use. Overall, however, the application of this model generally only explains a small amount of variance in help-seeking behaviour. Andersen (1995) noted that this may be because of the way in which the model has been applied rather than a failure of the model itself. However, the Behavioural Model of Health Services Use has also been criticized for relying too heavily on organizational factors (Mechanic 1979), failing to take the patients' perspective into account or ignoring the processes involved in decisions to seek healthcare advice (Stoller & Forster 1994). Using a health diary study, Stoller and Forster (1994) argued that rather than enabling, predisposing or need factors, it is the patients' interpretation of their symptoms that triggers consultation with a healthcare professional. The validity of predisposing factors has also been questioned, as a person may experience the same symptoms on separate occasions and may not seek help on one occasion but decide to seek help on another. This conundrum led Mechanic (1975) to state that insight from the behavioural sciences is required, in order to provide a way to account for the diversity of responses between different individuals and groups, and also within the life history of an individual.

The 'General Model of Total Patient Delay' (Andersen et al. 1995) is a stage model of help-seeking behaviour that is much more focused on the patient perspective and incorporates a patient's symptom interpretation as a key stage in healthcare use. The model offers a useful guide to understand the patients' decisions following the detection of a symptom (e.g. 'Am I ill?', 'Does the illness require healthcare?') and has been applied to a number of settings such as help-seeking for symptoms of myocardial infarction, cancer and sexually transmitted diseases (Hedges et al. 1998; Pitts et al. 2000; Walter et al. 2010). A recent amendment to this model (the 'Model of Pathways to Treatment'; Scott et al. 2013) (see figure 7.2) emphasizes the dynamic nature of the pathway into and through healthcare, and proposes processes that occur at each interval. The appraisal interval and the help-seeking interval are of most relevance to healthcare use. These are outlined below.

The appraisal interval

The 'appraisal interval' represents the time from detection of a bodily change to perceiving a reason to discuss symptoms with a healthcare professional. Reasons for discussing symptoms with healthcare professionals can include beliefs about symptoms (e.g. something is wrong/serious), the consequences of symptoms (e.g. interference of symptoms with one's ability to work; Zola 1973), perceived inability to cope with

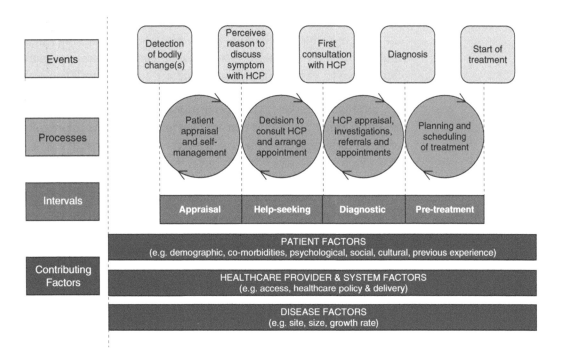

Figure 7.2 Model of pathways to treatment
Source: Scott et al. (2013)

symptoms (e.g. persistence, failure of self-medication) or emotional responses (e.g. anxiety, concern, need for reassurance).

During the appraisal interval, bodily changes are assessed and responses other than seeking help (e.g. self-medication) may be initiated. Patients' own understanding of their symptom episode will inform the selection of coping responses (e.g. if I believe my headache is due to dehydration, then I will drink water) (Mora et al. 2002). This self-management plays a key role in the pathway to diagnosis and has the potential to increase the time taken to seek help, as a patient may persist with self-medication for some time (Kaur et al. 2006; Mesfin et al. 2009). This was the case with Mr McNally in the case study. He thought he had a normal ulcer that needed mouthwash to help it resolve. His continued use of mouthwash meant he did not consult a healthcare professional about the mouth ulcer. Even when he mentioned his sore tongue at the appointment, he continued to believe he had an ulcer that needed a stronger form of mouthwash. Thus, his beliefs about his symptoms (symptom appraisal) was the main determinant of his behaviour. Indeed, patients' appraisal of their symptoms is crucially important in the decision to seek help, with misinterpretation being a key factor in delays in seeking help for symptoms of cancer and myocardial infarction (Smith et al. 2005; Corner et al. 2006; Turris & Finamore 2008).

Symptom appraisal is subject to a number of cognitive heuristics and biases such as the 'rate of change rule', the 'novelty rule', the 'age-illness rule' and the 'prevalence rule'. (Leventhal et al. 2007). For instance, those symptoms that are worsening, unstable or increasing in number, and/or have a sudden rather than gradual onset, are more likely to be perceived to indicate illness and provide motivation to seek help promptly (the 'rate of change rule'). Symptoms that are new or different rather than familiar, common or similar to a coexisting chronic illness are more often perceived to be a sign of illness and are a key motivator to seek help (the 'novelty rule'). As individuals grow older, they may increasingly attribute sensations to the ageing process rather than to illness (the 'age-illness rule'). Symptoms that are seen to be rare in the community are more likely to invoke concern, be perceived as a sign of illness and act as a motivator to seek help (the 'prevalence rule'). This indicates that the decision to seek help occurs within the social and cultural context (Andersen et al. 2010). Indeed, Cornford and Cornford (1999) found that patients spoke to up to 16 people prior to seeking help, with the average being three to four people. This lay referral network consisted of relatives, partners, workmates, friends, neighbours, nurses and pharmacists, and can influence symptom interpretations, perceptions of the need for care and persuasion or dissuasion to seek help.

The help-seeking interval

The 'help-seeking interval' describes the time from perceiving a reason to discuss symptoms with a healthcare professional to the first consultation with a healthcare professional about their symptoms. During the help-seeking interval, the decision to seek help is made and arrangements to do so are put in place. A person's self-efficacy (perceived ability) to discuss the symptoms and get help influences the use of healthcare (and the time it takes to seek help). If the barriers to seeking help appear insurmountable or help is perceived as unavailable, help will not be sought. Personal barriers may include a lack of time to visit a healthcare professional, problems arranging travel to a healthcare professional or general lethargy (e.g. due to depression) (Bunde & Martin 2006). Penchansky and Thomas (1981) suggested healthcare system barriers include:

- Accessibility: the location of services in relation to the location of patients.
- Affordability: the price of healthcare services/insurance in relation to patients' income and ability to pay.
- Availability: the volume and type of services/resources/specialist equipment/healthcare professionals in relation to the requirements of patients.
- Acceptability: patients' attitudes towards the healthcare services/providers and the healthcare providers' attitudes towards their patients.
- Accommodation: the organization of the healthcare services (e.g. opening hours, walk-in facilities) in relation to patients' needs.

On the other hand, opportunities such as having a pre-booked appointment or free health screening may encourage prompt help-seeking via making healthcare utilization easier and thus enhancing self-efficacy to seek help. In addition to self-efficacy, a person's expectations of what will happen as a result of seeking care – referred to by Bandura (1998) as 'outcome expectations': a person's perceived consequences of action – are also highly significant. Unless people believe that help-seeking can produce desired effects (e.g. a healthcare professional will be able to relieve symptoms), and seeking help will not result in ill-effects (e.g. will be ridiculed by the healthcare professional), they will have little incentive to consult a healthcare professional (Scott et al. 2013).

With regard to the dental setting, Finch et al. (1988) identified two main barriers to dental care: fear of dental treatment and the cost of dental treatment. These barriers continue to be relevant. Data from the 2009 Adult Dental Health Survey (an interview survey of 11,380 individuals living in England, Wales and Northern Ireland) demonstrated a relationship between dental anxiety and dental attendance. Those with high levels of dental anxiety were more likely to attend only when they have trouble with their teeth than for a regular check-up. Twenty-six per cent of respondents reported that the type of dental treatment they had chosen in the past had been affected by the cost of this treatment and 19 per cent said that they had delayed dental treatment because of the cost of treatment (Hill et al. 2013). Other barriers to dental care include: the reception and waiting room procedures; perceptions of a loss of control; the perceived personality of the dentist; the clinical smell of the dental practice; hearing sounds of dental treatment; white coats and bright lights; feeling vulnerable in the dental chair; being treated 'like a mouth and not a person'; and the time to travel to and attend a dental appointment (Finch et al. 1988). These are therefore important considerations when planning dental services. The qualities of a good dentist are perceived to be: friendliness; personal touch; good chair-side manner; explains what they are doing; explains what the cost of treatment is before starting; is caring, gentle and reassuring; inspires confidence; and good technical skills. Presence of these qualities will increase both satisfaction with dental services (Hill et al. 2003) and use of healthcare services (and also adherence to treatment and maintenance of a relationship between the dentist and patient).

Discussion Point

- When someone notices a change in their oral health, why may they decide to self-medicate rather than seek help? Consider both the appraisal interval and the help-seeking interval.

In summary, people frequently notice symptoms, yet healthcare use is relatively rare. In turn, healthcare professionals only see the 'tip of the iceberg' of the symptoms that are experienced.

Theoretical approaches have been applied to help-seeking research in order to understand why and when help-seeking occurs. These have identified two main processes that occur in the lead up to healthcare use: (i) appraisal of symptoms as requiring healthcare professional attention; and (ii) the decision to seek help.

The appraisal interval is influenced by a person's knowledge, their previous experience and social context, and a number of heuristics which guide symptom interpretation. The help-seeking interval is influenced by a person's perceived ability to get help, competing priorities, expectations about the healthcare visit and social and healthcare system barriers that may inhibit access. This is particularly pertinent to dentistry, where a number of barriers exist, including fear of dental treatment and cost of dental treatment.

Interventions to encourage healthcare use

For diseases such as cancer, finding ways to encourage prompt consultation for symptoms is vital. This is a difficult task as interventions need to target those most at risk in order to prevent over-burdening healthcare systems with people who are worried about symptoms that are unlikely to be signs of disease. This section considers the current evidence base for interventions that have aimed to promote timely healthcare use for symptoms of oral cancer.

Encouraging early presentation of oral cancer

Although many oral cancer awareness campaigns exist, few have been evaluated. Of those that have been evaluated, there have been mixed results. Some interventions aiming to encourage early presentation of oral cancer have been set within a dental practice. For instance, Boundouki et al. (2004) found an information leaflet given in dental surgery waiting rooms increased participants' knowledge of oral cancer by 4 per cent, and raised participants' intention to accept an oral cancer screen by the dentist. However, this study did not assess the impact of the intervention on help-seeking for signs of oral cancer (or intentions to seek help) and did not target those most at risk (e.g. those who use tobacco, drink alcohol and are over 45 years old) and only the short-term effects were monitored. As such the extent of its full usefulness is not known.

Other interventions have used a wider approach. Eadie et al. (2009) used a mass-media campaign consisting of TV and radio advertisements, news coverage, wall posters, leaflets and direct mail drops in target communities (individuals over 40 years old from lower socio-economic groups) in the West of Scotland. The intervention was guided by Social Cognitive Theory (see Bandura 1998) and the evaluation involved assessment of awareness, knowledge and behavioural intentions prior to and after the campaign. However, this intervention did not have a sizeable impact. This disappointing result has been replicated across other diseases. For instance, mass-media or community campaigns aimed at reducing delays in presentation for symptoms of myocardial infarction have also been largely unsuccessful (Caldwell & Miaskowski 2002; Kainth et al. 2004). The oral cancer intervention only had a short-term increase on awareness of oral cancer and had no impact on the perceived incidence of oral cancer or awareness of symptoms. The intervention did increase expected concern in situations where respondents experienced a persistent red/white patch, ulcer or sore and raised intentions to seek help from a general practitioner (but not a dentist) if these symptoms arose. The difficulties in assessing the impact of mass-media campaigns were demonstrated in that 23 per cent of participants in the control group were also aware of the TV advertisements.

Some community interventions do result in change, yet fail to achieve change in those most in need. For instance, a leaflet-based campaign to increase knowledge and awareness of oral cancer that was delivered throughout a Spanish town was shown to be effective in raising knowledge, yet the effect was highest among younger adults and those with a higher educational level (Petti & Scully 2007). As such, there has been a shift towards designing and implementing interventions that are targeted and/or tailored to particular groups (de Nooijer et al. 2004). This may involve targeting interventions at those most at risk of developing the disease in question or those who currently delay seeking help.

Scott et al. (2011) documented the development of intervention resources that were purposely designed for individuals at risk of developing oral cancer. The intervention was guided by theory and research evidence into the reasons for delayed presentation of oral cancer. The intervention involved a brief interactive discussion (with adjunct written information) of the importance of early detection, signs and symptoms to look out for, and making a plan (an implementation intention, see pp. 146–7) of when and where to seek help. The intervention was later found to be successful in raising awareness of oral cancer, confidence to seek help and intention to seek help for symptoms of oral cancer (Scott et al. 2012). Dentists are well placed to deliver this type of intervention during routine appointments, and dental patients are keen to receive this health advice. For example, in a survey of 184 dental patients, 92 per cent of respondents indicated that they would like their dentist to tell them if they were being screened for signs of oral cancer and 97 per cent indicated that they would like help from their dentists to reduce their risk (Awojobi et al. 2012).

7

Reflection Point

- How can dental practitioners encourage patients to seek help promptly for signs of oral cancer?
  What problems might they encounter in doing this?

In summary, encouraging early presentation of oral cancer is an important step in achieving better prognosis for this disease and dentists are well placed to deliver such interventions.

However, existing interventions to encourage early help-seeking for oral cancer have had mixed results. Those that have involved provision of information about oral cancer may increase knowledge and awareness of oral cancer but this may not translate into prompt help-seeking and the long-term success of these types of interventions needs to be investigated.

Interventions that are targeted at those who are most at risk of developing oral cancer or those who are likely to delay seeking help are likely to be most useful.

Conclusion

Symptom perception and seeking help from healthcare professionals are complex processes. They have implications for our health, quality of life and treatment options; they also have implications for healthcare systems, including the cost of healthcare services.

This chapter has highlighted the complexities of healthcare use. The presence of disease may or may not create bodily changes and those bodily changes may or may not be detected by individuals. People are relatively inaccurate at perceiving symptoms and this has implications for self-management of oral disease and disease detection if the responsibility for these is left with the patient. Psychosocial influences of symptom perception have direct implications for increasing patients' comfort whilst receiving dental care. For instance, using selective attention away from procedures may help patients cope with potential discomfort.

Symptoms are often the driver for healthcare use, but their presence is not sufficient to prompt a consultation with a healthcare professional. In fact, most symptoms do not result in healthcare use and some use of healthcare occurs in the absence of symptoms. The context of symptoms and various psychosocial factors influence the perception of symptoms and the perceived need for healthcare. Further, once a person perceives a need for healthcare, they must overcome barriers to care, including those of the health system and their own expectations about the consequences of visiting a healthcare professional. The barriers to healthcare are particularly relevant to dentistry and have implications for the way dental practices are arranged and managed and highlight the need for a patient-centred approach to dental care to achieve patient satisfaction and ensure prompt help-seeking for oral diseases such as oral cancer.

Adherence and Behaviour Change in Dental Settings

Koula Asimakopoulou and Blánaid Daly

IN THIS CHAPTER YOU WILL LEARN ABOUT:

▶ Competing definitions of the concept of adherence and some of their shortcomings

▶ Popular psychological theories of health behaviour change – their advantages and limitations

▶ Current thinking about behaviour change methods – in particular, the COM-B model of behaviour change and how it might be applied to dentistry

Introduction

Why do smokers carry on smoking when they know that it is bad for them? Why do overweight people find it hard to lose weight? Why won't people floss their teeth despite the dentist telling them about the importance of flossing and showing them explicitly what to do?

Advancements in healthcare have now made it possible for people to take advantage of health treatments which, if given in an appropriate manner, can help the person live a healthier, happier, longer life. However, the success of most of these treatments is not solely reliant on the administration of the treatment. They require patient cooperation and more often than not, at least some behaviour change on the part of the patient. For example, in order to benefit from the latest advances in periodontal treatment, the patient has to arrange and attend a dental appointment, listen, understand and recall the advice given by the dental team with regard to performing appropriate oral hygiene behaviours, undertake the treatment, believe that the advice they have been given will deal with their periodontal problem, have the opportunity, competence and confidence to carry out the brushing and flossing behaviours the dental team recommended, perhaps form an intention to perform them and, finally, appropriately engage in these behaviours at the correct time, using the correct equipment, for an appropriately sustained time period. Looking at this example, it should be obvious that although the medical and health advances are such that a patient's oral health *could* benefit, whether it actually does or not largely depends on behaviours that the patient performs on their own, outside the surgery and over which the dental practitioner has little if any direct control.

At the same time, prevention of disease has become a cornerstone of current health policy in the UK. The Wanless report (Wanless 2004) called for the public to become 'fully engaged with health' and stay healthy by optimizing their use of preventive and primary care services. A similar trend was observed in UK dentistry, where a more preventive model of care has been advocated by the Department of Health (2005, 2007). While we can now have confidence in the evidence base of advice patients are given (Department of Health 2014), it is probably true to say that supporting patients in changing and sustaining change in their oral health behaviours is one of the most difficult challenges the dental team faces. These difficulties may be because dentists are not always sure of the best way to encourage their patients to adapt their behaviour. Reviews of the effectiveness of dental health education (DHE), including chair-side DHE, have highlighted the lack of theoretical underpinning, particularly in relation to the psychological theories of behaviour change. Understanding the processes involved in behaviour change and how these changes may be sustained is essential if the dental team are to be successful in getting patients to engage in and continue with long-term lifestyle changes.

This chapter considers empirical and theoretical psychological work that underpins current understanding of two main areas of psychological enquiry: the issue of non-compliance (or non-adherence) with health advice; and the processes involved in people's attempts to change current health behaviours. Popular psychological models of behaviour change in health settings and advantages and limitations of each are outlined.

Before considering empirical evidence that explains how people go about engaging in behaviour change, take a look at the case study that follows, then think about the patient's potential for adherence with the dentist's advice.

Box 8.1: Case Study

Tony, a 50 year old Afro-Caribbean male patient, attends a dental surgery for a check-up. He says he doesn't have any major problems with his teeth but mentions his wife has told him he has bad breath. An initial examination shows signs of gingivitis.

The dentist explains for a third time in as many visits the many benefits of brushing and flossing, then proceeds to explore with the patient why he hasn't done as he was told. In an attempt to make the patient aware of the potential consequences of periodontal disease, the dentist further explains that Tony's plaque and gingival scores are very worrying. The patient replies that he brushes his teeth twice a day but doesn't like to use dental floss as it makes his gums bleed and surely that can't be a good sign. The dentist tells Tony that he needs to brush regularly and floss once a day, then book another appointment with the dentist. Tony is also advised that he needs to see a hygienist. He is sent home.

Tony leaves the dental surgery. He is not sure how he is supposed to floss and can't remember how often and when he is supposed to see the hygienist. He thinks that this dentist doesn't really know what he is talking about as he still doesn't know why he has bad breath – what is he to tell his wife? Everybody in his family has nice teeth and he never had problems before, so he reasons that as good teeth 'run in the family', he is going to be alright with the oral health routine he can currently manage rather than what he was told at the surgery. He remembers the dentist warning him about consequences but doesn't understand what he meant. He tells his wife that the dentist must have been very intelligent but was not much help with the bad breath problem so they should look for a new dentist.

Discussion Point

• Write down the advice you think Tony was expecting to receive from the dentist. Next to the list, write down the advice that he did receive. What seems to be the discrepancy here?

In this case study, the patient has come in to see the dentist hoping to get a solution to his bad breath problem. The dentist has addressed the problem by inviting the patient to brush, floss and see the hygienist. The consequence of the patient performing these behaviours is likely to be an improvement in the halitosis issue. However, whilst the patient has been educated about *what* to do, he has not been supported in working out *how* to do any of the prescribed behaviours. Behaviour change, as will be shown in this chapter, requires more than just telling patients they need to change a behaviour.

8

Why don't patients do what they are asked to do? The defining features of non-compliance and non-adherence

This area of research, looking to examine whether people normally do what healthcare providers (HCPs) ask them to do in order to improve their physical or oral health, is known as research into 'compliance' or 'adherence' with HCP advice.

Non-compliance is a term used to describe the extent to which 'a person's behaviour coincides with medical or health advice' (Haynes et al. 1979). There are several assumptions implicit in this statement. Firstly, the definition assumes that the person has been given one (rather than several) clear piece of health advice by an HCP. It assumes that there are the means to assess whether the patient has indeed behaved in ways that coincide with the given advice. It further assumes that the person has been able to behave in a way that matches the advice given. Finally, and quite importantly, it makes no room for considering the patient's views on the advice they have been given and the effect that such views are going to have on whether they follow the advice through.

The latter of these assumptions led researchers to suggest that the term 'non-compliance' should be replaced by the potentially kinder to patients 'non-adherence'. Non-adherence, according to the World Health Organization (2003) is about 'the extent to which a person's behaviour – taking medication, following a diet, and/or executing lifestyle changes, corresponds with agreed recommendations from a healthcare provider'. In line with recommendations that patients play some role in deciding their treatment regime (Department of Health 2012), the role of the patient in this definition is more readily acknowledged; an adherent patient is someone who has played some role in the process of accepting their HCP advice, as seen in the definition's emphasis on the patient's behaviour corresponding with '*agreed*' recommendations. So here, the patient is said to be complying with advice that they have had some role in shaping in collaboration with their HCP. Some researchers prefer to use the term 'concordance' to describe essentially the same process and one that acknowledges the active role patients (ought to) have in developing treatment plans and receiving HCP advice.

So what is non-adherence, or failure to concord with HCP advice, about? And what might it look like in the dental setting? Examples of non-adherence to treatment include:

1   failure to attend routine dental appointments or arriving late
2   not initiating a recommended and agreed course of dental treatment
3   failure to complete behavioural aspects of dental treatment, such as flossing regularly, either because of lack of competence/confidence or through conscious unwillingness to perform these behaviours
4   not taking medication as prescribed or varying the degree and dose of medication-taking prescriptions
5   ending a course of treatment prematurely
6   engaging in a different, non-prescribed, non-agreed course of action in order to correct an oral health problem.

It can be seen that non-adherence can take various forms and manifest itself in several ways. The one thing that all of these cases have in common, however, is the patient playing a central role in the non-performance of behaviours that have been agreed with an HCP in order to manage a health condition.

A review of adherence studies published between 1948 and 1998 (DiMatteo 2004) estimated that, on average, of the 760 million visits to HCPs that took place in the United States in 2000, around 200 million resulted in patients not following the advice they were given. It was concluded that across all work examining patient adherence that was published between the 1950s and 2000, about a quarter of all patients seeking HCP advice ended up not following that advice, with variations to this rate as a function of the illness patients were seeking to treat and patient characteristics.

Non-adherence is, potentially, a serious health problem. On a wider social level, patients who do not adhere to treatment and preventive regimens are said to use up scarce health resources and, by doing this, deny others the opportunity to benefit from healthcare. On an individual level, non-adherence with HCP advice has both financial and health consequences. Health consequences can range from the worsening of the current problem to the development of other, related, co-morbidities. This could affect the patient's overall quality of life, bring about or exacerbate psychological problems and result in further illness, disability, loss of function, loss of work and, as a result, more psychological problems. The financial consequences have to do with the costs associated with additional visits to correct a problem that would have been dealt with had the patient adhered to advice, and with the effects of reduced patient function or ability to be productive and earn a living. Overall, non-adherence to HCP advice can compromise recovery from a health condition, undermine the person's chances for a speedy and safe recovery from a health-threatening condition and may have a domino effect on other aspects of the person's livelihood.

What are the roots of non-adherence?

When asking any HCP why it is that their patients do not appear to be doing what the HCP has suggested they do, the first thing often raised is 'education'. It is easy to assume that people do not floss their teeth because they have not been shown the correct technique, or that they do not attend for dental check-ups routinely because they are unaware of the benefits of preventive dentistry. This is a somewhat naïve interpretation of the situation. When considering these behaviours further, evidence will be found as to why the idea that knowledge predicts health behaviour is a naïve one. Behaviours such as snacking on sugary foods, failing to floss twice a day, taking the lift rather than the stairs, smoking, eating an unhealthy, nutritionally unnecessary pudding on top of a big meal, being sedentary rather than engaging in a regular 20-minute daily exercise regime are extremely common. However, most people have sound information to suggest to them that these health-compromising behaviours are indeed health-compromising. It is proposed that knowledge is necessary to take up healthy behaviours, but in most cases is not sufficient in itself. There is more to non-adherence to healthy behaviours over and above lack of knowledge or skill. Behavioural scientists would argue that the performance of (or non-adherence to) a new health behaviour, is a function of knowledge, skills and a range of psychological factors that all work together.

As such, this chapter sees adherence and behaviour change as part of the same process.

> **In summary,** non-adherence with to advice is a widespread problem, seen not only in dentistry, but in medicine too. Giving people information about how to perform a health behaviour might increase their knowledge, but that in itself is unlikely to lead to sustained behaviour change.

The next section considers in detail some popular theories that have attempted to explain how people go about dropping an unhealthy behaviour and replacing it with a healthy alternative through a combination of factors. In particular, popular social cognition models (psychological theories) of behaviour change are reviewed and the evidence for each evaluated.

Health behaviour change and social cognition models

In an effort to be able to systematically predict behaviour, psychologists have attempted to come up with specific combinations of factors that are thought to be important in eliciting behaviour change in health settings. To this end, 'models' have been constructed that rely on 'social cognitions' – these are ways that people think about their social world. These social cognition models have been developed in order to try and define those features of behaviour that are important in helping people get to grips with behaviour change and, by definition, ignore those factors that are less important. Their basic premise is that information is not enough to change behaviour; the reasons why people adhere to new health behaviours are complex and cannot be explained by the amount of information they have been given. It is this complexity in the reasons behind behaviour change that these models have attempted to capture in trying to explain what factors are important in helping people change.

There are several social cognition models but this chapter reviews four of the most popular ones, namely:

- The Health Belief Model
- The Transtheoretical Model of Change
- The Theory of Planned Behaviour and
- Protection Motivation Theory.

The Health Belief Model

The Health Belief Model (HBM; Rosenstock 1966, 1990) has been studied extensively in various health settings and with an extensive sample of patients and health conditions. Researchers have used it to

The HBM
(Rosenstock, 1966)

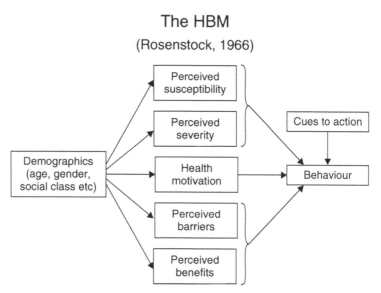

Figure 8.1 The Health Belief Model
Source: Adapted from Ogden (2012)

predict behaviour change in the uptake of diverse behaviours, from genetic screening, to the uptake of influenza vaccinations, to adhering to diabetes, hypertension and renal disease regimens, contraceptive use, smoking and drinking (Conner & Norman 2005; Jones et al. 2014). It is a comprehensive model aiming to break down the building blocks of undertaking a new health behaviour and to identify the interrelationships between those components. (See figure 8.1 for a diagrammatic representation.)

The model suggests that whether a health behaviour is likely to be performed depends on the patient's *beliefs* about that behaviour. In particular, it was suggested that it is of importance whether the patient perceives a particular health threat (in terms of how susceptible they are to an illness and how severe they perceive that illness to be) and believes that a particular health practice (conceptualized in a series of thoughts about the benefits and barriers associated with taking corrective action to control the illness) will be effective in dealing with the threat.

Although the HBM was not specifically developed for application in dental settings, its principles readily apply to such a setting. If we look back at the case study presented at the beginning of the chapter and consider the dentist's advice to Tony, the model would propose that the chances of Tony brushing his teeth would be influenced by a series of beliefs, as follows: Tony would need to believe that he was a likely candidate for gum disease (susceptibility to a health threat), that gum disease was a serious illness (severity of the health threat) and he was sufficiently concerned about gum disease to want to do something about it (health motivation). If he then thought that brushing was time-consuming (barrier) but that this behaviour would lead to fresher breath and avoidance of gum disease (benefits), Tony, the model predicts, would be more likely to brush his teeth. Should these beliefs also be supplemented by 'cues to action' (e.g. internal cues such as a foul taste in his mouth and/or external cues such as people telling Tony he had bad breath), the model suggests that Tony would be more likely to brush his teeth than someone who didn't think they were susceptible, didn't worry about gum disease and saw barriers but no benefits in brushing.

The model arose out of early work that included studies on dental patients (Kegeles 1963; Haefner 1974). In this early work, it was shown that perceived susceptibility to the worse imaginable dental problems, coupled with the belief that regular visits to the dentist might prevent these problems, were useful predictors of patients' frequency of dental visits over the next three years. Following this, a study assessing American women's success in engaging with preventive dental behaviour reported that such behaviour was strongly related to their health beliefs (Chen & Land 1986). These encouraging findings were taken as supportive of the role of health beliefs in predicting behaviour change and the Health Belief Model was put across as a viable predictor of the undertaking of healthy behaviours.

Although it sounds like a plausible set of predictors, studies using the HBM to predict adherence with oral hygiene instructions found that only some of the model's components, such as seriousness (Kuhner & Raetzke 1989), susceptibility (Barker 1994) and benefits (Kuhner & Raetzke 1989; Barker 1994), were successful in predicting adherence to daily plaque control assessed by plaque and bleeding scores. This means, that whilst *some* of the model's predictors may explain oral health behaviour, the model as a whole is unable to tell a convincing story that would explain a large amount of variance in oral health behaviour.

These findings are not surprising; critics of the HBM have suggested that it is inflexible in suggesting that people always consciously think about things such as seriousness and susceptibility before they perform simple health behaviours, such as picking up a toothbrush! It is easy to see that thinking about seriousness and how susceptible you are to illness may be processes that people undertake when considering some serious illnesses (e.g. heart disease or cancer), but perhaps they are not that salient a construct for other less serious, non-life-threatening conditions (e.g. periodontal disease). In addition, the model ignores the role of emotional or environmental influences. It treats people as rational, logical and coherent thinkers rather than people who might at times be subject to emotional (e.g. frustration, anger) or environmental (e.g. tiredness after a long day) consequences. The model further fails to consider that beliefs may change in response to experience; for example, think about a situation where a person's oral health is suffering despite the person's conscious efforts to adhere to oral hygiene instructions. The model is not helpful in telling us what would happen to the patient's beliefs at that point and how these modified beliefs might now predict their brushing behaviour.

So, overall, whilst appearing useful and potentially practical in predicting whether someone is likely to engage in a health behaviour (e.g. taking up brushing following a dental consultation), the model *as a whole* does not seem to be that strong in explaining the various reasons that may be behind people's reluctance to take up and adhere to routine, ongoing, simple health behaviours.

The Transtheoretical (Stages of Change) Model

A second, very popular model in the field of adherence and behaviour change is the Stages of Change Model (Prochaska & DiClemente 1984). This argues that differences in the rate and speed by which people take up a new behaviour or adhere to HCPs' recommendations can be attributed to differences in how prepared people are to take up health-care advice (see figure 8.2).

Originally developed in the 1980s, the model was arrived at through theoretical work in psychotherapy and also in smoking cessation. Since then it has been applied in an attempt to explain a range of behaviours from drug use and drinking alcohol, to condom use and attendance at mammography screening appointments (Sutton 2001).

The Stages of Change Model proposes that in assessing people's readiness to change their health habits, HCPs need to assess which of these stages people are at: a motivation-based stage where they have not considered taking up a health behaviour (pre-contemplation), a stage where they are only just starting to think about it (contemplation), a stage where they are making concrete preparations in changing the behaviour (preparation), or an action-based stage where they are actively performing the newly adopted behaviour (action) or indeed have been doing so successfully for some time (maintenance). The model also includes a consideration of the person's confidence in undertaking the behaviour change, as well as the pros and cons of changing (Prochaska et al. 2002).

○ Not all people are at the same point of adopting a specified behaviour.

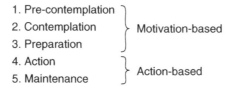

1. Pre-contemplation ⎫
2. Contemplation   ⎬ Motivation-based
3. Preparation   ⎭
4. Action   ⎫
                      ⎬ Action-based
5. Maintenance   ⎭

Figure 8.2 Stages of Change Model

Source: Adapted from Prochaska and DiClemente (1984)

The idea proposed by the model is that people at different stages of the process will require different HCP input in order to help them move from an early to a later stage in the process of change. That is, it is argued that it is pointless talking to a patient who has never considered giving up smoking (so is at the pre-contemplation stage) about ways to give up smoking; instead, communication should be focused on moving them from a pre-contemplation stage to the next one up, i.e. to contemplating a change. Once the person has moved up through the various stages to being ready to consider smoking cessation (e.g. they are at a preparation stage), it may then be sensible to support them in behaviour change by explaining about the different methods of giving up smoking. However, some work has shown that smokers who were not 'ready to change' according to the Stages of Change Model responded favourably to offers of help to quit and went on to become ex-smokers (Pisinger et al. 2005), contrary to what the model would predict. Similarly, in a study of flossing in patients who were either ready to change or not (Suresh et al. 2012), it was found that an intervention consisting of keeping a simple flossing diary led to improvements in flossing frequency, plaque and bleeding scores in both people who had reported that they were not ready to change and in those who were considering change.

At the same time, work using the Stages of Change Model to predict attendance at dental check-ups (Coulsen & Buchanan 2002) revealed some interesting findings. Students' self-reported intentions and behaviour with respect to dental check-up attendance, which were subsequently classified by the Stages of Change Model, predicted their perceptions of positive and negative aspects of visiting the dentist; students classified as being in the action stages of the model (stages 4 and 5) were more likely to agree with statements in favour of visiting the dentist than students who were in the motivation stages (stages 1–3) of the model, with this latter group focusing more on the negative aspects of dental visits. This study would suggest that people's attitudes to a health behaviour, in this case attending the dentist, will change depending on where in the process of change they might be. It would thus appear that the Stages of Change Model may be helpful in predicting adherence to dental appointments and give some insight into the attitudes underpinning dental attendance behaviour.

Critics of the model (e.g. Ogden 2012), however, have identified a few difficulties with the main ideas it proposes. For example, it is argued that it is not clear whether behaviour really does change according to distinct stages, or along a continuum. So the stage boundaries are perhaps in reality more fuzzy and less clear-cut than the model would suggest. The model also makes no predictions about the speed by which people can move up (and down) the different stages, nor does it elaborate on the concept of relapse and its relation to the different proposed stages. Finally, as reported in the example of the smokers' study and the flossing diary study, people who, according to the model, should not benefit from behaviour change because they are not ready for it, actually do change, making the Stages of Change theory rather weak. So, although conceptually helpful, the Stages of Change Model may not be as robust a theory of behaviour change as originally thought, especially when it comes to complex behaviours.

Theory of Planned Behaviour

Key to the Stages of Change Model is the idea that most behaviour change will probably happen through a transition between the proposed stages. Inherently important in this scheme is the concept of intentions, i.e. people are unlikely to change their behaviour unless they have spent some time contemplating the change and forming an intention to do so at the contemplation and preparatory stages. The Theory of Planned Behaviour (TPB) (Ajzen 1985), the third model examined here, considers intentions in a systematic and detailed way and proposes that they are central in determining whether a particular health behaviour is performed or not.

The Theory of Planned Behaviour (TPB) arose in the late 1980s as an extension of previous theoretical work, which had placed central emphasis on the role of people's attitudes in predicting engagement with a health behaviour. The basis of this work was that people's attitudes are formed after careful consideration of all information that is made available to them and that such carefully constructed attitudes may be good predictors of subsequent behaviour (Conner & Norman 2005). Since its inception, TPB has become a particularly popular model, which has been applied in an extensive number of contexts and has been the subject of numerous meta-analyses and systematic reviews (Armitage & Conner 2001; Hardeman et al. 2002).

According to TPB, the most important, primary determinant of a behaviour is the person's intention to perform the behaviour. So, in this model, actual behaviour is predicted by one's intentions to perform the said behaviour, which in turn are determined by attitudes, subjective norms and perceived behavioural control. Attitudes consist of an evaluation of how positive (or pleasant) the particular behaviour is and beliefs about the outcome of the behaviour (e.g. going to the dentist is fun and it will improve my health). Subjective norms are beliefs about important others' attitude to the behaviour and the person's motivation to comply with others (e.g. my family and friends think that going to the dentist is important and I want to please them). Perceived Behavioural Control is the person's belief that they can carry out the behaviour. This judgement is made on the basis of internal factors (e.g. skills; 'I know where there is a dentist and I know how to get there') and external factors (e.g. barriers and obstacles; 'going to the dentist is expensive and time consuming'). These variables, the model argues, are themselves, respectively influenced by the person's behavioural beliefs (i.e. consequences of a behaviour; e.g. 'going to the dentist improves oral health'), normative beliefs (i.e. what important others think about the behaviour; e.g. 'going to the dentist is a generally encouraged behaviour') and control beliefs (i.e. beliefs about the factors that will encourage or hinder performing the behaviour; e.g. 'I can access a dentist quite easily by picking up the phone and making a convenient appointment'). These are influenced by demographics, personality and environmental variables.

However, the central tenet of the Theory of Planned Behaviour – the role of intentions in predicting behaviour – has not always been backed up in practice; the problem here is what is generally known as the 'intentions–behaviour gap'. Although people are usually very efficient at forming good intentions of behaviour change, these often do not get translated into actual behaviour. For example, in a study by Lavin and Groarke (2005) looking at TPB variables in an intervention aiming to enhance the frequency by which participants engaged in dental floss use, TPB variables were moderately good at predicting 46 per cent of the variance in intentions to use dental floss. This means 46 per cent of the variability in people's intention to use dental floss could be related back to variables such as attitudes, perceived behavioural control, etc. However, when the researchers looked at the participants' *actual* dental floss use through inspecting dental floss diaries kept by the participants, rather than their self-reports of their intended use, TPB components predicted only 29 per cent of actual flossing behaviours. Recently, in a review of the application of popular social cognition models to behaviour change in dental settings, it was reported that whilst TPB constructs explained around 30–50 per cent of variability in intentions to engage in a given behaviour, this dropped to only 20–30 per cent when the theory was used to explain actual behaviour (Renz & Newton 2009). The inability of TPB to actually make worthy behavioural predictions in behaviour change studies has been demonstrated very convincingly in systematic review (Hardeman et al. 2002) leading to the premise that 'the majority of behavioural intentions do not lead to behaviour change' (Sniehotta 2009b, p. 262). The theory's inadequacy in being a sensible behaviour change tool has recently been extensively discussed (Sniehotta 2009a, 2009b), leading to Sniehotta quite appropriately suggesting that we 'retire the TPB from our research for good' (cited in McDonald 2013).

Given the weak link between intentions and actual behaviour, Gollwitzer (1993) proposed the idea of 'implementation intentions'. His work has attempted to bridge the intentions–behaviour gap by proposing ways of helping people translate intentions into behaviour. The way to do this is by negotiating with people the precise situational context where the behaviour will be implemented; when, where and how the behaviour will be performed are some of the factors that Gollwitzer proposes will help people turn their intentions into actual behaviours. Sniehotta et al. (2007) carried out a study aimed at enhancing dental floss use. Participants were either given a flossing guide and a packet of floss, or they received these and also took part in a 1.16 minute discussion where they formed a concrete plan of where, when and how each one of them was going to floss. The latter group was more adherent to flossing at 2-week and 2-month follow-up. This provides evidence that a quick and simple intervention, aiming to put people's good intention into a personal context for them, can significantly improve adherence with oral self-care behaviour instructions.

It would appear that TPB alone may not be as strong a model to predict behaviour change as it is with the addition of the concept of implementation intentions. In practical terms, it is suggested that whilst it may be important to assess people's attitudes, ability to perform a behaviour and normative beliefs surrounding a new behaviour, it is also important to be aware that these constructs may explain small increases in intentions to perform the behaviour but are unlikely to be translated into actual behaviour, unless the person has been 'helped into' contextualizing their intentions in their personal circumstances by making plans, such as implementation intentions.

Protection Motivation Theory

The models reviewed so far have one characteristic in common; they seem to ignore the fact that often people make decisions about their health not on the basis of rational, logical, factual thinking, but rather on the basis of how they *feel* about a particular health threat. For example, it could be that some people have terribly negative attitudes about dentists (attitude), that they feel they could possibly get away with not visiting for some time as they are not prone to oral health problems (susceptibility) and hence never quite move themselves from a stage where they are thinking about visiting the dentist (contemplation stage of change) to one where they make arrangements to visit the dentist. But what is it that changes and makes this person finally engage in the health behaviour and arrange to see their dentist?

One area that has been considered by psychologists is that of the effects of *fear*. Here, the role of fear of (further or more serious) ill-health has been investigated as a variable that might explain how people are motivated into the uptake of health behaviours. It is research into the effects of fear campaigns on people's health behaviour that gave rise to what is now known as Protection Motivation Theory (PMT) (Rogers 1983) or, in other words, people's innate desire to protect themselves from harm. The theory has been used to predict uptake of health services such as screening and provides a framework for understanding the cognitive, emotional and behavioural responses to receiving information threatening to health, such as being informed that one is susceptible to developing a disease. It has been the subject of several meta-analyses (Floyd et al. 2000; Milne et al. 2000) and has

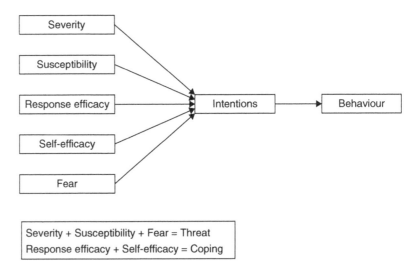

Figure 8.3 Protection Motivation Theory

Source: R.W. Rogers (1983) Cognitive and physiological processes in fear appeals and attitude change: a revised theory of protection motivation. In J. Cacioppo and R. Petty (eds) *Social Psychophysiology*. New York: Guilford Press. (Reprinted with the permission of Guilford Press.)

attracted attention from researchers in fields as diverse as adherence to treatment, sexual behaviours, screening and binge drinking (Conner & Norman 2005).

Protection Motivation Theory (figure 8.3) proposes that when people receive health information that they may find threatening, this process initiates two forms of thinking patterns: a threat appraisal process, i.e. where the person works out how much they feel threatened by the information they have received (e.g. 'how threatening do I think periodontal disease is'), and coping appraisal, where the person, in parallel, evaluates the extent to which they feel they can cope with the threat (e.g. 'what can I realistically do to minimize the threat of periodontal disease'). These appraisals are in turn said to result in an adaptive or a maladaptive response. Whilst thinking about threat and coping, people consider the severity of the threat (e.g. 'how life-threatening do I think periodontal disease is?'); their perceived vulnerability to the threat (e.g. 'how likely is it that I will develop it?'); intrinsic (e.g. pleasure) and extrinsic (e.g. social approval) rewards which may accompany a maladaptive response; costs (e.g. 'periodontal treatment takes time') or barriers (e.g. 'I don't like the dentist doing the treatment') which may inhibit an adaptive response; response efficacy (the belief that the adaptive behaviour will be effective in reducing the threat); and self-efficacy (belief in one's own ability to perform the adaptive behaviour). Protection motivation (the intention to perform the adaptive behaviour) results from this appraisal process and in turn directs and sustains behaviour.

The model suggests that when people find a health threat serious, but also feel they have the resources to deal with it, they will form the intention to engage in a threat-minimizing behaviour and then, accordingly, perform the behaviour.

Reflection Point

Look back at the case study presented at the start of the chapter. Which components of Protection Motivation Theory has the dentist addressed in his consultation with Tony?

It would appear that, often, consultations with patients may focus on some aspects of the PMT model but not others. In the case study presented earlier, the dentist's communication may well have tackled the 'threat appraisal' component of the model (i.e. increasing fear of serious consequences arising from Tony developing periodontal disease at a future date, unless he changed his oral hygiene behaviours), but did not really address the 'coping appraisal' aspect, i.e. assessing issues such as Tony's self-efficacy. The model would thus suggest that in this case Tony is unlikely to form an intention to protect himself from the potential harmful effects of periodontal disease.

Although arising from an area that had been neglected by previous models, that of fear about adverse health consequences motivating the uptake of health behaviours, like TPB, PMT also treats people like rational processors of information who make logical judgements about their health, form intentions to engage in health behaviours and then behave according to those intentions. There is probably more to how people make decisions about their health and to this process, so it is perhaps important to build in the role of behavioural complexity. This is discussed below.

Social cognition models – and behavioural complexity

The models reviewed so far make a lot of sense from a theoretical point of view in that they combine a lot of potentially relevant factors that may be explanatory as to why people change their behaviour and/or adhere to HCPs' advice. When tested in practice, though, the results are not always as encouraging as the models predicted.

It is suggested that the reason why this might be the case has to do with the fact that these models tend to take on a 'one size fits all' approach to explaining health-related behaviour; they tend to focus on socio-cognitive processes, which may play a necessary, but not sufficient, role in predicting health behaviours; however, they tend to reliably ignore the *type* of behaviour people are asked to adhere to. Thus, whilst a short-term, fairly mundane behaviour such as tooth-brushing might well be explained by one model, it is not necessarily the case that

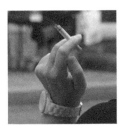

Image 8.1 Non-adherence to health advice is a widespread problem

Source: By Oxfordian Kissuth. Wikimedia Commons.

more long-term, complex behaviours, such as following a healthy diet, will also be the result of the same social-cognitive processes.

Additionally, none of these models seem to be allowing for whether the behaviour is old and habitual or whether the person is being asked to take up an altogether new health behaviour. What is more, the models pretty much ignore the social context in which the behaviours are being undertaken. These are important issues which need more careful behavioural research in order to demystify the concepts of behaviour change and adherence.

In summary, traditional behaviour change models have offered a way to break down behaviour change into its potential constituent components. The Health Belief Model, Stages of Change, Theory of Planned Behaviour and Protection Motivation Theory have all been considered in traditional medical and also dental settings. Although some models are better than others at explaining behaviour change and adherence, there has been no single, universally accepted model that may be used to understand and support behaviour change with both simple and complex behaviours.

A new paradigm of behaviour change: the COM-B model

Some time ago, a group of behavioural scientists based at University College London (Michie et al. 2005) started working on a project aimed at identifying simple behavioural components that might be relevant in shaping behaviour change in health settings. So, rather than aiming to combine lots of potentially relevant but also unrelated factors, as seen in the attempts encountered in some popular social cognition models, the aim was to list theoretical domains that *may* be involved in behaviour change. These factors have been put together in a 'taxonomy', as shown in table 8.1.

According to this list of domains, knowledge and skills are important, but, as suggested earlier, not sufficient, to help patients adhere to advice from the HCP. So, patients need to know what it is they are being asked to do (e.g. floss twice a day after meals) and have the skills to be able to undertake the behaviour (e.g. be in a position to buy and use dental floss). Social standards, social influences and environmental context and resources are also important in helping patients adhere to HCP advice. For example, the importance of a perfect smile in current Western societies and the environmental context in which such treatment can nowadays take place are different from what they were two or three decades ago; a patient who is undertaking orthodontic treatment within current Western trends and within a privately funded, aesthetic dentistry paradigm, might be more likely to adhere to orthodontic treatment recommendations now, than they might have been had they lived in a society which did not place as much emphasis on 'perfect'

Table 8.1 Michie et al.'s (2005) taxonomy of potential factors implicated in behaviour change	
Theoretical domains that *may* underpin adherence	
1.	Knowledge
2.	Skills
3.	Social standards
4.	Beliefs about capabilites
5.	Beliefs about consequences
6.	Motivation
7.	Memory, attention, decision process
8.	Environmental context and resources
9.	Social influences
10.	Emotion
11.	Behavioural regulation (ability to set goals, monitor, feedback)
12.	Nature of behaviours

Source: Adapted from Michie et al. (2005)

smiles and did not make such treatment readily available, within and outside a state-funded dental context.

The person's beliefs about their own ability to perform the behaviour, as well as their beliefs about the consequences of performing (or indeed failing to perform) the agreed healthcare behaviour, will further influence the chances that the person will adhere to a recommendation from an HCP according to this taxonomy (Michie et al. 2005). For example, where a dental patient is advised to have a routine dental appointment every 6 months, the person may well know that attending for preventive dental care is important. They may have the skills to make an appointment and turn up at the surgery. All their friends and family might also be of the opinion that looking after one's oral health is important. However, if the person believes that attending for preventive treatment is not essential to their life, or that, even if they made an appointment to attend, their ability to attend would be compromised by a very heavy work schedule, they may choose not to take up the advice.

Motivation to adhere to oral health instructions is another interesting factor. Here, there are two theories that go some way towards explaining how motivation may underpin behaviour change and adherence with health instructions. The first theory, proposed by Miller and Rollnick (2002), suggests that most people are generally ambivalent about most things, and in particular about behaviours to do with their health. So, for example, they might be wishing they could keep to a healthy weight, but are also tempted to snack on high-calorie foods such as sweets and chocolate. It is the balance between competing demands (in this case, the need to be of an acceptable healthy weight, versus the short-term pleasurable effects experienced from unhealthy snacking) that will put the person in a highly/less motivated state to perform a behaviour that is likely to compromise health. Motivation to perform a health-enhancing behaviour can be affected by a myriad of factors, including the person's ideas about how important the behaviour is to them (e.g. 'Being of normal weight is the most important thing in my life'), how competent they feel in undertaking it (e.g. 'I feel completely and totally able to resist snacking'), and how confident they are about performing it (e.g. 'I can resist snacking most of the time but I do not trust myself to not snack on holiday').

In a second theory, the PRIME (Plans, Responses, Impulses/ Inhibitions, Motives, Evaluations) Theory of Motivation (West 2006), it is suggested that behaviour is primarily driven by *automatic* processes, mainly revolving around a system of basic needs and wants that are competing for the person's attention and for gratification. For example, the need to eat when the brain detects hunger signals is one such automatic process. The theory suggests that the motivation to meet this basic need will guide behaviour first and foremost, in a pretty automatic, stimulus-response (e.g. hunger-eat) fashion. At the same time, there is a *reflective* system of motivation that is more advanced and stores things such as the person's beliefs about what is good or bad, or pre-formed plans. This is the system where, for example, one's knowledge that sugary snacks are bad for them might be stored. PRIME Theory suggests that this second, reflective motivation system will only come into action if it can overcome the messages the person is getting from their automatic, basic needs/wants system. That is, the automatic stimulus-response behaviour described earlier (hunger-eat) will be stopped by the reflective system storing one's knowledge that the sugary snack sitting in front of them and which can potentially satisfy their 'hunger-eat' need may be bad for them, only if the reflective system can generate a new need/want (e.g. the desire to have good oral health or be of a healthy weight) that can replace the basic, reflective one. As such, according to this theory, people's beliefs about what is good or bad and their plans to behave according to those beliefs will only influence their behaviour if they can generate sufficiently strong new needs/wants which can replace the basic competing, automatic needs or wants.

Both theories of motivation clearly show that the concept is complex and tapping into it with the view to change it will probably require time and effort. The taxonomy of behaviour change techniques (Michie et al. 2005) suggests that memory, attention and decision-making processes are also paramount in determining whether a patient will adhere to recommendations received in a dental setting. Not only is it essential that the patient has encoded and can retrieve information about the proposed treatment plan, but their decision to adopt the recommendation needs to have been strengthened within this setting, if they are to follow through with the recommendations. Our team (Misra et al. 2013) recently found that dental patients' memory of consultation content was not particularly sound; we showed that whilst most patients could recall the reasons that brought them to the consultation (e.g. need for restorative work) and the technical procedures of the visit (i.e. dental injection followed by drilling), their memory for future actions that were agreed with the dentist (e.g. avoiding sugary snacks) and also dental health education (e.g. brush and floss twice daily) were not frequently recalled. It follows that poor memory for dental advice and agreed actions is likely to compromise patients' efforts to adhere to dental advice.

It is further known that patients' emotional profile (e.g. depression and anxiety) are also likely to undermine their efforts to adhere to HCP advice. To this end, it is pointless agreeing a plan of care with a patient, where the patient's emotional profile is such that they will feel unable to see the plan through. Dentally anxious patients, for example, are unlikely to benefit from planning a set of complex dental treatments where it is likely that they would find a simple routine consultation too stressful and thus be unlikely to attend.

Related to this issue is Michie's idea surrounding behavioural regulation (Michie et al. 2005). It is known that patients who are helped into setting specific, measurable, agreed, realistic, time-specific (also known as SMART) goals, who are then monitored in their attempts to achieve them, and are supported by feedback in doing so, are more likely to adhere to a set of recommended health behaviours than those who are poor at behavioural regulation processes. It then follows that setting such goals and monitoring them with patients is likely to be helpful to patients engaging in behaviour change or seeking to adhere to a new health behaviour.

Finally, it goes without saying that the type of behaviour the patient has to adhere to is going to play some role in the extent to which it is followed. Some oral health behaviours (e.g. brushing) may be easier to adhere to than others (e.g. giving up smoking) and by definition will have a higher success rate than behaviours that are complex and require sustained and prolonged effort on the part of the patient.

To complete this discussion of factors that are likely to predispose to non-adherence, we have seen that a variety of elements, from lack of education and skill, to lack of goal-setting and monitoring, can all undermine people's efforts to adhere to oral health advice.

So what behavioural factors should be targeted when tackling non-adherence in a dental patient? A recent model of behaviour change suggests that there are three areas that should be tackled. This model is known as the COM-B (Capability, Opportunity, Motivation- for Behaviour) model (Michie & West 2012). The COM-B model of behaviour change asks three main questions:

1 Does the patient have the C-apability to perform the behaviour of interest?
2 Do they have the O-pportunity to perform it?
3 Do they have the M-otivation to do it?

Depending on the answers to these three questions, the HCP should be in a position to assess what sort of intervention they need to work on to help the patient with behaviour change. For instance, thinking back to the case study at the beginning of the chapter, it might have appeared that Tony needed support to change his flossing habits. A goal might have been set to help Tony floss once a day after his evening meal. In this instance, the COM-B model could have been used to support the consultation. That is, having checked that Tony knew how to floss (Capability), the dentist might have given a packet of floss to Tony to use. This could have been supplemented by a discussion about when, where and how Tony was going to fit flossing into his evening routine (Opportunity). Any barriers with this plan would have been considered at this stage. Finally, the next area to have considered would have been the Motivation part of the model. Here, the attempt would have been to try and understand whether there were Importance, Competence, Confidence issues with Tony (see Miller & Rollnick's (2002) theory of motivation) that interfered with his potential adherence or whether there were PRIME model issues (i.e. Tony being unable to overcome the automatic need to relax by, e.g. sitting on the sofa and eating chocolate before going to bed) that might have fuelled his difficulty to adhere to flossing recommendations. In Tony's example, discussing his views of how important flossing was to him, how confident he felt about performing it and how competent he felt he was at the actual flossing behaviour, would have provided a platform for the dentist to explain away the worries that Tony was having with regard to the bleeding he was observing when flossing.

Once the dentist had a better idea of the area that needed intervention, the next step would have been to decide what behaviour change technique (BCT) would be necessary to help the patient take up flossing. Amongst the many BCTs a dentist might consider are:

- increasing Tony's knowledge by going over the importance of flossing during the appointment and showing him, again, what he needed to do;
- initiating a fear campaign by, for example, showing Tony images of teeth that people have lost as the result of periodontal disease;
- promising a reward (e.g. a fee-free or reduced-fee visit next time) if the patient's plaque score improved.

Obviously, some of these BCTs would be more appropriate in one setting and with some patients rather than in others, and the idea explored earlier that 'one size does not fit all' still applies in this context. Ongoing work by Michie et al. (2013) has identified 16 clusters of BCTs that can be used when people are supported in behaviour change. These clusters vary from simple BCTs such as highlighting to people the rewards/'threats' associated with change, to more complex interventions such as developing cognitive dissonance, or an elaborate behavioural contract. It is beyond the scope of this chapter to go into detail here about the various BCTs, but the reader is referred to Michie et al.'s (2013) work for a complete list of these techniques and for detailed descriptions of what each entails.

> **In summary**, given the difficulties faced in using traditional behaviour change models, current thinking about behaviour change has aimed to consider three major aspects of the process: Capability, Opportunity and Motivation. Whilst traditional consultations in the dental setting may routinely focus on whether patients are Capable of performing a behaviour by, for example, having the technical skills and equipment necessary to perform it, the model suggests that the O and M aspects of behaviour change also need to be tackled and considered, if behaviour change is to take place. Different patients and different behaviours will require different behaviour change techniques (BCTs) according to this model, and work is currently under way to establish a taxonomy for different BCTs for different health behaviours.

Conclusion

Being aware of the behaviour change and adherence messages described in this chapter might help dentists better engage with patients and therefore help patients to engage in the health behaviours prescribed. What is clear from a review of current research and theoretical models of behaviour change is that behaviour change is a multi-faceted combination of educating, supporting and reviewing behaviour, all of which contribute to patients' engagement with health advice.

8

Discussion Points

- Why might information be necessary to increase knowledge but not sufficient for behaviour change?
- What does COM-B stand for, and which factor should be tackled first in supporting people in changing their health behaviours?
- 'It is pointless tackling smoking cessation with a patient who is not ready to give up'. Discuss with reference to empirical work.

Stress and Health

Jessica Walburn and Suzanne E. Scott

Introduction

Think about the last time you felt 'stressed'. What had happened? What were you thinking about? How did your body feel? How long did you feel this way? Did anything happen as a result of your stress? How may stress affect the way you work? Could stress affect or be affected by your health?

Now think about your patients. Try to recall the last patient you saw who was stressed. How did you know they were stressed? How did their stress impact the appointment or their care plan? What did you do? We all experience stress at some point in our lives and within our careers. Further, patients may be stressed at their appointment or about their appointment. Consider the following case study and discussion point to see how stress may arise with the dental practice. How the dental team recognize, interpret and manage their own stress and that of their patients is an important aspect of dentistry. Further, the study of stress and health has particular relevance to the dental setting, as there is evidence linking stress to the rate of wound healing, as well as various oral/dental conditions such as periodontal disease, apthous ulcers and oral lichen planus.

This chapter explores the link between stress and health and investigates the potential of psychological stress to be a determinant of health and disease. It discusses the conceptualization of stress and theoretical approaches developed to help us understand the causes of stress and its consequences. The chapter also considers how stress is measured and how the association between stress and health or disease is assessed. The chapter concludes with an overview of stress management techniques that could be used to alleviate or prevent stress in dental patients or the dental team.

Box 9.1: Case Study

Ashley is a dentist in a busy dental practice. He has worked there for 3 years. He lives with his girlfriend, who is training to become an accountant. She is about to take her exams so spends most nights studying. She says she is feeling 'run down' and has a cold coming on. Indeed, she was coughing and sneezing in the night, which disturbed both their sleep.

Today, as usual, Ashley has had a full day of appointments. One patient had previously made a complaint about him. Although the issue was resolved, Ashley was nervous that this appointment may be awkward and it had been on his mind last night.

Also this morning, at least two appointments overran by over 15 minutes. A child he was treating felt faint, and Ashley had to ensure he was fully recovered and reassure his parents. Another patient was extremely anxious and required extra care before and during her treatment.

Ashley had a very short lunch break to try to make up time. Whilst he ate his sandwich, he completed some administrative forms that his manager had requested last week.

Ashley now has three patients left to see, one of whom is getting very annoyed about waiting so long and is becoming quite vocal in the waiting room. The other two patients include a woman who is pleasant and very chatty and an elderly gentleman who has difficulty hearing.

Ashley is feeling stressed. He can't wait to finish work and go to the pub.

9

Discussion Point

Why does Ashley feel stressed? Try to identify all the possible sources of his stress.

Who else mentioned within this case study may feel stressed?

What is stress?

'Stress' is a commonly used word and you no doubt have a notion of what it means. However, 'stress' is actually multifarious and not easy to 'pin down'. It has been construed by researchers to mean both a threat to the individual, something that happens to you (e.g. divorce, bereavement, financial difficulties, getting a parking ticket, going to the dentist), and the emotional reaction (e.g. anxiety, distress) to the threat (Vedhara & Nott 1996). That is, it is used interchangeably to mean 'the agent, the process and the response' (Le Moal 2007). This conceptual ambiguity has translated into substantial variation in how it is measured (Monroe 2008). A significant body of research has focused on the stressor, by measuring life events in large samples of people and relating these to negative health outcomes (morbidity and mortality). In contrast, stress has also been studied as a response, namely a non-specific state of physiological arousal which occurs in response to a threat. This fight/flight response, described by Cannon (1914), was perceived to be an adaptive reaction promoting survival by preparing the body to fight or escape from a dangerous situation (Bartlett 1998). Selye (1956) developed this idea into a theory of stress, General Adaptation Syndrome, which highlighted that the generic response had three progressive phases (Alarm, Resistance and Exhaustion) regardless of the stressor. However, there are some limitations to this way of conceptualizing stress. For instance, the same stressor may not elicit a response in all individuals. Further, people differ in the degree of their response or reactivity (e.g. Kudielka et al. 2004). In addition, different stressors (e.g. sleep deprivation, prolonged physical exercise, electric shock, academic examinations) may produce a unique physiological response rather than general non-specific arousal (Pacak & Palkovits 2001). In light of these limitations, the response-based approach has been superseded by the 'Transactional Model of Stress' (Lazarus & Folkman 1984), which is able to accommodate individual differences by the inclusion of the salient psychological variable: appraisal. Lazarus and Folkman (1984) define stress as 'a particular relationship between the person and the environment that is appraised by the person as taxing or exceeding his or her resources and endangering his or her well-being' (p. 19).

The Transactional Model of Stress – see figure 9.1 for an updated transactional model (Steptoe & Ayers 2005) – proposes that a stress response occurs as a result of two stages of appraisal. In the first stage, a primary appraisal process is implemented whereby a situation is evaluated to see if it is going to be a challenge to the individual ('Am I in trouble or being benefited, now or in the future, and in what way?'; Lazarus & Folkman 1984: 31). The potential stressor is appraised as either irrelevant, or relevant and positive, or relevant and negative. For example, imagine someone trips and falls and thinks they have broken a tooth. If appearance is very important to them, this would be appraised as a relevant and negative threat. A secondary appraisal also occurs where an individual assesses the potential resources available to meet the requirements of the event ('Can anything can be done about it?'; Lazarus & Folkman 1984: 31). Resources can include personal characteristics (e.g. confidence, prior experience, coping strategies) and external factors (e.g. financial, social support or context). In the example of the broken tooth, if the person feels that they have access to dental care (and the tooth can be fixed relatively easily), they may not interpret the situation as stressful. On the other hand, if the person is not registered with a dentist and is doubtful as to the prognosis of the tooth, they may feel extremely stressed by the event. Therefore, stress concerns a transaction between the individual and their environment which, if the individual thinks that there is an imbalance between the demands and available resources, results in a stress response (Ogden 2007). These stages do not happen sequentially but work in parallel, that is appraisal of the level of threat posed by an event will be influenced by whether or not the person thinks they have the resources ready to deal with the threat (Bartlett 1998; Steptoe & Ayers 2005). Appraisal is the mainstay of the transactional approach; however, certain characteristics of the stressor have been identified which could increase the likelihood of a stress response. Circumstances that are salient, uncontrollable, ambiguous, requiring 'multi-tasking' and with social consequences have been reported to be particularly salient (Dickerson 2008; Ogden 2012).

The transactional approach to stress and its focus on the cognitive process of appraisal is supported by experimental research by Lazarus and colleagues, whereby participants' reactions to potentially disturbing films were influenced by manipulation of the appraisal of the footage (Lazarus & Folkman 1984). A series of experiments showed that those who received training before exposure designed to change

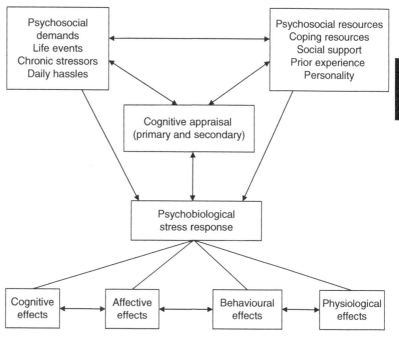

Figure 9.1 Transactions model of stress
Source: Adapted from Steptoe and Ayers (2005)

the meaning of what they were about to see (e.g. that protagonists in the film did not really experience pain) experienced a weaker physiological and self-reported stress response than those who watched the film without training (e.g. Lazarus & Alfert 1964; Folkins et al. 1968). Therefore, participants had different responses to the same stimuli due to differences in their cognitive appraisal of what they were seeing.

Discussion Point

According to the transactional model of stress, people feel stressed if they believe that they do not have the ability or resources to cope with a situation. Reconsider the case study in box 9.1.

Towards the end of the day, Ashley is faced with two patients whom he usually enjoys seeing. Mrs Greene, a woman who is pleasant and very chatty, and Mr Lyone, an elderly gentleman who has difficulty hearing.

Why might the prospect of these patients make Ashley feel even more stressed? Consider the following:

- What is the 'threat' that he appraises as relevant and negative?
- What resources may he feel he is lacking to be able to meet the needs of this situation? Consider both personal resources and environmental factors.

Ashley normally enjoys seeing these two patients. What makes today different?

The stress response is understood to have physiological, cognitive, behavioural and emotional dimensions (Sapolsky 2004; Steptoe & Ayers 2005). These are each outlined in turn. A summary of how stress can affect you is displayed in figure 9.2.

The physiological stress response

The physiological stress response involves an interrelationship between the central and autonomic nervous systems as well as the endocrine system. The following description of the classic stress response focuses upon the functioning of two neuroendocrine systems: the sympathetic adrenomedullary (SAM) axis controlled by the sympathetic branch of the autonomic nervous system (SNS); and the hypothalamic-pituitary adrenal (HPA) axis controlled by the hypothalamus and the pituitary gland (Lovallo 2005). Be aware that this is an oversimplification: the physiological responses involved in and associated with the stress response are highly complex, involving multiple interacting processes (Rabin 2007).

The sympathetic adrenomedullary axis (SAM)

The SAM is the primary instigator of the rapid, evolutionary adaptive, behavioural and physiological responses to an acute stressor, designed to safeguard survival (Sapolsky 2004). Activation of the SAM response

The Effect of Stress on:				
Emotional state	**Mental activity**	**Health**	**Physical reactions**	**Behaviour habits**
• Nervousness • Edginess • Anxiety (phobias, panics) • Depression (apathy and fatigue) • Sadness • Lowered self-esteem • Guilt and shame • Moodiness • Loneliness	• Difficulty in concentrating • Difficulty in making decisions • Frequent forgetfulness • Increased sensitivity to criticism • Negative, self-critical thoughts • Distorted ideas • More rigid attitudes	• Coronary heart disease • High blood pressure • Strokes • Stomach upsets, indigestion and nausea • Diarrhoea • Migraines and headaches • Worsens asthma and hay fever • Skin rashes	• Increased heart rate • Rapid, shallow breathing • Muscle tension • Fidgeting and restlessness • Hot most of the time • Cold hands and feet • Numbness and tingling sensations • Increased blood glucose levels • Dilation of pupils • Frequent urination • Increased blood and urine catecholamine and corticosteroids	• Impulsive and impatient • Excessive eating or loss of appetite • Excessive drinking • Heavier smoking • Accident-prone and clumsy • Disorganised or over-organised • Disturbed sleep – insomnia, early awakening, or excessive sleeping

Figure 9.2 Effects of stress

Source: Adapted from Sage et al. (2008)

occurs within seconds of encountering a stressor (Kaye & Lightman 2005). This fight or flight response includes an increase in heart rate and blood pressure and breathing, lower flow of saliva, dilation of pupils, chills, sweating and trembling. Non-essential processes such as digestion and reproduction are inhibited. These physiological changes are orchestrated by the catecholamines (adrenaline and noradrenaline) (Bartlett 1998; Kaye & Lightman 2005). See figure 9.3 for a summary of physiological changes associated with the fight/flight response. You may be able to see some of these physiological signs in yourself, your patients or colleagues in times of stress.

9

The hypothalamic-pituitary adrenal axis (HPA)

The HPA axis forms the parallel branch of the neuroendocrine stress response, which is slower than the SAM to react, relying on hormonal rather than neural transmission (Bartlett 1998). Corticotrophin releasing factor (CRF) is released and stimulates the release of adrenocorticotrophic (ACTH) hormone. ACTH acts on the adrenal gland eliciting the release of corticosteroids, such as cortisol, into the blood stream. Cortisol has a number of functions associated with the stress response; however, the primary function of cortisol is to regulate and modulate other aspects of the stress response. It does this by a number of negative feedback loops, acting upon, for example, the hypothalamus and the pituitary gland to terminate the stress response when it

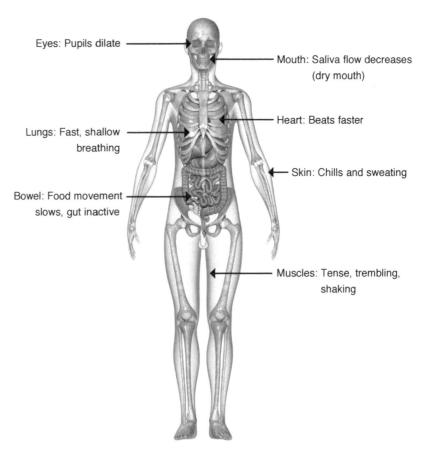

Eyes: Pupils dilate

Mouth: Saliva flow decreases (dry mouth)

Lungs: Fast, shallow breathing

Heart: Beats faster

Skin: Chills and sweating

Bowel: Food movement slows, gut inactive

Muscles: Tense, trembling, shaking

Figure 9.3 Summary of physiological changes associated with the fight/flight response
Source: 7activestudio

is no longer required (Tsigos & Chrousos 2002). The peak of cortisol response occurs approximately 20–30 minutes after the initiation of the stress response. Cortisol also has multiple functions during 'peace time', to enable normal cellular functioning (Lovallo 2005). Its secretion follows a cycle whereby it is highest in the early morning, gradually reducing during the day. In the dental setting, this slower physiological stress response may arise in a dentally anxious patient in the weeks leading up to their appointment. A systematic review of 62 studies investigating the magnitude of this 'cortisol awakening response' supports a relationship between psychosocial factors and cortisol awakening response. The most robust finding showed that greater background life stress and job stress was related to increased cortisol awakening response (Chida & Steptoe 2009). This association was robust and maintained after controlling for methodological quality. However, as the studies were predominately cross-sectional (studying both stress and cortisol awakening response at one time point), it cannot be said for certain that stress causes the change in cortisol awakening response.

Cognitive changes associated with the stress response

Stress has been reported to be associated with a variety of changes in terms of attention, memory, retrieval and recognition. A review of the literature using both human and animal models concluded that there is generally an inverted U relationship (Lupien & McEwen 1997) between stress and cognitive performance, whereby moderate levels of stress are associated with better performance and too much or too little are detrimental. This has implications for dental practices: if patients (or the dentists themselves) are very stressed (due to the dental visit or something else in their life), their ability to think clearly, make decisions, concentrate and remember key facts may be compromised. Remember that giving informed consent, adhering to treatment and dental attendance all involve cognitive elements and as such may be affected in times of stress.

Behaviours associated with the stress response

It is difficult to discern which behaviours are associated with the stress response and which are part of the coping arsenal (Steptoe 2000). One approach is to investigate the behaviours specifically associated with the 'fight or flight' response (e.g. escape, combat, freezing). A broader perspective is to assess the association between stress and specific behaviours (e.g. smoking, alcohol intake and fat consumption). The results are mixed, dependent on the specific behaviour. Stress has been shown to increase maladaptive health behaviours such as smoking, alcohol consumption (Steptoe et al. 1996), eating behaviour and fat consumption (Ng & Jeffery 2003; O'Connor et al. 2008) and inhibit adaptive behaviour, such as adherence to treatment regimes (French et al. 2005, 2011) and exercise (Ng & Jeffery 2003). In addition, stress is reported to be associated with disturbed sleep (Hall et al. 1998). Thus, indications that a patient is under stress may include tiredness, increased tobacco use or alcohol consumption, poor diet or a lapse in maintaining oral hygiene. This also applies to the dental team. In the case study in box 9.1, recall that Ashley was keen to get to the pub when feeling under pressure at work. Ashley had also worked during lunchtime, which may have impacted his eating behaviour. Further, the previous night's sleep was disturbed by his anticipation of seeing a patient who had previously complained about him and this may have been exacerbated by his girlfriend's illness.

Lazarus and Folkman (1984) proposed that coping behaviours can also be separated into strategies used to ameliorate the unpleasant emotions of the stress response (emotion-focused coping) and those to tackle the source of the stress (problem-focused coping). It is likely that it is the degree of flexibility in selecting appropriate strategies and the ability to integrate different strategies that may be important in coping with stress (Cheng & Cheung 2005; Sideridis 2006).

Problem-focused coping is best suited to stressors perceived as controllable and emotion-focused coping to those beyond control (Chesney et al. 1996). For example, if you feel under stress because you need to cancel a patient's appointment due to a family commitment, it would be more helpful to cope with this by talking to your manager/receptionist in order to let the patient know and reschedule, rather than reducing your negative emotions by having a moan to friends. However, there are circumstances where you may have little control, such as the progression of a chronic illness. In this situation, seeking support to cope with the negative emotions will be helpful. In the example of the case study, Ashley attempted problem-focused coping by trying to deal with a late-running clinic by reducing his lunch break. However, as he continued to work during his break (doing administration), this may have inadvertently added to his stress levels, as he did not get a chance to rest and recover from the busy morning.

Emotions associated with the stress response

Negative mood (e.g. distress, anxiety, sadness, fear, nervousness) is the familiar, tangible experience of stress (Steptoe & Ayers 2005) and it is often assumed that these negative emotions will be present if the stressor is present (Vedhara & Nott 1996). A review of experimental studies investigating emotional responses to laboratory-induced stressors (e.g. giving a speech, tracing a star-shaped figure given the mirror-image, holding a handgrip for a period of time) confirmed a small positive association between exposure to an acute stressor and an increase in negative emotion (Feldman et al. 1999). That fact that the relationship was small indicates that the relationship is not so straightforward and that other factors (e.g. appraisal, coping style, social support) are likely to be important in determining the degree of emotional distress associated with exposure to a stressor (Vedhara & Nott 1996). Interestingly, recent studies looking at a naturalistic stressor (academic examinations) indicate that a variety of negative and positive emotions can emerge during a stressful event (Spangler et al. 2002).

In summary, stress is an amorphous construct with no accepted definition. Researchers have studied stress by focusing on the stressor (e.g. a negative life event) or the response (e.g. negative emotion or physiological arousal) or both. These approaches are tied to different models of stress. The transactional model of stress, which interprets stress as an interaction between the event and the individual's appraisal of the event and their coping resources, is widely used. The stress response occurs when there is a mismatch between the perceived demands of the event and available resources. The stress response has physiological, cognitive, emotional and behavioural dimensions.

Stress and health

The biopsychosocial model (Engel 1977) proposes that the biological, psychological and social contexts of an individual interact to influence and be influenced by health status (Sarafino 2002). Psychoneuroimmunology (PNI) is the study of the complex interrelationships between the central nervous system, the neuroendocrine and immune systems (Glaser & Kiecolt-Glaser 2005). Research to date has focused on the investigation of the impact of stress on a variety of health outcomes. The ability to draw conclusions about the precise role of stress (e.g. whether it is an aetiological factor that is influential in the progression of a condition) is hampered by methodological weakness that arises due to limitations imposed on human research by ethical considerations (Kasl 1987). For example, researchers may hit regulatory barriers if they designed a study that involved random allocation of dental students to extreme chronic stress for a number of years to see whether they developed heart disease! Instead, the literature has to rely on observational paradigms and animal models.

There is evidence linking stress to increased mortality, morbidity and aggravation of symptoms for a wide variety of conditions including chronic heart disease, autoimmune disease, oral health (see box 9.2), some cancers, multiple sclerosis, upper respiratory infection, HIV, childhood lung function, skin conditions and muscular functioning (Buljevac et al. 2003; Cohen 2005; Rozanksi et al. 2005; Steptoe & Brydon 2005; Kemeny & Schedlowski 2007; Chida et al. 2008; Finestone et al. 2008; Suglia et al. 2008; Chida & Vedhara 2009). The most consistent and reliable evidence exists for stress being an

9

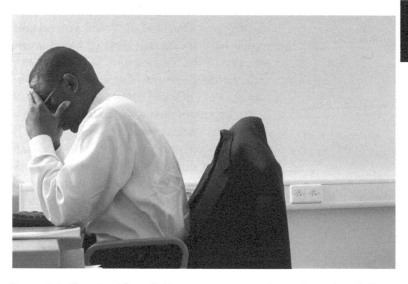

Image 9.1 There is evidence linking stress to increased mortality and morbidity
Source: Thomas_EyeDesign

Box 9.2: Examples of links between stress and oral health

Stress has been linked with periodontal disease (Rosania et al. 2009).

- Individuals suffering from a heavy workload, those experiencing marital difficulties, occupational dissatisfaction and high psychological strain have more periodontal destruction than those not under such stresses (Croucher et al. 1997).
- Patients under psychosocial stress have been shown to have a poorer outcome following non-surgical periodontal treatment as compared to patients who were not stressed (Bakri et al. 2013).

Links between stress and oral health have been reported for recurrent apthous stomatitis (Zadik et al. 2012) and auto-immune diseases such as oral lichen planus.

- Patients with oral lichen planus often cite stress as a cause of their disease (Burkhart et al. 1996)
- Patients with oral lichen planus appear to have higher stress levels than those without an oral disease (Chaudhary 2004; Lundqvist et al. 2006; Shah et al. 2009).
- Those with more severe lichen planus appear to have higher perceived stress levels (Mohamadi Hasel et al. 2013).

Longitudinal data is required to understand the impact of stress over time.

---

aetiological factor in chronic heart disease and having an exacerbatory impact in autoimmune conditions (Steptoe & Ayers 2005).

In addition to the research linking stress to disease outcomes, there is evidence that the physiological stress response, although adaptive in the short term, becomes maladaptive if the response is 'left on', resulting in physiological 'wear and tear' or 'allostatic load' (McEwen 1998). Allostasis is an umbrella term to describe the multiple physiological processes that are required to maintain stability within a changing environment and that allostatic load is the physiological cost of achieving this goal (Korte et al. 2005). For example, experimental animal studies have shown that elevated blood pressure and increased heart rate, part of the SNS response to stress, when prolonged, is associated with the development of atherosclerosis, which can be initiated by manipulation of social contact (Kaplan et al. 1991; Watson et al. 1998).

An important theme behind allostatic load is that chronic activation of the stress systems make it less likely for the body to return to its pre-chronic stressed state as the stress response itself is altered. For example, a number of studies have reported a dysfunction in the negative feedback of cortisol in patients with post-traumatic stress disorder (PTSD), resulting in an altered cortisol response to stress (Wessa et al. 2006).

Life events and health outcomes

Researchers have looked at the incidence of stress (as indexed by critical life events such as moving house, divorce, financial difficulties) and related these to mortality or to the occurrence of specific health outcomes. Life events have been measured by self-report instruments composed of predetermined lists of events (e.g. schedule of recent experiences; Holmes & Rahe 1967) and by semi-structured interviews (e.g. the interview for recent life events; Paykel 1997). A number of large epidemiological studies with prospective designs have reported a relationship between stressful life events and all-cause mortality as well as morbidity and mortality related to specific conditions, particularly heart disease (Rosengren et al. 1993; Matthews & Gump 2002; Kriegbaum et al. 2008). However, there are a number of specific concerns about the assessment of stress caused by life events, including:

- that they do not measure everyday stress;
- they do not account for individual differences in appraisal of events;
- if measured retrospectively in those who are ill, they are vulnerable to recall bias from current psychological and physical states;
- different people can interpret items on a checklist differently (i.e. some people may consider a minor illness to fall under the category 'serious physical illness or injury');
- life events differ in duration, some are short term and others long-lasting (Dohrenwend 2006; Ogden 2012).

Despite these drawbacks, the life events approach is widely used in understanding the impact of human life stress on health (Monroe 2008).

Perceived stress and health outcomes

An alternative approach involves measuring the degree of perceived stress experienced (reflecting the theoretical perspective of the transactional model). Researchers have modified the life events approach by recording the individual's perceived degree of stress associated with the events or by capturing the experience of stress using other methods, such as diaries (e.g. Mitsonis et al. 2008). A widely used measure of perceived stress is the perceived stress scale (Cohen et al. 1983) (see box 9.3).

Prospective studies across a range of conditions have reported a negative association between perceived stress and specific health outcomes such as breast cancer incidence (Helgesson et al. 2003), cardiovascular disease (Iso et al. 2002), genital herpes recurrence (Cohen et al. 1999), as well as all-cause mortality (Nielsen et al. 2008). However, this approach is especially vulnerable to the difficulties of temporally separating the stressor and the health outcome and ensuring that stress is measured before the health outcome (Leventhal & Tomarken 1987).

Box 9.3: The perceived stress scale

PSS-14

INSTRUCTIONS:

The questions in this scale ask you about your feelings and thoughts during THE LAST MONTH. In each case, you will be asked to indicate your response by placing an 'X' over the circle representing HOW OFTEN you felt or thought a certain way. Although some of the questions are similar, there are differences between them and you should treat each one as a separate question. The best approach is to answer fairly quickly. That is, don't try to count up the number of times you felt a particular way, but rather indicate the alternative that seems like a reasonable estimate.

	Never	Almost Never	Sometimes	Fairly Often	Very Often
	0	1	2	3	4
1 In the last month, how often have you been upset because of something that happened unexpectedly?	◯	◯	◯	◯	◯
2 In the last month, how often have you felt that you were unable to control the important things in your life?	◯	◯	◯	◯	◯
3 In the last month, how often have you felt nervous and stressed?	◯	◯	◯	◯	◯
4 In the last month, how often have you dealt successfully with day to day problems and annoyances?	◯	◯	◯	◯	◯
5 In the last month, how often have you felt that you were effectively coping with important changes that were occurring in your life?	◯	◯	◯	◯	◯
6 In the last month, how often have you felt confident about your ability to handle your personal problems?	◯	◯	◯	◯	◯
7 In the last month, how often have you felt that things were going your way?	◯	◯	◯	◯	◯
8 In the last month, how often have you found that you could not cope with all the things that you had to do?	◯	◯	◯	◯	◯
9 In the last month, how often have you been able to control irritations in your life?	◯	◯	◯	◯	◯
10 In the last month, how often have you felt that you were on top of things?	◯	◯	◯	◯	◯
11 In the last month, how often have you been angered because of things that happened that were outside of your control?	◯	◯	◯	◯	◯
12 In the last month, how often have you found yourself thinking about things that you have to accomplish?	◯	◯	◯	◯	◯
13 In the last month, how often have you been able to control the way you spend your time?	◯	◯	◯	◯	◯
14 In the last month, how often have you felt difficulties were piling up so high that you could not overcome them?	◯	◯	◯	◯	◯

Source: Cohen et al. (1983)

Stress and the immune system

A significant factor supporting a direct physiological association between stress and disease is that the neuroendocrine stress response also has consequences for the immune system. Research from human (naturalistic and acute laboratory-induced stressors) and animal studies consistently demonstrates that stress is related to dysregulation of the immune system (Segerstrom & Miller 2004; Glaser 2005). Immune dysregulation has been reported across a range of natural human stressor scenarios, including short-term stressors (e.g. examinations) and longer term stressors (e.g. bereavement, divorce and marital conflict, care giving). Human experimental studies have also reported altered immunity associated with laboratory-induced acute stressors (e.g. mental arithmetic, public speaking or marital conflict discussions) (e.g. Kiecolt-Glaser et al. 2005; Rohleder et al. 2006).

A systematic review of over 300 studies concluded that acute laboratory stressors (lasting minutes) were associated with up-regulation of natural immunity and down-regulation of specific immunity, whereas chronic stressors were associated with a more global suppression of both types of immunity (Segerstrom & Miller 2004). Although there is consistent evidence showing that immune dysregulation is associated with stress, it is less clear how these changes translate into poorer outcomes across the range of disease states.

Stress and infectious disease

Have you ever got a cold after or around the same time as you have been feeling stressed? Could the two be linked? The following evidence about stress and infectious disease may support your anecdotal experience.

Evidence from a series of studies focused on infectious disease (e.g. the common cold) supports the association between stress and health and adds greater weight, due to their prospective design and greater control over the health outcome (e.g. type of virus, previous exposure to virus, timing of exposure to virus) as well as control of potential confounding variables (e.g. age, gender, allergic status) (Miller & Cohen 2005). The studies have reported a positive association between degree of stress prior to exposure to a number of cold viruses and rates of clinical illness (Cohen et al. 1991, 1993, 1998). For example, Cohen et al. (1991) assessed the relationship between frequency of common colds and stress in individuals deliberately exposed to the cold virus. Using a prospective design, 394 healthy volunteers were assessed for their levels of psychological stress and two days later nasal drops of five different cold virus/placebo were administered. Participants then stayed in a residential laboratory for one week (in order to control the influence of the environment), at which point presence of infection and clinical symptoms were assessed by a clinician blind to the participant's exposure condition. The results of this study indicated that rates of infection and clinical colds increased in a dose response manner to level of stress (i.e. the more stress experienced, the greater the risk of an individual developing an infection).

Stress and wound healing

A (now classic) study by Kiecolt-Glaser et al. (1995) aimed to investigate the impact of chronic stress (e.g. caring for a dementia patient) on the rate of wound healing. In this study, 13 female carers of dementia patients were all given biopsies on their upper arm and the rate at which this healed was compared with those of age-matched controls. Healing took significantly longer in carers (48.7 days) than in controls (39.3 days) and this difference persisted after controlling for a number of confounding variables.

A number of studies have looked at stress and healing within the mouth. For instance, Marucha et al. (1998) investigated the effects of academic exams on mucosal wound healing. Healthy male and female dental students were given a 3.5 mm punch biopsy on the hard palate at different times during the academic year. Students took significantly longer to heal (mean = 10.91 days) during the examination period compared to the holidays (mean = 7.82 days). In addition, wound size over the first five days post-healing was significantly smaller during the holidays compared to the examination period.

A systematic review (Walburn et al. 2009) examined 22 articles that had investigated stress and wound healing in a variety of tissue types and clinical and experimental settings. The majority of studies (17 of the 22) found that psychological stress was associated with impaired healing or dysregulation of a biomarker associated with wound healing. A sub-sample of 12 out of the 22 studies included in the systematic review were entered into a meta-analysis (statistically pooling all the available data) which resulted in a significant effect of stress: greater levels of psychological stress were associated with impaired wound healing. However, there were differences in conceptual interpretations of stress, methodology and measurement between studies, which made comparison between studies problematic and diminished confidence in the accuracy of certain findings, in particular the use of surrogate measures of healing (re-hospitalization rates, inspection of clinical notes) or the lack of objective standardized measures of wound healing.

Stress and health behaviours

As discussed earlier in this chapter, certain behaviours are associated with the stress response, and it is proposed that these behavioural consequences form an alternative pathway by which stress further influences health. The importance of measuring the behavioural pathway, when assessing the relationship between psychosocial factors and health outcomes, is highlighted by two prospective studies which reported that the impact of personality traits (hostility, neuroticism and extraversion) on all-cause mortality, was significantly reduced once health behaviours were controlled for in the analysis (Everson et al. 1997; Shipley et al. 2007).

It is proposed that the detrimental impact of the behaviours on health outcomes will increase if individuals engage in multiple behaviours (e.g. drinking alcohol, lack of exercise and smoking), as these behaviours alone and in combination have multiple physiological consequences (Kiecolt-Glaser & Glaser 1988). The physiological and behavioural pathways are commonly perceived as distinct and separate routes for stress to impact on health; however, this is perhaps a simplistic interpretation as there is accumulating evidence of interrelationships between the two (Ogden 2012). For instance, greater HPA-axis activation (cortisol reactivity) to stress is associated with increased intake of snack foods (Newman et al. 2007).

> **In summary**, it is widely acknowledged that there is a cost to the individual when the stress response is maintained over a long period of time. This is thought to be responsible for the association between stress and poor health. There is evidence linking stress to increased mortality, morbidity and aggravation of symptoms for a wide variety of conditions, including oral health. There are two pathways by which stress may impact on health:
>
> (i) directly as a result of physiological changes associated with the stress response
> (ii) indirectly as a result of unhealthy behaviours which increase at times of stress.
>
> Psychoneuroimmunology (PNI) is the discipline which studies the interrelationship between neuroendocrine stress response and the immune system. To date there is robust evidence indicating that stress is associated with dysregulation of the immune system. PNI researchers have shown how these processes interrelate to impact on specific clinical areas, such as wound healing and infectious disease. It is less clear how these changes translate into poorer outcomes across the range of disease states.

9

Stress management

Stress in dentistry

In addition to treating patients who may be feeling stressed, members of the dental team are likely to experience periods of stress themselves from time to time. Indeed, there is mounting evidence that dentists experience high levels of stress throughout their career. Dentists have been noted to feel stressed due to:

- fear of litigation
- fear of physical violence from patients
- financial concerns

- time pressures
- business problems.

Dental students can also experience stress throughout their studies and their concerns often reflect those of qualified dentists. Humphris et al. (2002) found that levels of emotional exhaustion were higher among dental students compared to medical students. Chronic occupational stress may lead to 'burnout'. Maslach et al. (1996) describe burnout as a combination of emotional exhaustion (mental fatigue), depersonalization (psychological distancing from others) and reduced personal accomplishment. Burnout can become debilitating and dentists who experience burnout may be unable to continue to work. Freeman et al. (1995) noted that stress-related disorders are a common cause of early retirement from dentistry. It is therefore important for the dental team to be familiar with ways to manage their own stress in addition to that of their patients.

What can be done to manage stress?

Researchers have investigated different ways of tackling stress. There are a wide variety of stress management approaches reported in academic publications and lay self-help books. These include:

- relaxation training based on breathing, imagery or muscular tension (see box 9.4);
- massage;
- yoga and meditation;
- psychoeducation skills training based on a cognitive behavioural therapy approach;
- problem solving;
- planning and time management skills;
- communication skills and assertiveness techniques;
- emotional expression (whereby stressful events are written or spoken about)
- improving access to social support;
- making lifestyle changes (e.g. increasing exercise or changing diet).

All of these stress management techniques can be defined as interventions designed to help people manage stressors, the associated negative emotions and/or physiological arousal (Kenny 2007). It can be helpful to use this definition to categorize the interventions into those that are more likely to target the appraisal processes and those designed to 'dampen down' the physiological responses to stress. For example, a cognitive behaviour therapy-based approach, which looks at how our thoughts can influence our emotions and behaviour, would focus on changing how we perceive an event from something that is

Box 9.4: Relaxation exercise to target muscle tension

Relaxed breathing:
- Fill up the whole of your lungs with air, without forcing. Imagine you're filling up a bottle, so that your lungs fill from the bottom.
- Breathe in through your nose and out through your mouth.
- Breathe in slowly and regularly counting from one to five (don't worry if you can't reach five at first).
- Then let the breath escape slowly, counting from one to five.
- Keep doing this until you feel calm. Breathe without pausing or holding your breath.

Deep muscle relaxation:
This technique takes around 20 minutes. It stretches different muscles in turn and then relaxes them, to release tension from the body and relax your mind.

Find a warm, quiet place with no distractions. Get completely comfortable, either sitting or lying down. Close your eyes and begin by focusing on your breathing; breathing slowly and deeply, as described above.

If you have pain in certain muscles, or if there are muscles that you find it difficult to focus on, spend more time on relaxing other parts.

You may want to play some soothing music to help relaxation. As with all relaxation techniques, deep muscle relaxation will require a bit of practice before you start feeling its benefits.

For each exercise, hold the stretch for a few seconds, then relax. Repeat it a couple of times. It's useful to keep to the same order as you work through the muscle groups:

- Face: push the eyebrows together, as though frowning, then release.
- Neck: gently tilt the head forwards, pushing chin down towards the chest, then slowly lift again.
- Shoulders: pull them up towards the ears (shrug), then relax them down towards the feet.
- Chest: breathe slowly and deeply into the diaphragm (below your bottom rib) so that you're using the whole of the lungs. Then breathe slowly out, allowing the belly to deflate as all the air is exhaled.
- Arms: stretch the arms away from the body, reach, then relax.
- Legs: push the toes away from the body, then pull them towards the body, then relax.
- Wrists and hands: stretch the wrist by pulling the hand up towards you, and stretch out the fingers and thumbs, then relax.

Source: http://www.nhs.uk/conditions/stress-anxiety-depression/pages/ways-relieve-stress.aspx

9

potentially threatening to more neutral. It would also alter our perception of the ability to cope with the event (secondary appraisal) which in turn would reduce how threatening we thought the event was. In contrast, relaxation training would provide techniques to target the shallow breathing and muscular tension associated with the physical stress response. Box 9.5 outlines how some of the stress management techniques could be used in combination.

Assessing the effectiveness of stress management techniques is difficult because there is little consensus as to what constitutes a stress management intervention; there are also the multiple approaches to measuring stress itself. Research has looked at stress management interventions for employees in the workplace, for those with physical health conditions (Kenny 2007) as well as the general population (Van Daele et al. 2013). Although the research is hampered by methodological

Box 9.5: Example of stress management

Imagine you have a heavy workload and are feeling under stress. You have been asked to give a presentation and you are dreading it. You keep imagining yourself stumbling through the presentation and being unable to deliver it in full. The feelings of stress are stopping you from working on the presentation. Every time you sit down to work on it you end up fretting, procrastinating and eating chocolate and crisps. You are feeling tired because the thought of the imminent presentation is keeping you awake at night.

What might help?

- A cognitive behaviour therapy-based stress management intervention could focus on your appraisal of the event (e.g. aiming to move from 'There is no way I can do the presentation, it will be absolutely awful' to a less threatening thought such as 'It may be challenging, but it does not need to be perfect'. This may involve reminding yourself of your previous achievements. For example, 'I have delivered presentations in the past and they were OK. If I prepare and practise, I will be able to do the presentation').
- You could boost your coping skills by ensuring that you will do enough preparation by improving your time management.
- A social support intervention could involve practising in front of friends to give you confidence, or talking about your concerns to friends to vent negative emotions.
- You could reduce your physical feelings of anxiety by regularly practising a breathing relaxation technique in order to instil a sense of calm.

limitations, there is consistent evidence that stress management can improve the psychological well-being of patients with a physical illness (e.g. Antoni et al. 2006; Brown & Vanable 2008) and lower stress levels in healthy people (Van Daele et al. 2013). Although there are studies that show physiological parameters can be altered by stress management interventions (e.g. McGregor & Antoni 2009), evidence demonstrating that these changes lead to health improvements is less consistent. Thus stress management techniques may be reliable in helping a dentist, or their patient feel better, but may not be sufficient to impact on (oral) health.

Reflection Point

Reconsider the case study in box 9.1. Which stress management techniques might be useful for Ashley?

Social support, stress and health

Many stress management interventions include an 'accessing social support' component. This is because it is widely accepted that social support moderates the relationship between stress and health by forming a protective buffer during stressful periods (Cohen 2004). This is referred to as the 'buffering hypothesis'. Social support is perceived to have at least two dimensions: the structure and size of a social network (i.e. number and type of social contacts) as well as aspects of the function of the network (i.e. the nature and perception of the support available)

(Wills & Ainette 2007). Thus some people may only have a small number of social contacts, but those they have are available, dependable and close, thus providing social support. Alternatively, someone may have a lot of social contacts, but no one who is there to share problems and help when needed, leading to low perceptions of social support.

A number of large prospective epidemiological studies have reported a beneficial impact of structural support on mortality rates across a range of diseases (Berkman et al. 2000), and there is prospective evidence that functional support has a protective effect and facilitates recovery from illness (Brummett et al. 2005). Reduction in the physiological stress response is a potential mechanism by which social support may diminish the impact of stress (Uchino 2006). However, understanding the impact of social support is complex and made more challenging by differing conceptualizations and measures (O'Donovan & Hughes 2008).

The stress-buffering hypothesis is supported by cross-sectional and prospective epidemiological surveys of the relationship between stress and all-cause mortality, which report a relationship between life events and mortality but only for those participants with inadequate social support. Thus a good starting point in times of stress is to ensure your patients (or you) are not 'suffering in silence', and that there is a support network that is capable of offering guidance, assistance and compassion when needed.

> **In summary**, everyone is likely to experience periods of stress, which can be related to events in our personal as well as professional lives. There is evidence that dentists can experience high levels of stress throughout their career. Therefore, it is useful for dentists to be aware of ways to manage stress. There are a variety of approaches, some focus on changing our appraisal of events and coping resources whilst others target the physiological symptoms of the stress response. Despite methodological limitations, there is consistent evidence that stress management can improve psychological well-being. Having good social support can act as a buffer during times of stress and has been shown to protect against the detrimental impact of stress on health.

9

Conclusion

The link between the mind and body is not new but the scientific study of psychoneuroimmunology is relatively recent. Stress is a nebulous concept, which has been construed both as a stimulus and a response. More recently, it has been understood as a dynamic process involving an interaction between the individual and their environment, including a perception of imbalance between the situation and resources available to cope. Stress incorporates physiological, cognitive, emotional and behavioural dimensions that occur when the demands of a situation outweigh the resources available to meet the challenge. The stress response is perceived to be adaptive in the short term, but maladaptive if the stressor is chronic due to the price the body must pay to continually respond to the stressor, namely allostatic load. This allostatic burden is the primary direct pathway by which stress is proposed to impact upon health. An alternative indirect behavioural route exists as a consequence of the maladaptive behaviours (e.g. smoking, drinking, consumption of unhealthy snacks), which are hypothesized to increase during a stressful period. Further, the relationship appears to be moderated by the social context of stress, with social support acting as a protective buffer against the negative effects of stress.

There is a significant body of animal and human research indicating that experience of 'life events' and perceived stress is associated with the development and exacerbation of a wide range of diseases and health outcomes, including those of oral health, although it is often difficult to demonstrate causality. The link between stress and health is supported by data indicating that stress is associated with dysregulation of the immune system, with chronic stresses associated with a global suppression of both natural and specific immunity and immune-related health outcomes. However, it is less clear how these changes translate into poorer outcomes across the range of disease states. Dentists need to be aware of the impact that stress can have on themselves, their colleagues and their patients. Whilst we do not know which stress management intervention is most effective, there are a wide variety of options available and there is research evidence indicating they are efficacious in improving psychological well-being.

Discussion Points

- What are the difficulties in studying the relationship between stress and health?
- What makes it difficult to investigate which stress management technique is the most effective?

Issues in Social Psychology

Koula Asimakopoulou

IN THIS CHAPTER YOU WILL LEARN ABOUT:

▶ Seminal work in social psychology showing that
  ▶ people tend to conform to group and other pressures
  ▶ unrealistic optimism about ill-health can fuel and support unhealthy behaviours
  ▶ obedience to authority and to social context expectations can shape patients' expectations and behaviour in the dental surgery.

Introduction

People, and this includes dentists, dental healthcare professionals and patients alike, are social beings. This means they live and work and are surrounded by others. From pre-historic times, people have lived in social groups. They have worked together, hunted together and co-existed. This chapter considers some of the ways in which people who find themselves in the same social space might, directly or indirectly, wilfully or without awareness, influence the behaviour of those who surround them.

In particular, this chapter considers key studies in social psychology that may explain behaviour in the dental practice. It is not the purpose of the chapter to introduce the reader to every aspect of social psychology. Rather, the chapter aims to take the reader through a journey of interesting social psychology experimental and survey work that explains what makes people behave in fairly predictable ways, in the social context in general and in dental settings in particular. As with previous chapters, the bulk of this research work has taken place in non-dental settings and with young, healthy, student participants. So, the extent to which the findings of the studies described here may be confidently generalized to dental settings has not been demonstrated; to the extent that dental settings are, however, parts of society, it is proposed that much of this work applies to the dental surgery too.

The chapter considers some of the general principles that seem to govern people's social behaviour. These include ideas about conformity, obedience to authority and automatic errors and biases in people's thinking that may lead to unhealthy behaviours. We shall consider these issues by taking a look at the case study that follows.

Box 10.1: Case Study

Mrs Goldsmith is a mature lady who has been a good attender at her local dental practice for many years. She says she does not particularly enjoy visiting the dentist but sees it as a necessary event in her life; at interview about her local practice and the staff who treat her there, she tells us:

> 'Well. . . . You know, no one likes going to the dentist, do they . . . but it's one of those things. If you go regularly, you avoid the pain later on. I have been going to the dentist regularly since I was a child. So have all my family, most of the people I socialise with and most people I know really.'

Her regular attendance has been, she feels, helped by the fact that when visiting the dentist not much dental work needs to take place:

> 'I am of course very lucky because all my family have really good genes, so good teeth run in our family. In fact, good health runs in our family, we are generally very healthy people who do not often get sick . . . you know, properly sick, needing time off work. It just doesn't happen to us! We might get the odd cold, but generally speaking, we are a healthy lot!'

When asked about the reasons for visiting her local practice, Mrs Goldsmith explains:

> 'They are very good. But my dentist, Mr Lucas, well, he is not just very good . . . he is fantastic. He is very gentle, personable and a true expert. He knows of all the latest techniques to make sure that anything he does on my teeth is totally pain-free – he has a very gentle touch. I am sure some dentists are better than others with their hands and I suppose Mr Lucas just has a natural talent that I doubt others have. I am very very lucky to have him as my dentist.'

Discussion Point

There are a lot of 'common sense' ideas in the case study above. Jot down those instances of behaviour that you think psychologists might be able to explain using psychological theory. Then, as you read through the chapter, check your notes as the answers to this exercise are revealed.

Conformity

The idea of people conforming in groups has been a topic that social psychologists have been looking at for some time. Conformity, in general, can be described as the tendency of people to give into group pressures. These pressures can vary from implicit societal norms surrounding expectations of people with regard to, for example, dress code, appearance and acceptable behaviour in public, to more subtle yet formal requirements for conformity such as conforming to the General Dental Council (GDC) guidelines on how they should conduct their professional life as a dentist. Either way, it is accepted that a lot of the time, much of human behaviour is normally in line with group pressures, whatever the relevant 'group' might be.

Some of the best-known work on this innate psychological pressure that people find themselves under, to 'blend in' with groups and conform with the group norm, was carried out in the United States by Solomon Asch (Asch 1955). In his now famous study, he set up an experiment where a group of seven people were asked to sit together and look at a display. Their task was apparently simple; they had to say out loud which of three straight lines on the display was the same length as a fourth line (let's call it X) when asked by the researcher. The interesting thing about the three lines and the comparator line X was that it was pretty obvious which of these matched the stimulus line (see figure 10.1).

The slight deception inherent in the experiment was that all but one of the people taking part in the experiment were actually confederates of the experimenter. These confederates had all been instructed prior to the start of the experiment to confidently give out loud the *wrong* answer, when asked about their judgements of line length. The one real participant was always placed in the room in a place where s/he would be asked for their line judgement only *after* they had heard what the confederates' answers were. The point of the experiment was to find out if the participant would deny the evidence of their own eyes and conform with the group's obviously wrong, but strongly held view about the lines' length.

The study yielded some surprising results: 75 per cent of all real participants went along with the obviously wrong group answer at least some of the time. Only 25 per cent of those people stuck to what they were actually seeing and refused to yield to group pressure. In a variation of the experiment, one of Asch's confederates gave the right answer. In this situation, 95 per cent of participants resisted the need to conform and gave the right answer, in line with the single other confederate. It would seem that conformity can break down when there is at least one other person who shares the same version of reality as the person who is asked to make a judgement.

So what other factors can break down conformity? *Cohesiveness* is one such factor. Cohesiveness refers to the degree of attraction people

10

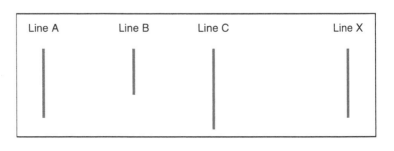

Figure 10.1 An example of the type of line display with which participants in the Asch experiment were presented

feel towards the group. The greater the attraction, the more likely people are to conform to group pressures. In terms of dental setting work, these observations would propose that, for example, the more a dentist sees themselves as an important member of the GDC and the more they respect the GDC's principles, the more they are likely to want to conform to the GDC's guidelines than if they simply thought the GDC was a body that they did not really see themselves as being a part of. So, it is argued that the more people admire and respect a group that they are part of, the stronger the pressures are going to be for them to want to conform to the group's behaviour or standards.

Group size is a second factor. Some early research (Thomas & Clinton 1963) showed that, generally speaking, the larger the group the greater people's tendency to go along with it, even if this meant behaving differently than they would normally do, outside the group. So, for example, if a person found themselves amongst a crowd of students being disruptive in a lecture that they felt was not up to their expectations, they might find themselves more likely to join in with the disruption, rather than if they were in an equally uninspiring tutorial with only a few people present.

It has been argued that 'conformity is a basic fact of social life' (Baron & Byrne 2003: 357). Most people conform most of the time to the norms of the groups they feel associated with. But why is this the case? Why does conformity occur?

Discussion Point

Think back to the case study. Did you notice any implicit conformity in the situation that was described there?

You might have answered here that Mrs Goldsmith seems to have conformed all her life to the implicit instruction that she should visit the dentist regularly.

So why does conformity occur? It has been suggested (Baron & Byrne 2003) that there are *normative influences* and *informational influences* on people's social behaviour. The first refers to people's innate desire to be liked and accepted by others. It is argued that people have learnt, through interactions with others, that the more like them they are, the more they all agree with one another's views and, ultimately, the more these people like one another. So, one explanation for group conformity is people's psychological need to 'fit in' and be liked by those they perceive as being part of the same group. In a family setting, if all the family are regular attenders at the dental practice, it would be harder for individual members not to attend.

A second explanation rests on another innate need, that people have to be right. From an evolutionary point of view, people have always wanted to 'be right' about things in their lives; not being right about how fierce a lion is might have got the hunter-gatherer savaged in the jungle. Not being right about what the presence of dark clouds in the sky could signal might have got them soaking wet in the pouring rain and subsequently ill. So, generally, it pays in terms of evolutionary principles, to 'be right' about life events. But unlike variables that may be objectively measured, such as one's weight or height, judgements about life and general life events are not that easy to verify. In those cases, people rely on other people and use other people as a gauge to tell them if their own opinions are right. It is this need to rely on others to confirm one's own ideas that sometimes (as in Asch's study) backfires and gets people to agree with obviously inaccurate group views.

These studies on conformity can be used to explain patient behaviour in the dental surgery. For instance, where patients wait in a waiting room, they are momentarily all members of the social group of 'dental patients awaiting treatment'. It would only take a small group of patients to express a view about dentistry, their dentist, their experience in the practice and so on, for the rest of the patients to all wish to join in with agreeing about the accuracy of the view. The more the patients associate with the group, the more likely they will be to wish to be seen to be conforming to it. Equally, it would only take one dissident, as has been shown in Asch's work, to make those who disagree with the group view feel able to voice their dissenting view.

A note of caution is needed here; not everybody conforms all of the time! Research has shown that the 'Asch effect', as group conformity is often referred to by psychologists, is more prominent in cultures that emphasize the importance of being part of a group (collectivist cultures) rather than those that highlight the importance of the person themselves (individualistic cultures). Typically, Western cultures are considered to be individualistic in their nature and, as such, might

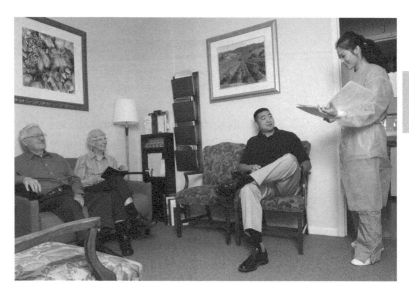

Image 10.1 Most people conform to certain rules dictated by their social setting
Source: leezsnow

put their members under less pressure to be seen to be conforming to group behaviour than otherwise expected (Bond & Smith 1996).

> **In summary**, conformity is a psychological phenomenon with evolutionary roots that shapes a lot of human behaviour. Although not everyone conforms all of the time, it has been suggested that the human need to appear to 'fit in' can sometimes produce very powerful conformity effects.

Unrealistic optimism

Another key finding about people's social judgements, this time about themselves as individuals, comes under the term 'unrealistic optimism'. This phenomenon refers to people's tendency to think they are less likely than others to have negative events happen to them. This is the case for a wide variety of negative events ranging from divorce, to car accidents, to lung cancer, to a tooth extraction. The belief usually leads people to take risks or engage in unhealthy behaviours, simply because they do not consider themselves to be at risk or their judgements of personal risk are inaccurate. In practice, these are the people who will talk about being at a lower risk from lung cancer because they smoke less than 'properly' addicted smokers, or those who do not consider they need to see the dentist preventively because they have 'good teeth running in the family'. The work that led to the proposition of this term by Weinstein (1980, 1984) was grounded in studies showing that people have difficulties accurately estimating risks, and that in doing so, they engage in inaccurate social comparisons that reflect best on the self rather than the people they are comparing themselves to.

> **Discussion Point**
>
> Think back to Mrs Goldsmith. Would you say she was a case of unrealistic optimism? Did her risk-taking profile fit in with the main tenet of the theory?

Unrealistic optimism is mainly used to explain (unhealthy) risk-taking in health psychology. As such, whilst Mrs Goldsmith exhibits the unrealistic optimism about 'good teeth' that 'run in the family' because of her 'good genes', what is not seen in this case is the risk behaviour that usually follows these irrational thoughts.

In what is now considered as seminal work in the field of health, Weinstein collected data from American university students, rating the likelihood that they would experience a series of positive (e.g. living past 80, having a mentally gifted child, graduating in the top third of their year) and a series of negative (e.g. getting divorced, developing a drinking problem, having a tooth extracted, not finding a job for 6 months) life events, compared to other students at the same university.

Overall, the sample rated their chances of experiencing positive events as much higher than the 'average student', whilst they rated their chances of experiencing the series of negative events much lower (Weinstein 1980).

Similar data were obtained in a second study using a similar paradigm, but this time asking students to rate their chances of experiencing a series of health hazards, ranging from suicide, cancer and drug addiction to catching a cold. Again, students consistently rated their chances of experiencing a range of health hazards as much lower than those of the 'average student'. It was concluded that, generally, people tend to favour their own chances of experiencing good things in life, but seem to believe they are in a somewhat more advantageous position than others when it comes to experiencing negative events, including physical illness (Weinstein 1982).

So why are people so wrong in their estimates of personal hazard? What is it that fuels this optimism about the future? Four reasons have been proposed that might explain people's tendency to believe they are less at risk than others (Weinstein 1987).

The first factor has to do with *a lack of personal experience with the negative event*; this goes back to how people judge the frequency of events and work on what psychologists call 'cognitive heuristics'. It is known that the less experience people have with an event, the less likely they believe it is to happen. Equally, the more they hear about an event, and the more experience they have with it, the more frequent they judge it to be (Tversky & Kahneman 1974). For example, it is known that women are more worried about their risk of dying from breast cancer, a much publicized illness, than dying from heart disease (a less discussed illness), when in fact heart disease kills five times more women than does breast cancer (Covello & Peters 2002).

A second explanation for unrealistic optimism has to do with *people's inaccurate beliefs about control*: that is, people tend to think that their own actions can prevent the potential negative event from happening, a belief that they do not hold for their 'average other' person. For example, someone might think they are less at risk from caries because, although they eat lots of sugary foods, their tooth brushing technique is exceptional. Here, their belief about others would be that those people who do get caries (i.e. the 'average other' they compare themselves to) must be less proficient in their oral health routine.

A third explanatory factor has to do with people's beliefs about *negative past events*: that is, if something negative has not yet happened so far, people tend to reason that it is unlikely to happen in the future. For instance, someone who has not visited the dentist for a year and is not experiencing any oral health problems, is likely to use the absence of a problem as a reason to carry on avoiding the dentist: 'I have not been to the dentist for years and my teeth are fine, so why would this change now?'. In parallel to thinking that because ill-health has not happened yet, it is unlikely to happen now or in the future, the lack of oral health problems might often be used as a reinforcing factor in people's lack of dental visits.

A fourth explanation of the optimistic bias phenomenon proposes that optimistic bias is fuelled by inaccurate beliefs about the problem *frequency*. That is, people who are unrealistically biased towards an event tend to think that the event is rare and as such unlikely to take place. 'Tooth loss is rare – when was the last time you saw people without their front teeth?' is the sort of thought that would sustain an unrealistic optimism tendency.

Finally, it is argued that one of the most basic needs that people have is to maintain self-esteem, that is, people strive to feel good about themselves. One way that people can achieve this, temporarily at least, is to focus only on positive things happening in one's life and play down the risks of negative events occurring. It might not be a long-term winning strategy, but it helps to maintain self-esteem, which is one of the most basic human needs.

The combination of all the factors above probably explains why people tend to take risks with their life in general and with their health in particular. Unrealistic optimism research suggests that people carry on with unhealthy behaviours such as smoking, unhealthy eating, etc., or fail to take up health-enhancing behaviours such as preventive visits to the dentist or giving up smoking, as a result of an interplay between the factors we have described above, all of which put them in a state of mind that 'protects' them from thoughts that they are actually at risk.

So what are the implications of this work for dental practice? It is useful to remember that when people visit the dentist, they do not come in as carriers of a *tabula rasa* (a 'blank slate'). If the research described here is reliable, patients are likely to think that they are less at risk than the 'average other' patient for any negative health consequence to happen to them.

How might knowing about 'unrealistic optimism' be helpful to a dentist? Firstly, knowing generally about this interesting research should help in understanding one's fellow human beings a little better. So, when a dentist wonders why is it that the patient who has been explicitly told that their caries profile is high and that they are at risk of losing teeth, fails to attend a follow-up appointment, unrealistic optimism may help explain their visiting pattern.

Secondly, knowing about unrealistic optimism work should help dentist–patient communication. It is advisable for the dental team to know the nature of patient's ideas about how at risk they feel they are and hence be able to tackle any potentially unrealistic thoughts before offering dental health education and advice. The dentist's communication style and content might need to address several unhelpful beliefs. For example, where a patient unrealistically thinks that (i) they are not at risk of losing their teeth because tooth loss is rare and only happens to 'old' people, or (ii) that their brushing is superior to anybody else's, both these thoughts are unrealistically optimistic, both are likely to be hurdles in any expectations a dentist has for the patient to adhere to their advice, and both need to be dealt with before dental health education is offered. Offering dental health education and support, whilst being unaware of what the patient's thoughts about their oral health are in the first place, is likely to be an unhelpful exercise, likely to result in non-adherence and difficulties with behaviour change, as we have discussed in chapter 8.

> **In summary**, unrealistic optimism or optimistic bias is people's tendency to think that adverse events are less likely to happen to them (and more likely to happen to others). These thoughts can often explain poor dental attendance patterns and are explained through ideas about control, adverse event frequency and self-esteem. Unrealistic optimism may be a barrier to regular dental attendance and/or adherence to oral health advice.

The fundamental attribution error, the actor–observer effect and self-serving bias

Another piece of seminal work that has attempted to explain errors in how people make judgements about their social world has been proposed by social psychologists working in the area of attributions – by attributions, psychologists refer to 'causal explanations'. In particular, this area of psychological enquiry examines how people go about explaining the causes of other people's behaviour in an attempt to gain knowledge of their stable traits and dispositions. It has been suggested that people tend to prefer living in a world that they can predict (Fiske & Taylor 1991). At the same time, people have been described as 'cognitive misers' (Fiske & Taylor 1991). They tend to find using cognitive resources strenuous and they would rather save their time and cognitive effort for thinking about situations that are truly worth it rather than about everyday, mundane events. The idea proposed is that people develop strategies to try and understand why other people behave the way they do and what they are likely to do next, and this will save them having to think about these processes at length on each occasion.

As an example, a dental nurse works with the same dentist every Tuesday morning. She finds that over 6 months of working with this dentist, their first appointment has always started 10 minutes late because the dentist never manages to arrive at the surgery and be ready in time. It is Tuesday morning and the dentist is, once again, not there – what will she do? Will she spend cognitive resources (i.e. time thinking) to wonder where the dentist might be? Or will she assume, albeit perhaps in the back of her mind, that they will be late as usual, and get on with her Tuesday morning routine? Chances are that the longer this behaviour pattern on the part of the dentist has been going on for, the more likely it is for the nurse in this hypothetical example to take it for granted. The nurse may assign a general explanation to the dentist's behaviour. For example, thinking that:

1 the particular dentist is generally unreliable, or that
2 Tuesdays are a problem for this, otherwise perfectly reliable dentist, or that
3 the dentist values and trusts the nurse's work so much that they know she will get everything ready without the need for them to be present, or that
4 they are totally unprofessional and have no regard or respect for their 9 a.m. patients.

The strategies that the nurse may use to attribute causes to the dentist's (and others') behaviour have been examined in detail by psychologists and have developed into a body of work known as 'attribution theory'. It is beyond the scope of the chapter to provide a detailed explanation of various theories of attribution, but the reader might wish to look at work on Kelley's co-variation model (Kelley 1973) and Jones and Davis' Correspondent Inference theory (Jones & Davis 1965). What is of more interest in terms of application of this work to the dental practice, is the *errors* that we make whilst trying to make causal attributions about people's behaviour and the reasons behind such attributions.

Fundamental attribution error

The fundamental attribution error (Ross 1977) refers to the human tendency to exaggerate people's dispositions or personality influences as explanatory factors of their behaviour and, at the same time, to minimize the impact or influence of the situation that people find themselves in when trying to explain a particular event. For instance, the first reaction on seeing a periodontal patient return to clinic with unacceptable levels of bleeding and plaque scores might be to conclude that the person has been non-adherent to treatment recommendations because they haven't tried hard enough. The next thought might be to question their non-adherence and move on to a dental health education campaign to 'get the person to comply'. In this example, the dentist would appear to have made a judgement about the person *per se*, rather than consider the possible situations the patient may have found themselves in since leaving the surgery last time. Dentists may benefit from thinking about the person's situation that might have prevented them from brushing and flossing their teeth after leaving their last appointment. Could it be, for example, that the person's circumstances were such that they did not understand the instructions the dentist gave them on the day? Or that they did attempt to brush their teeth but their technique was not particularly efficient? Or that the person has since developed diabetes or some other medical condition beyond their direct control that might have influenced their oral health? All these are *situational* factors, outside the person's stable personality and disposition, that may well have affected behaviour.

However, people tend to ignore situation factors when explaining others' behaviour. This tendency to wish to explain a behaviour in terms of stable, personality or dispositional features rather than the situation the person has found themselves in is known as the Fundamental Attribution Error. One of the original studies that gave rise to the observation was conducted by Jones and Harris (1967). These American researchers gave participants two sets of essays to rate. These essays were either in favour or against the Fidel Castro government in Cuba (Castro's politics and thinking were at odds with 1960s US government policy). In one set of essays, students were told that the essay author had freely chosen whether to write a pro- or anti-Castro essay. For the other set, the students were told that the essay author had been randomly assigned (by the toss of a coin) to write either for or against Castro. So, in the first instance, the essay writer may well have chosen to take a stance that reflected their own personal views about the politician, whilst in the second group, their personal views were probably redundant as they were explicitly told which stance to take in their writing. The study participants' task was to gauge how much in favour or against Castro the essay author was, simply by reading the essay the person had written and knowing whether the author was writing under the 'free choice' or the 'assigned essay' conditions.

What the researchers found was that when the participants believed that the essay writers had freely chosen the positions they took, for or against Castro, they naturally rated the people who spoke in favour of Castro as having a more positive attitude towards him compared to those who spoke against him. However, when the raters were told that the writer's essay stance was determined only by a coin toss, they *still* rated writers who spoke in favour of Castro as having, on average, a more positive attitude towards him than those who wrote essays against him. In other words, the participants were unable to see the influence of the situational constraints placed upon the writers; instead, they attributed the writers with a pro- (or anti)-Castro disposition and belief even in the condition where the writers had no choice over what to write about. This tendency to feel the urge to make 'person' rather than 'situation' statements about people is an important psychological tendency which has implications for work in the dental surgery – these are discussed next after a short explanation of the reasons behind the Fundamental Attribution Error.

So what leads to the Fundamental Attribution Error? 'Perceptual salience' is one explanation that is favoured by psychologists. Or, to put it in Heider's (1958) words, 'behaviour engulfs the field' – where the field is any situation people find themselves in and the person is seen as an 'actor' behaving in the field. What is suggested here is that

10

someone's behaviour is more salient or prominent and hence more noticeable and likely to be used in causal judgements than the situation they are in. The result of this is that people are routinely tricked into making *dispositional* (i.e. to do with the person *per se* and their individual characteristics), rather than *situational* judgements about behavioural events.

Discussion Point

What evidence is there in the case study of Mrs Goldsmith perhaps committing a Fundamental Attribution Error?

In the case study, Mrs Goldsmith seems to have total trust in her dentist, describing him as *fantastic . . . gentle . . . personable . . . a true expert . . . has a natural talent. . . .* An alternative explanation of course could be that the situation that Mr Lucas finds himself in, for example, having been trained at a top dental school rather than inherent talent, might have had some influence in his treatment skill. So, in this case the influence of the context is ignored; rather, Mrs Goldsmith attributes the high-quality dental treatment she receives to the personal, stable characteristics of the dentist.

It is worth noting that the Fundamental Attribution Error does not always yield positive interpretations of realiity; thus a similar process may go on in the patient's mind when they are having treatment; whatever event takes place at the time of treatment is very likely to be attributed to one's skill as a dentist rather than the situation. So, for example, where an anaesthetic top-up is required, the event might be judged as the dentist being a poor judge of the situation and failing to administer enough in the first place (rather than something about the fact that the patient may be anxious and their anxiety is making them more prone to notice, focus on and respond to pain). Equally, where a hygienist may complete treatment without any discomfort experienced by the patient, they are likely to be judged positively as a dental professional, rather than by the patient considering the situation (e.g. that the treatment in itself was unlikely to cause discomfort).

The Actor–Observer Effect and Self-Serving Bias

Another two errors closely related to the Fundamental Attribution Error concern how people make judgements about others as opposed to themselves. Interestingly, people have a tendency to attribute others' behaviour to dispositional causes, as discussed, but when it comes to explaining their *own* behaviour, they more often than not attribute their behaviour to situational causes. This is known as the Actor–Observer Effect or the Actor–Observer Discrepancy (Jones & Nisbett 1971). Actors, that is, people explaining their own behaviour, tend to do so by offering situational explanations (e.g. 'I was late for an appointment because the traffic was bad'), but when they attempt to explain others' behaviour they tend to attribute it to stable, dispositional characteristics (e.g. 'He was late for an appointment because he is unreliable and did not leave in time'). The reasons for this are not particularly clear, but it has been suggested that where one is asked to judge their own behaviour, the salience of the circumstances is prominent, whereas situational judgements are not that obvious to others (Fiske & Taylor 1991).

Related to the Actor–Observer effect is an error known as 'Self-Serving Bias' (Baron & Byrne 2003). This is the tendency to attribute positive events and outcomes to *internal* causes such as one's own ability, personality and skill, but negative outcomes to causes *outside* one's personal control such as chance or task difficulty. So, generally, where a dental student may have been particularly successful in extracting a tooth causing minimal pain, the theory would propose that the student would explain the event by making some sort of internal, dispositional judgement ('oral surgery was always my forte'). On the other hand, if a patient complains that an extraction was painful or in some way unsatisfactory, the theory would propose that the first explanation to come to the student's mind would be that the patient is being too anxious or critical, or that the student had difficulties with the particular tooth, or equipment or environment and so on (i.e. they would make external judgements). The reason for this self-serving bias has to do with human beings' innate expectation that they will succeed in whatever task they are performing. As such, where the person expects to succeed and they do, it is perfectly normal to take responsibility for this success. Another explanation comes from the idea that people have an innate desire to maintain self-esteem and appear good to others; as such, they are motivated to claim success and attribute it to themselves rather than the situation around them (Fiske & Taylor 1991).

So what are the implications of this research for working as a dentist? It is hoped that psychology will have given the reader some information about people's basic psychological states that might explain their behaviour in general and more specifically in the dental setting. So, it is now known that people will be more likely to make dispositional judgements about their dentists than situational judgements. It is known that this tendency will be more pronounced when explaining others' behaviour rather than their own. It is also known that people are generally motivated to maintain self-esteem, and to do so they will engage in self-serving biases that may or may not reflect reality but which will go a long way towards maintaining self-esteem. In essence, people are inaccurate judges of reality, and have a process of attributing causes for behaviour that is not foolproof; being aware of these circumstances might help our understanding of patient behaviour a little better than if the assumption was made that people are rational, logical judges of the social world.

In summary, this section has shown that people are not always logical, rational, objective judges of the causes behind (i) their own and (ii) other people's behaviour. Psychologists have offered theories in the form of the Fundamental Attribution Error and related concepts that explain why some dental patients' judgements about the dental team and their own oral health might not always be accurate.

Obedience to authority and social power: the Milgram and Stanford Prison experiments

The final, yet equally important area of psychological research that will be explored in this chapter has to do with how people respond to authority figures. Society is designed in such a way that most people will find themselves in one position of authority or another at some point in their lives, and it is interesting to know what research says about the way that people tend to respond to authority figures. 'Authority', in this case, is not necessarily synonymous with 'high status' or 'high wealth', so although a prime minister or a High Court judge is evidently and quite obviously a person that would reasonably be classified as being of high authority, there are other everyday roles which involve power/authority and which people experience; for example, relationships such as those of a parent–child, teacher–pupil, doctor–patient, bank manager–customer are all situations where one member of the pair is quite likely to be in a position to exercise some power over the other.

Authority relationships do not normally cause problems and people are 'programmed' to accept them as involving certain expected behaviours. So, for example, patients in a hospital bed receiving treatment would probably not question a stranger walking them up in the middle of the night and insisting they took some tablets. Equally, people would probably not question the divulging of personal information about their finances to a person they had never met before as long as that was a bank manager assessing their application for a loan. Authority figures are often implicitly trusted, listened to and obeyed; as a result, they are rarely questioned.

Psychologists have been interested in what happens when the process of obeying an authority figure goes wrong. Under what circumstances will people question authority figures? How far are people prepared to go in their obedience to authority? What happens when people are asked by a person in authority to do something that they believe is wrong? Stanley Milgram, a Yale University professor, designed a series of experiments to examine precisely these questions.

In what is now considered ground-breaking work into the human psyche (Russell 2011), Milgram (1963) recruited participants by advertising in a newspaper for 'subjects' to take part in a memory experiment. The study told participants that, supposedly, it was going to look at the effects of punishment on learning. Participants believed that having been put in pairs 'randomly', one would be a 'teacher' and the other person would be the 'learner'. In fact, the unsuspecting participant always drew the 'teacher' card whilst an associate of the experimenter was always the 'learner'. The 'teacher' was asked to sit in front of a machine that looked as if it was capable of delivering electric shocks of ever-increasing magnitude (unbeknown to the study participants, this was a fake machine).

The 'learner' was in theory sitting behind this machine, but out of view of the 'teacher'. The 'teachers' were told that every time the 'learner' made a mistake during the memory task at hand, the 'teacher' would be instructed to administer an electric shock to the 'learner' by pressing a button. The instructions were such that every time a mistake was made, the 'teacher' was ordered to move up one notch on this 'electric shock administrator'. So, where a 'learner' made a lot of mistakes, they were at risk of receiving fairly substantial electric shocks. The shock scale ranged from 15 volts to 450 volts. The experiment was prearranged so that the 'learner' always made a lot of mistakes. The point of the experiment was to see how far the unsuspecting 'teacher' participant would go in punishing the 'learner' with these increasing, 'painful' and ultimately life-threatening electric shocks.

The experimental set-up was obviously not quite as the 'teacher' was led to believe. The learner, always an associate of the experimenter, was sitting out of view, in an adjacent room, and never really received any shocks. They *acted out* the role of someone who had just been shocked, however. So, they responded as if they were in pain when a supposed shock was 'administered' and their reaction got more severe and louder, the higher the 'shock' they had supposedly received. The 'teacher', on the other hand, sat in a room with a man in a white coat, the study researcher, giving the command '*you must continue*' in varying forms. Where the participants hesitated, the researcher in their white coat pressured them with the following commands:

1 *Please continue*
2 *The experiment requires that you continue*
3 *It is absolutely essential that you continue*
4 *You have no other choice – you must go on.*

Milgram was interested to see the reaction of the 'teacher' participants when put in a situation in which they were being asked by a person in an obvious position of power and authority (a researcher at Yale) to cause potentially serious harm to another human being.

In this study, it is reported that participants found themselves in quite a dilemma. Should they carry on punishing this person with what they believed to be painful shocks, simply because they were making mistakes on the test? Or should they refuse to go on? The participants complained and questioned the researcher. They protested against the instructions they were being given. But in the end, 65 per cent of all those tested showed total obedience, that is, they proceeded through the entire series of shocks up to the 450-volt mark. They carried on with this, even when the 'learner' was demonstrating behaviour that they would have interpreted as him banging at the wall in severe distress (at about 300 volts) and when the 'learner' stopped responding altogether.

Milgram (1963) also found that manipulating the extent to which the 'teacher' was exposed to the learner (by, for example, being in the same room as the 'learner', or the 'learner' not making any noise at all) affected the obedience rates in the direction that would be expected: where the 'teacher' could see the 'learner' suffer, the participants were less likely to obey; where the 'learner' was not very vocal about the supposed pain they were in, the participants were more likely to obey. Having the research take place in an ordinary city office (rather than at Yale University) brought down the percentage of people obeying the researcher to the end by around 20 per cent. Having the authority figure give the instructions to the 'teacher' to carry on over the phone rather than in person further reduced obedience to just over 20 per cent. Where the 'teacher' had free choice as to whether to continue or not, only 2.5 per cent of all people obeyed the original instructions to the end (Milgram 1963). This indicates that the presence and persistence of the authority figure was crucially important for the obedience reactions.

What are the implications of this work for dental settings? Firstly, this work was carried out in the 1960s and it is possibly the case that people are more questioning and less worried about standing up to authority figures than they were back then. Obviously, to be sure that this is the case, Milgram's work would need to be replicated and to do so nowadays would probably be considered highly unethical due to the potential distress the study would cause to unsuspecting volunteers. Although it may be the case that obedience to authority figures is not as pronounced as in the 1960s, the general inclination of the human psyche to obey people who are perceived to be in positions of authority is probably an innate one.

Why might that be the case? Why are people 'tuned' to follow directions from people in authority? Generally speaking, it makes evolutionary sense; so, for example, young children learn that it is a good idea to do as their parents tell them rather than, for example, crossing the road and risking getting knocked down by a bus during an outing, or getting scalded by a hot iron or boiling water. So, in many respects people learn to obey authority because doing so in the past has contributed to their survival.

A second explanatory factor in the need to obey authority has to do with previous experiences of negative consequences when failing to do so. For example, pupils may have had to have uncomfortable meetings with their headteacher after an episode of failing to obey the authority figure at school – thus obedience deviation might have been punished. Or, a person may have vicariously learned by, for example, observing other children having to have an unpleasant discussion with the headteacher that it is sensible not to disobey what the school authority tells them. So, it is a process of positive reinforcement (e.g. listening to parents and avoiding accidents) but also punishment (e.g. being made to feel uncomfortable when disobeying teachers at school) that may partially explain why people are 'set up' to wish to obey authority figures.

Milgram's obedience experiment is, of course, slightly more complex than what has been described above, in that here, obeying authority was going against the participants' learnt beliefs and ideas and probably their most basic instincts about what is 'right' and what is wrongful behaviour. Theorists have written a lot about how it was possible for Milgram's participants to engage in potentially really harmful behaviour. It is beyond the purpose of the chapter to go through the complex social psychological theory that might explain the experimental participants' behaviour, but the simplest explanation has to do with the idea of 'transfer of responsibility'; that is, where the individual believes that they themselves are not individually responsible for the harm they are causing by obeying, but rather that the person in the position of power and authority who is actually issuing the orders must bear overall responsibility. This raises a larger social question that is still very relevant, yet unanswered, to date (Baron & Byrne 2003).

It follows from the discussion so far that knowledge of Milgram's work places a huge sense of responsibility on those in positions of authority not to explicitly or implicitly abuse their power. In the dental setting, dentists and their teams are generally likely to be perceived as being in positions of power; patients will tend to do what dentists ask them to do without questioning it while they are in the dental chair, as dentists are often seen as authority figures. Two things follow from this observation; either there needs to be a change in ethos in the dental surgery, whereby patients are made to feel that there is no one powerful figure dominating the setting, and in that sense power is equally distributed between dentist and patient (Asimakopoulou & Scambler 2013). Or, where the dentist and their team do find themselves inherently being perceived as in a position of power, they need to be aware that the position comes with great responsibilities.

This discussion, of how the social context of a dental setting may be construed by patients as one where a non-authority figure obeys an authority one, leads the discussion to consider the power of the social situation. The idea here is that people in a position of authority have 'social power', that is, the power to effect change in other people's behaviour or attitudes through their perceived position in the particular social setting.

In summary, this section has introduced you to a key study in psychology that demonstrates how people respond to authority. Although there are caveats attached to the work regarding how generalizable the findings might be in today's society, the key point is that where people perceive that they are in a position where a high-authority figure instructs them to take action, they will often act without feeling particularly responsible for their actions and will not question that authority.

The Stanford Prison experiment

Another piece of major psychological research that took place in the United States in the 1960s highlighted the importance of the power of the social situation in making people behave in ways that were not in their usual behavioural repertoire, but which they felt they had to enact because of the social situation (rather than explicit orders from an authority figure) they found themselves in. This study is known as the Stanford Prison experiment (Zimbardo 2007) and was carried out by Philip Zimbardo. What he set out to show was that, where the social context that people find themselves in has rigid power structures inherent in its set-up, people's behaviour will be subject to these power structures in ways that are concordant with the behaviour the power structures suggest should be exhibited. Zimbardo, working from Stanford University, set up a mock prison situation within a laboratory setting at Stanford. He recruited young volunteers who were randomly allocated to being either 'prisoners' or 'wardens' to spend just over two weeks in this mock prison. Zimbardo wanted to see whether the publicized cruelty and hostile behaviour that is often associated with prisons is the unfortunate result of

(i) a group of angry, violent and aggressive people having to interact with people who are naturally attracted to be controlling of others' lives (as in the stereotypical prisoner and warden), or

(ii) whether it was something about the social power and role expectations inherent in the particular social situation seen in a prison environment that made ordinary young people on both sides perhaps behave differently to normal.

In Zimbardo's mock prison study, there were rigid rules in place. Prisoners had to ask permission to write letters or use the bathroom. They ate and were 'locked up' at predetermined times. They generally had to ask permission to do anything much in that environment, in line with what often happens in prisons. So, although this was very much a mock environment with people in it who were neither true prisoners nor real wardens, the realism of the study was quite high.

The study findings were utterly unexpected. The violence and fighting that ensued within a couple of days of the start of the experiment were so great that it was deemed unsafe for the study to continue into the planned full two weeks. There were riots between prisoners and wardens that were of a truly violent nature. The two seemed to have been immersed in their roles, and taken on behaviours they believed the context expected them to take on, to such an extent that worryingly ill-health was soon very evident in the 'prisoners'. As such, for ethical but also for health reasons, the study was abandoned after only six days.

Zimbardo had shown that when completely 'normal', psychologically stable, law-abiding strangers are put in a situation with a rigid power structure and inherent expectations on how its members should behave, they will often unquestioningly internalize those expectations and demonstrate behaviours that they would not have considered acceptable under normal circumstances.

So what are the implications of Zimbardo's work for dental settings? After all, the dental surgery is neither a prison, nor are there rigid structures present that might give people cues about what is and is not acceptable behaviour.

The dental surgery is a social setting, however, which comes with inherent structures that give patients and staff clues as to what is considered normal, expected behaviour. So, for example, there are expectations placed on patients and staff as to what their roles in the setting might be, what they are allowed to express and do, and what behaviour they are or are not expected to demonstrate. For example, most patients will expect to sit in a waiting room before their appointment, will know that once the dentist has finished talking to them, s/he will want to tilt them back in the dental chair and sit in close proximity to them. These are currently accepted social norms that fit in with patients' expectations about the dental situation (often referred to as 'scripts' in cognitive psychology).

At the same time, a dentally phobic patient will often have quite an elaborate script of the pain they fear they will endure whilst in that setting. Or, indeed, their script may contain ideas about how little control they will have of the situation, how the dentist may fail to stop even if asked to do so, and so on. These social expectations will be supported by the social setting in a way similar to that seen in the participants of the study by Zimbardo, and are going to guide much of a patient's behaviour in the dental surgery. These expectations, however, are malleable such that both dentist and patient might change them in order to be comfortable with them. For instance, patients may learn, after repeat exposure, that a visit to the dentist involves being tilted on a chair, no loss of control, a pain-free experience and classical music played in the background. Or, they may learn that a particular dentist does not follow a model of telling patients what to do, but adopts a more patient-centred style where patients are not necessarily objects in the power relation between themselves and the dentist. Such social cues can be communicated to patients by, for example, inviting them to choose amongst several treatment options, scheduling appointments that fit in with their lives, and treating them generally as more equal

10

partners than the traditional biomedical model of care would suggest is expected in dental settings.

The final message from the studies on obedience to authority and Zimbardo's Prison experiment is that, although people have expectations about their role and position in relation to power figures and specific settings, being aware of this should help dentists to help patients have as good an experience in the dental surgery as is possible.

> **In summary**, this section has introduced you to a key study in psychology that tries to explain how people respond in situations carrying inherent 'rules of expected behaviour'. Here, the key point is that where people perceive that they are in a situation that comes with rigid, society-dictated, widely accepted rules, they are likely to follow these societal rules and fail to question them.

Conclusion

This chapter has presented key social psychological ideas that have shaped the foundations of the discipline and are considered key work in the area. Obviously, the studies have not been carried out with dentists and dental settings in mind and their findings are not always neatly translated into such settings. Equally, they have generally been carried out on young, US students of the 1960s, so it is arguable that their findings are not readily applicable to people living outside the US and in modern times. But what these studies have succeeded in is to uncover some of the most basic, innate psychological states that most people might experience at least some of the time. In this sense, they have demonstrated the general principles that guide human behaviour in social settings and which probably remain broadly the same, whatever the setting.

Discussion Points

- What reasons may explain smokers' psychological resistance to giving up smoking?
- What factors influence how likely people are to conform to group pressure?
- How might the social context influence patient expectations in the dental surgery?

Pain and Dental Anxiety

Suzanne E. Scott and Tim Newton

IN THIS CHAPTER YOU WILL LEARN ABOUT:

Pain
- ▶ What is pain?
- ▶ Mechanisms of pain
- ▶ Measuring pain
- ▶ Non-pharmacological interventions to reduce pain

Dental anxiety
- ▶ What is dental anxiety?
- ▶ The consequences of dental anxiety
- ▶ Reasons for dental anxiety
- ▶ Measuring dental anxiety
- ▶ Interventions to reduce dental anxiety

Introduction

What do patients mean when they say they are in pain? What causes the pain? How can you assess how much pain someone is in and whether your efforts to alleviate pain are working? If someone finds a dental procedure to be painful, will that make them anxious about visiting a dentist in the future? Do anxious patients feel more pain? These are just some of the questions that arise when considering the social and behavioural aspects of dental anxiety and pain.

Although an aim of dentistry is to alleviate or prevent pain, patients may enter the dental practice in pain, or in the expectation of feeling pain. Furthermore, dental procedures have the potential to be painful. As such, as a member of the dental team, it is important to understand the concept of pain and learn about ways to help patients avoid and lessen dental pain. Patients often expect pain during dental treatment and this can contribute to dental anxiety. Further, feelings of anxiety

Box 11.1: Case Study

Mrs Kilpatrick is a 36-year-old woman who is extremely anxious about visiting the dentist. She has trouble sleeping in the days leading up to her appointment. She has cancelled her two previous appointments because of her anxiety (although she was embarrassed about this, so when she called the receptionist to cancel she said she had family commitments which would prevent her attendance). She considered cancelling today's appointment but has had bad toothache for the last two months and really wants it to end. She feels she can't cope with the pain any longer. The pain is a dull ache that is there all day and taking painkillers and her attempts to distract herself from it aren't working.

She is now in the waiting room and has the feeling of butterflies in her stomach, which is making her feel nauseous. Her arms, hands and legs are tense and she has a dry mouth.

Mrs Kilpatrick doesn't mind the actual procedure of a check-up with a dentist, but is panicking about what the dentist might find. She believes the dentist will say she needs at least one filling – this petrifies her. Just the thought makes her imagine the size of the needle, and the pain of the local anaesthetic procedure. She says she 'isn't good with needles' and will faint if she has an injection. The last time she had an injection (a vaccine) she recalls it being extremely painful and feeling like an intense 'burn'.

may heighten experiences of pain. Anxiety and apprehension are uncomfortable (and sometimes debilitating) feelings that often arise from uncertainty about the future or, conversely, fearful beliefs of what will happen. Consider the case study in box 11.1 as an example.

This chapter will discuss models of pain, assessment of pain and non-pharmacological techniques that can be used to help reduce the experience of pain. The chapter will then outline the concept and consequences of dental anxiety and present its possible causes, including learning from previous experience and learning via observation. Ways to measure dental anxiety will be presented with reference to how they could be used in the dental setting. Non-pharmacological techniques to reduce dental anxiety will be outlined, providing an introduction to evidence-based practical solutions for the dental setting.

Pain

What is pain?

Through accidentally trapping our finger in a door, standing on a sharp object, having a headache or indigestion, we all know what pain is and what it feels like. Nevertheless, pain is a difficult concept to define. There is a location aspect of pain in terms of where the pain is felt. There is also an emotional aspect of pain, for example, pain is unpleasant. There are also different characteristics of pain. For instance, with regard to duration, pain can be acute (hours or days), sub-acute (months) or chronic (years) (Turk & Okifuji 2001). The International Association for the Study of Pain defined pain as 'an unpleasant sensory and emotional experience associated with actual or potential tissue damage, or described in terms of such damage' (Merskey & Bogduk 1994), whereas Pasero and McCaffery (1999) described pain as 'whatever the experiencing person says it is, existing whenever the experiencing person says it does'. As evidenced by these rather vague definitions, it is difficult to explain exactly what pain is. The difficulty in defining pain may arise because pain is a subjective, private experience, so unlike other bodily phenomena (e.g. temperature) it cannot be measured without asking the individual to describe the experience.

Dental pain can result from a whole range of conditions including a lost filling, caries, infection, sinusitis, a fractured tooth, burning mouth syndrome, oral lichen planus, recurrent aphthous stomatitis, and temporomandibular joint disorders. Furthermore, receiving dental treatment has the potential to result in discomfort or pain. Many patients report that they *expect* to feel pain during their visit, and up to 77 per cent report that they do feel pain, even though dentists generally report their patients have a pain-free experience (see Kent & Croucher 1998). Whilst pain can be a motivating factor to visit the dentist in order to obtain pain relief, the anticipation of pain experienced during a dental visit can lead an individual to avoid or delay attending (as seen in the case study in box 11.1, Mrs Kilpatrick cancelled her two previous appointments because she thought she needed dental treatment that would involve a painful local anaesthetic injection). Learning about the mechanisms of pain and how it is measured is important in order for a dental practitioner to understand how to alleviate pain and to reduce the likelihood of it occurring.

Reflection Point

How would you define dental pain? Why might this be different from someone else's definition?

Mechanisms of pain

There have been a number of conceptualizations of the mechanisms of pain. These include single factor theories that select a particular cause of pain (e.g. biology) and multidimensional models that propose a number of factors that contribute to the experience of pain (e.g. gate control theory) (Turk & Burwinkle 2007).

Biomedical models of the mechanisms of pain claim that the underlying cause and mechanism of pain is damaged tissue (see figure 11.1). The model suggests there is a linear relationship between the size of the injury and the extent of pain: the greater the tissue damage, the more pain. However, this biomedical approach to understanding pain does not account for a number of issues associated with pain. For instance, sometimes people have a large amount of tissue damage yet feel relatively little pain. Jensen et al. (1994) reported that up to 35 per cent of people with observable pathology have no symptoms of pain. In contrast, sometimes people have a minimal amount of tissue damage (or in fact no detectable tissue damage) yet experience intense pain. The shortcomings of the biomedical model of pain are also demonstrated by the placebo effect. For instance, if a person is given medication that

11

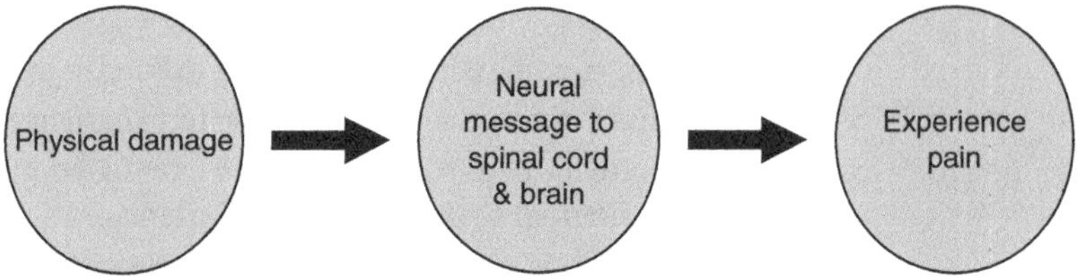

Figure 11.1

Biomedical model of pain

is actually inert but that they believe is a painkiller, they may find that the medication reduces their pain. This placebo effect has been demonstrated extensively (Kirsh 2007), yet the biomedical model of pain cannot account for this phenomenon.

The shortcomings of the biomedical model of pain has led to the development of other, more complex (but more realistic), ways of understanding pain. One seminal model is the Gate Control Theory of pain, which was proposed by Melzack and Wall (1965). They suggested that the experience of pain is the result of a combination of three components: (1) a physical aspect – the 'sensory-discriminative component'; (2) an emotional aspect – the 'affective-motivational component'; and (3) a cognitive or belief-based aspect – the 'cognitive-evaluative component'. The theory goes that these components interact to determine how much pain a person feels and how they react to it. The main implication of Gate Control Theory is that pain is not either solely physical or psychological, but instead is a combination of three interdependent factors:

1 *Sensory-discriminative component*: This component gives information about the location, type and intensity of the pain stimuli, i.e. the sensory qualities. In addition to the information from sensory nociceptors, there are also descending pathways from the brain centre that influence our perception and experience of pain.
2 *Affective-motivational component*: This component is connected to the emotional responses to pain (e.g. anxiety, fear, distress) and the urge to respond via escape or eradicating the stimulus (Godfrey 2005).
3 *Cognitive-evaluative component*: This component is the interpretation or meaning of the sensory experience to the individual. In a way it is the conscious appreciation of the pain. The meaning of the experience will be influenced by the situational context and the memories of past experiences, the presence of psychological co-morbidities (e.g. depression) and the individual's expectations.

Melzack and Wall (1965) provided an account of *how* these components interact via the peripheral and central nervous system. They proposed that the dorsal horn on the spinal cord acts as a 'gate' to the

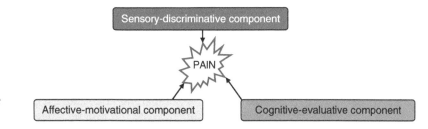

Figure 11.2 The components of pain as identified by Gate Control Theory

peripheral fibres and brain. When the gate is open, the nerve fibres can send 'pain messages' and thus pain is experienced. When the gate is closed, these pain messages are blocked. The gate can be opened and closed (i.e. the cells are excited or inhibited) by small fibres from the location of injury. The gate can also be opened and closed by the brain stem. As the brain stem is affected by cortical activity, it means that cortical activity can indirectly open and close the gate. The sensory-discriminative component, the affective-motivational component and the cognitive-evaluative component interact to form an experience of pain (see figure 11.2).

Measuring pain

As pain is a subjective experience, measurement tools are needed to assess this experience in order to find out whether individuals are in pain, the extent of this pain, and whether interventions intended to alleviate pain have been successful. There are two main categories of pain measurement: behavioural and self-report. These are each discussed in turn.

Behavioural measures of pain

Behavioural measures of pain include monitoring facial expressions (e.g. grimacing) and measuring handgrip pressure. These measures can be used during dental procedures (see Humphris et al. 1991). Other behavioural measures of pain include requests for pain relief, or recording the amount of analgesic administered. However, these behavioural measures of pain are likely to be influenced by factors other than pain and as such may not be wholly reliable or valid (Kent & Croucher 1998).

11

Discussion Point

Aside from the level of pain, what else may influence these behavioural measures? Consider:

• What may affect facial expressions?
• Why might two people experiencing the same amount of pain administer differing handgrip pressure or request different amounts of analgesic?

Self-report measures of pain

As pain is a personal experience, it may be more valid to use a self-report measure of pain in combination with a behavioural measure. Patients can be asked to report their levels and types of pain in a number of ways. A popular method is the use of a visual analogue scale. This is simply a line (usually 100 mm in length) with labels at each end such as 'no pain at all' and 'the worst imaginable pain'. The patient is asked to report how much pain they are experiencing by making a mark corresponding to the level of pain they feel. Visual analogue scales are a useful measure of pain as they are simple and quick to implement in the clinical environment.

Visual analogue scales only give an overall rating of the level of pain, they do not assess the multidimensional aspects of pain (Newton & Buck 2000). To assess the different components of pain, the McGill Pain Questionnaire (Melzack 1975) can be used. This questionnaire asks respondents to indicate which of 78 adjectives describes their pain. The adjectives represent the three components of pain. For instance, the sensory component is represented by words such as 'throbbing', 'shooting', 'gnawing' and 'aching'. The affective component is represented by words such as 'exhausting', 'punishing' and 'frightful' and the cognitive component is represented by words such as 'annoying' and 'unbearable'. Another way to assess pain via self-report is to ask patients to complete a diary for a set period of time. Pain diaries allow a more detailed assessment of the pain experience and to assess the pattern of pain over time (Humphris & Ling 2000). Although these offer a more comprehensive measure of pain, they may not be as practical as a visual analogue scale due to the length of the questionnaire and the demands of keeping a diary. They may therefore be more suited to research than clinical use.

Non-pharmacological interventions to reduce pain

There are a number of chair-side non-pharmacological techniques that can be used to reduce the pain and discomfort associated with dental treatment. These include reducing anxiety (e.g. by using relaxation techniques), distraction from the painful stimulus, increasing perceptions of control, and attention to language used in the dental setting. Each of these non-pharmacological techniques are discussed below. The non-pharmacological techniques are often used in combination with each other and with pharmacological methods (e.g. local anaesthetic) in order to achieve maximum comfort.

Reducing anxiety

Just as pain (or the expectation of pain) is one of the contributing factors to the development of anxiety, anxiety is a contributing factor to pain. This may result from anxiety increasing sensitivity to pain, exacerbating physiological reactions, or by increasing expectations of pain.

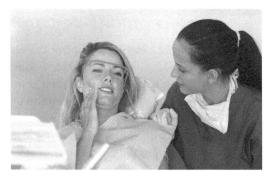

Image 11.1 There are a number of non-pharmacological techniques that can be used to reduce the anxiety and discomfort associated with dental treatment
Copyright: wavebreakmedia

If anxiety is a contributing factor to pain, a reduction in anxiety should lead to a reduction in pain (Kent & Croucher 1998). Relaxation techniques such as controlled breathing, progressive muscle relaxation or even hypnosis (self- or dentist-led) can be used to reduce anxiety and pain. In terms of Gate Control Theory, the anxiety reduction techniques operate on the effective-motivational and sensory-discriminative components of pain. Further details of techniques to reduce anxiety are discussed later in this chapter.

Distraction

By using distraction, a person focuses their attention on the environment rather than their body, and in turn they are more likely to process the environmental details rather than incoming bodily (pain) information. Distraction in the dental setting may be achieved by having interesting wall displays, playing music or video in the clinic, asking patients to perform puzzles, or imagine a desired, relaxing scene (e.g. guided imagery of a beach holiday). Conversely, if a patient focuses on their body and the potential for pain, they are likely to notice and process bodily information and, in turn, experience pain (see pp. 123–4) Indeed, Mullen and Suls (1982) conducted meta-analysis of distraction and attention techniques and found that distraction from acute (short-lived) painful stimuli results in better adaptation (i.e. greater ability to stand the pain) than strategies of attention to painful stimuli.

However, distraction only seems to be appropriate for acute pain. If pain is chronic, then attention to the physical sensation (but not the emotional or cognitive components) may be more effective (Cioffi 1991). This ties in with Gate Control Theory: if fewer components of pain are activated, less pain will be experienced. Focusing on just the sensory experience (i.e. the sensory-discriminative component) without the negative emotional qualities of pain (i.e. the affective-motivational component) or the negative meaning (i.e. the cognitive-evaluative component), the pain experience will be reduced and thus make it more manageable.

11

Increasing perceptions of control

Having a feeling of control can affect the experience of pain (Thrash et al. 1982; Croog et al. 1994; Feldner & Hekmat 2001). Stop signals (e.g. asking patients to raise their arm when they wish the dentist to stop) can give patients the perception of control. For instance, Wardle (1982) found that only 15 per cent of those patients who were told to use stop signals during dental treatment reported some pain compared to 50 per cent of patients who were not invited to use stop signals. There are individual differences that moderate this effect, however. Increasing perception of control is found to be more effective for those who feel they have a sense of control in general and for those who would like to be in control during dental treatment (McNeil et al. 2006). It is likely that the effect of increasing perceptions of control on pain is the result of reduced anxiety, but it may also be due to increased pain tolerance.

Language

It has been suggested that the language used in the dental setting may have negative meaning or emotional connotations, which in turn lead to heightened anxiety and pain. For example, the words 'drill', 'pain', 'hurt', 'inject' may alarm people or imply the experience will be unpleasant. Similarly, even using phrases such as 'this might hurt a little' or 'you may feel some pain' may create an expectation that pain will occur. Thus using terms that are less likely to activate the cognitive-evaluative or affective-motivational components of pain (e.g. 'discomfort' rather than 'pain') may result in less pain.

> **In summary**, dental pain is a difficult concept to define. Multidimensional models of pain such as Gate Control Theory (which considers the emotional, sensory and cognitive components of pain) are more useful ways of understanding pain than single factor theories such as the Biomedical model of pain. Pain can be assessed via behavioural measures and self-report measures. Non-pharmacological techniques that can be used to reduce the experience of pain include reducing anxiety, using distraction, increasing perceptions of control, and paying attention to language in the dental setting.

Dental anxiety

What is dental anxiety?

Anxiety is the term used to describe feelings of apprehension, dread and uneasiness. Kagan and Havemann (1976) described anxiety as a 'vague, unpleasant feeling accompanied by a premonition that something undesirable is about to happen'. Anxiety may be general across situations or it can be specific, focused on a particular event or object. This is the case with dental anxiety – anxiety that is specific to aspects of dentistry. A related term, 'fear', is a reaction to a specific event or object. For instance, a person may be anxious about looking under the sofa in case they see a spider, and experience fear when they actually see a spider. With regard to dentistry, a person may be anxious about visiting the dentist and fearful when they hear a dental drill. The term 'phobia' is reserved for an anxiety disorder, comprising a marked and specific fear that is excessive or unreasonable. For those people who have a phobia, the anxiety-provoking situation is avoided and this avoidance interferes with the person's daily life for at least six months (American Psychiatric Association 2000). Thus, dental phobia is an extreme form of dental anxiety. Anxiety has three components (see figure 11.3): physiological (how the body changes), behavioural (what we do) and cognitive (what and how we think).

1 *Physiological elements* of anxiety are changes in the body such as an increased heart rate, sweating, raised blood pressure, nausea, muscle tension, palpitations and breathlessness. Thus there may be signals that your patient is anxious before you have started to talk to them.
2 *Behavioural elements* of anxiety include avoidance of the anxiety-provoking situation or escape from the situation. Thus, patients who are anxious may avoid visiting the dentist or cancel

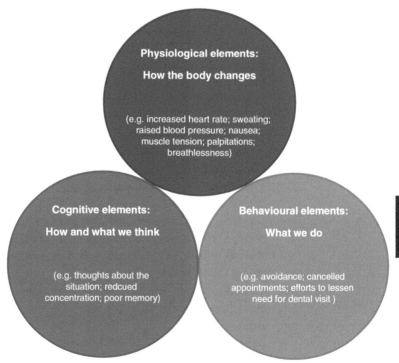

Figure 11.3 The three elements of dental anxiety

appointments at the last minute. Behavioural elements of dental anxiety may also include attempts at meticulous oral hygiene in order to maintain oral health and therefore lessen the need for visiting a dentist.

3 *Cognitive elements* of anxiety include both the thoughts about the situation (e.g. 'the scale and polish will be unbearably painful') and also the impact of anxiety on our thinking processes. For instance, anxiety can reduce a person's ability to concentrate or to remember. This has implications for the dental practice as an anxious patient may find it difficult to concentrate on discussions regarding their oral health, care plans or oral hygiene advice, and may not be able to recall the content of these discussions after the appointment. It is therefore important to consider a patient's mind-set and comfort before holding these discussions. For instance, a patient may prefer to sit in a normal chair rather than the dental chair to talk about their care plan.

Reflection Point

Reconsider the case study in box 11.1. Try to identify the physiological, cognitive and behavioural elements of Mrs Kilpatrick's dental anxiety.

It is highly likely that you have already met a patient who is dentally anxious. This is because dental anxiety is common. Data from the 2009 Adult Dental Health Survey (an interview survey of over 11,000 adults living in England, Wales and Northern Ireland) found that 36 per cent of adults reported moderate levels of dental anxiety, and 12 per cent reported extreme dental anxiety (Nuttall et al. 2011). The same survey found that women are more likely to report high levels of dental anxiety than men (17% vs. 8%). Further, a greater proportion of adults from lower socio-economic groups report high levels of dental anxiety compared to those from higher socio-economic groups.

In a survey of 1959 Dutch adults, Oosterink et al. (2009) found that fear of dental treatment was more prevalent (24%) than fear of blood (9%), injections (16%), darkness (8%), thunder (10%), flying (12%), spiders (23%) and enclosed spaces (17%). The fears that were more prevalent than fear of dental treatment were fear of snakes (35%), fear of heights (31%) and fear of physical injury (27%). When looking at the severity of each of these fears, fear of dental treatment was rated more severe than any other fear.

Some people who are dentally anxious are apprehensive about everything to do with dentistry. However, it is more often the case that people are fearful about specific aspects of dentistry. These aspects differ between individuals and, as such, dental anxiety is really a broad term used to describe a range of different anxieties. Box 11.2 highlights a range of stimuli for dental anxiety.

> ## Box 11.2: Different aspects of dentistry that may underlie dental anxiety
>
> **Embarrassment or crying**
> People sometimes believe that their poor oral health is embarrassing and they will have the worst teeth the dentist has ever seen. They may feel ashamed of this and fear the dentist's reaction or their own reaction (such as crying) to hearing about the state of their oral health.
>
> **Loss of control**
> Dentistry involves handing over control to the dentist. People often fear that the dentist will 'take over' and won't stop, even if a procedure is painful.
>
> **Needles, drills and other equipment**
> The sights, sounds and smells of dental equipment, the dental practice or the dentist are common aspects of dentistry that provoke anxiety. For example, the sight of a needle, or the sound of a dental handpiece are often the source of a patient's anxiety.
>
> **Pain**
> A common reason for dental anxiety is the expectation of pain from dental procedures. Related to this is a fear that the anaesthetic will not work and in turn the patient won't get numb and will feel pain during a procedure.
>
> **Gagging, choking, panic attacks and fainting**
> Some patients are fearful that they will gag and/or choke during, or because of, a dental procedure or find that they gag when anxious and find this very upsetting. Relatedly, sometimes patients believe they will suffer a panic attack or faint during a visit to the dentist and are frightened about what may happen in this circumstance.
>
> **Reactions to local anaesthetics**
> Some patients believe they will have an allergic reaction to the local anaesthetic, which will initiate a medical emergency. Alternatively, they may believe the effects of the local anaesthetic will be irreversible and they will permanently loose sensation in that area of the mouth.
>
> **Extensive treatment and cost**
> Patients who are dentally anxious often believe that their oral health is poor and they require a large amount of dental treatment. This can invoke presumptions (and associated fear) that a visit to the dentist will be very expensive.

The consequences of dental anxiety

Although uncomfortable, anxiety can be a useful response that alerts people to possible dangers (e.g. a spider may bite) and in turn trigger self-protective strategies (e.g. run away). However, if anxiety becomes excessive, it can be maladaptive. Dental anxiety can have a number of negative consequences in people's lives. For instance, people who are anxious may postpone visiting the dentist, skip or cancel their appointments, or not visit a dentist at all. Todd and Lader (1991) found that 45 per cent of those surveyed rated fear of the dentist as the most important barrier to dental care. The 2009 Adult Dental Health Survey indicated that adults who reported high levels of dental anxiety were more likely to visit a dentist only when they have trouble with their teeth (22%) than for a regular check-up (8%) (Nuttall et al. 2011). This survey also found that those adults who reported high levels of dental anxiety were less likely to have visited a dentist within the last 12 months (9%) than those who had last visited a dentist more than 10 years ago (24%).

11

Without regular dental care, the oral health of dentally anxious individuals is compromised and can result in gingivitis, tooth loss and persistent dental pain (Berggren & Meynert 1984). Those who are able to attend may have postponed treatment to such an extent that conservative treatment options are no longer viable (Newton et al. 2012). Further, due to the cognitive effects of anxiety, patients who are anxious may not recall or comprehend advice given by the dentist.

Dental anxiety can also have more wide-ranging effects on people's lives. For instance, the anxiety surrounding an imminent dental visit may disturb sleep in the lead up to a dental appointment and affect concentration at work. Dental anxiety can also have social consequences. Cohen et al. (2000) interviewed a group of dentally anxious patients to get an insight into the impact of dental anxiety on their life. They found that relationships and interactions with friends and family can be affected due to embarrassment, shame and misunderstanding. Look back at the case study in box 11.1: Mrs Kilpatrick did not want to admit she was cancelling her dental appointment due to dental anxiety because she felt embarrassed about feeling anxious. She had also had trouble sleeping in the nights before her appointment.

Reasons for dental anxiety

There have been a number of explanations as to why people may feel anxious about dentistry. These range from evolutionary theories, whereby we are biologically predisposed to fear objects or events that may harm or hurt us, to implicit learning theories, whereby people may learn to fear dentistry because of a negative image of dentistry portrayed in the media. However there are two main explanations as to why people become dentally anxious: learning from previous experience and learning via observation. These are now considered in turn.

Learning from previous experience

People may become anxious by learning from previous encounters with the dentist that visiting the dentist is something to be fearful of. If someone experiences an unpleasant, painful or traumatic event at the dentist, this could lead a person to believe similar future events may also be unpleasant, painful or traumatic and they are therefore fearful of them. The theory of learning, whereby people learn to associate events or objects with specific responses, is called 'classical conditioning' (Pavlov 1927). Physiologist Ivan Pavlov studied digestive processes in dogs and noticed that they began to salivate while he was preparing the food rather than whilst they were eating the food. On investigating this further, he found that the dogs could learn the signals that indicated food was about to be dispensed and salivate in response to the signals rather than the food. See box 11.3 for a description of classical conditioning.

Box 11.3: Classical conditioning

For classical conditioning to happen, there must first be an unconditioned stimulus and unconditioned response – an event/object that triggers a natural, automatic reaction (a reaction that does not need any learning or 'conditioning' to occur). In the case of Pavlov's dogs, the unconditioned stimulus was the bone and the unconditioned response was salivating.

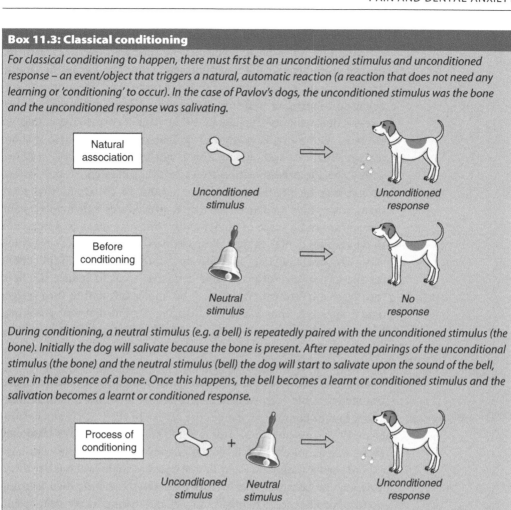

During conditioning, a neutral stimulus (e.g. a bell) is repeatedly paired with the unconditioned stimulus (the bone). Initially the dog will salivate because the bone is present. After repeated pairings of the unconditional stimulus (the bone) and the neutral stimulus (bell) the dog will start to salivate upon the sound of the bell, even in the absence of a bone. Once this happens, the bell becomes a learnt or conditioned stimulus and the salivation becomes a learnt or conditioned response.

When considering reasons for the development of dental anxiety, classical conditioning can be applied to those circumstances in which patients have had a negative experience at the dentist as an explanation of the emergence of dental anxiety. For example, imagine a child experienced a painful dental procedure. A natural response to pain is fear. Here, there is an unconditioned stimulus (pain) and an unconditioned response (fear). Through classical conditioning, the dentist, the dental surgery and the dental equipment (all neutral stimuli) are paired with the event of a painful procedure, and in turn any of these aspects of dentistry or a dentist may become associated with the response of fear. As such, any future encounter with a dentist, the dental surgery or dental equipment (conditioned stimuli) may

11

lead to fear (conditioned response). With Pavlov's dogs, for classical conditioning to occur, repeated pairings were required with the neutral stimulus and the unconditioned stimulus. Yet in the case of dental anxiety, it would appear that one unpleasant event may be sufficient to trigger fear of future dental visits. This may be explained by 'preparedness theory' (Seligman 1971). This theory suggests that we are born with a predisposition or 'preparedness' to be anxious about certain situations and objects. This is not to say that people are born with a specific predisposition to fear visiting the dentist, but instead people may be predisposed to be cautious of situations that leave them susceptible to harm. As dental procedures can involve pain, discomfort and a sense of vulnerability, this may make us susceptible to developing dental anxiety. Preparedness theory offers a suggestion as to why dental anxiety is relatively common. This has implications for the importance of preventive dentistry, so as to reduce the need for invasive treatment (which may be unpleasant and in turn trigger dental anxiety). Thus water fluoridation, a good diet and good oral hygiene are key to minimizing the likelihood of a patient becoming anxious in the first place.

The classical conditional theory of learning is supported by the finding that many people who are dentally anxious have experienced traumatic events (e.g. considerable pain, invasive treatment, humiliation, loss of control) at the dentist earlier in their life (Lautch 1971; Shaw 1975; Vassend 1993). This is not to say, however, that a traumatic event will definitely lead to dental anxiety – many people who have experienced a traumatic event do not become anxious about dentistry. This may be because other factors moderate how and when learning occurs. For instance, a dentist's rapport and manner is very important: pain inflicted by a dentist who is perceived as caring is much less likely to result in dental anxiety (Bernstein et al. 1979; Milgrom et al. 1992).

Dental anxiety may also develop from learning from experiences in other (non-dental) settings. For example, as in the case study, Mrs Kilpatrick is anxious about needles following a painful vaccination and is now also anxious about receiving dental injections. Likewise, someone who is scared of medical equipment may also be scared of dental tools. This process, by which a fear of one object or situation transfers to another, is called *generalization*, and indicates that people may become fearful of dental procedures without having had a painful dental procedure in the past.

It has been proposed that another form of learning, 'operant conditioning' (Thorndike 1901; Skinner 1938), may help to maintain fear and avoidance of dentistry (Mowrer 1939). Operant conditioning is the term used to describe how behaviour is shaped and maintained by its consequences. For example, positive reinforcement involves provision of favourable events (rewards) to increase the likelihood of the behaviour happening again, whereas negative reinforcement involves removal of an unfavourable event to increase the likelihood of the behaviour. As seen with Mrs Kilpatrick in the case study in box 11.1, a person may become increasingly anxious as their appointment becomes closer. They may become so anxious that they cancel their appointment. This would lead to an immediate feeling of relief. Here, avoidance of the dental appointment resulted in the person's anxiety levels reducing. From an operant conditioning perspective, this relief (i.e. the removal of the anxiety) negatively reinforces subsequent avoidance of dentistry. The patient has learnt that cancelling an appointment and avoidance of dentistry feels better than keeping an appointment and, as such, the next time the person will be more likely to cancel their appointment again.

Most of the research into the impact of traumatic dental experiences and development of dental anxiety has been retrospective, asking people about what has happened to them in the past. This is problematic as retrospective research relies on participants' accurate recall of events. The recalled traumatic event may just be an artefact of the anxiety itself: those people who are dentally anxious may just be more likely to *remember* negative aspects of dental visits than those people who are not anxious. Or, those people who are already anxious may be more likely to interpret events more negatively than those who are not anxious.

A further criticism of learning theory comes from research that suggests that cognitions (thoughts) surrounding uncontrollability, unpredictability, dangerousness and disgust create a feeling of vulnerability that in turn leads to dental anxiety (Armfield et al. 2008). De Jongh and colleagues have reported that negative thinking patterns and catastrophic thoughts play a crucial role in dental fear, with frequency of negative cognitions and perceived degree of control accounting for 75 per cent of the variance in dental trait anxiety scores (de Jongh & Ter Horst 1993; de Jongh et al. 1994). Learning theories do not incorporate the role of cognitions (thoughts) and, as such, do not offer a complete explanation for the emergence of dental anxiety.

Vicarious learning: learning from others

Some people who are anxious cannot remember a traumatic event. If indeed they have not experienced a traumatic event (rather than merely failing to recall one), why are they anxious about visiting a dentist? An alternative explanation to learning from experience is learning from others. Learning from others has been termed 'vicarious learning' (Bandura 1977). A person may become fearful of dentists because their parents, siblings, friends or the media teach them (intentionally or unintentionally) that dentistry is something to be feared. Indeed, Johnson and Baldwin (1968) found that mothers whose dental anxiety was high were more likely to have children who demonstrated negative behaviour in the dental chair (as observed by the researchers) compared to mothers who were not anxious. Similarly, Shaw (1975) found that children who were anxious about visiting their dentist were more likely to have anxious mothers compared to children who were low in dental anxiety. Unfortunately, parents' attempts to reassure their children may inadvertently teach their children that a trip to the dentist may be something to worry about. For example, a parent who suggests to their child that 'it's going to be OK and won't hurt' may create expectations that the dental visit may be painful – something they had not considered before the 'reassuring' statement was issued.

Who is anxious? Measuring dental anxiety

All patients may have some level of anxiety about their treatment; after all, receiving dental work is rarely an enjoyable experience. In turn, dental anxiety should not be viewed as something which is present or absent – with patients either anxious or not. Instead, it would be better viewed as a continuum. Thus patients may be relaxed about dental treatment, nervous about visiting the dentist but fully able to cope, or so anxious that they are suffering dental phobia and avoid visiting a dentist at all costs. Newton et al. (2012) suggested that it is essential that the dental team are aware of the patient's level of anxiety in order to tailor any intervention to the patient's degree of anxiety. In order to permit this to happen, valid and reliable ways of measuring dental anxiety are required. Some examples of measures of dental anxiety are discussed below.

General measures of dental anxiety ask people to rate how anxious they are about going to the dentist or various aspects of the dental visit (e.g. sitting in a dental chair or having a dental injection). For example, the Modified Dental Anxiety Scale (MDAS) (see figure 11.4; Humphris et al. 1995) asks respondents to indicate their level of anxiety (ranging from 'not anxious' to 'extremely anxious') for five separate procedures. Scores range from 5 to 25, with scores over 19 indicating dental phobia. There is also a version of the MDAS for use with children (Wong et al. 1998). The MDAS is suitable for use in the clinical setting as it is quick to complete, has extensive evidence of reliability and validity and is acceptable to dental staff and patients (Humphris et al. 2006). Recent research into the use of the MDAS has indicated that if patients complete the MDAS prior to their appointment and share (and discuss) their scores with the dentist, their dental anxiety is reduced on completion of the appointment (Hull & Humphris 2010).

There are also more comprehensive measures of dental anxiety that address the physiological, behavioural or cognitive components of dental anxiety. However, the three components are not always correlated. For example, a person may feel very anxious and have an increased heart rate (physiological component) but will be totally compliant and cooperative in the dental chair (behavioural

Please tell us how anxious you get, if at all, with your dental visit. Each item is about different aspects of visiting a dentist. The scale ranges from 'Not anxious' (1) to 'Extremely anxious' (5). For each item we would like you to circle the number that represents how anxious you get. The more anxious you feel, then the higher the number you circle.	Not anxious	Slightly anxious	Fairly anxious	Very anxious	Extremely anxious
1 . If you went to your dentist for **treatment tomorrow**, how would you feel?	1	2	3	4	5
2 . If you were sitting in the **waiting room** (waiting for treatment), how would you feel?	1	2	3	4	5
3 . If you were about to have a **tooth drilled**, how would you feel?	1	2	3	4	5
4 . If you were about to have your **teeth scaled and polished**, how would you feel?	1	2	3	4	5
5 . If you were about to have a **local anaesthetic injection** in your gum, above an upper back tooth, how would you feel?	1	2	3	4	5

Figure 11.4 The Modified Dental Anxiety Scale

Source: 'The Modified Dental Anxiety Scale: validation and United Kingdom norms', in Community Dental Health (Humphris et al. 1995)

component). Therefore it may be misleading to rely on measuring one component (Kent & Croucher 1998). Some measures of dental anxiety do include all three components. An example is the Index of Dental Anxiety & Fear (Armfield 2010). This is a 23-item self-report questionnaire. To address the physiological component of dental anxiety, questionnaire items include 'My heart beats faster when I go to the dentist' (Disagree – strongly agree). Questions such as 'I think that something really bad would happen to me if I were to visit a dentist' (Disagree – strongly agree) address the cognitive component of dental anxiety. Behavioural aspects of dental anxiety are monitored with questions such as 'I delay making appointments to go to the dentist' (Disagree – strongly agree).

Interventions to reduce dental anxiety

11

Once a patient's level of dental anxiety is known, an intervention can be delivered that is proportionate to that level of anxiety. Newton et al. (2012) have suggested three categories of dental anxiety (low, moderate and high) and corresponding interventions (see figure 11.5), although it could be argued that the 'low level interventions' should be a part of routine practice with all dental patients.

The outline of approaches suggested by Newton et al. takes into account the urgency of the need for treatment. This is important,

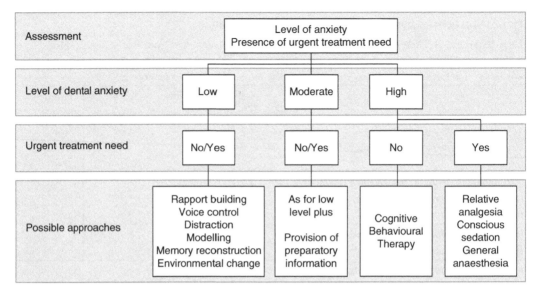

Assessment	Level of anxiety Presence of urgent treatment need			
Level of dental anxiety	Low	Moderate	High	
Urgent treatment need	No/Yes	No/Yes	No	Yes
Possible approaches	Rapport building Voice control Distraction Modelling Memory reconstruction Environmental change	As for low level plus Provision of preparatory information	Cognitive Behavioural Therapy	Relative analgesia Conscious sedation General anaesthesia

Figure 11.5 Matching approach to anxiety management with patient's needs

Source: Newton et al. (2012)

because if a highly anxious patient is in pain, relieving the patient of their discomfort is the priority rather than reducing anxiety in the long term. Pharmacological interventions (such as conscious sedation or general anaesthesia) are more suitable in such circumstances. The management strategies suggested by Newton et al. (2012) are outlined below.

Rapport building

As emphasized in the chapter on communication in the dental surgery (see pp. 218–35), forming a trusting relationship with patients is vital. Building a relationship with patients and developing rapport can help put a patient at ease. Silverman et al. (2004) suggest that rapport can be developed by accepting the legitimacy of patient's views and feelings; being careful not to be judgemental; expressing empathy and support to communicate understanding and appreciation of the patient's feelings or predicament; showing a willingness to help; and by dealing sensitively with embarrassing and disturbing topics and physical pain. Peretz and Gluck (2005) demonstrated how performing a magic trick helped to put children at ease and increased cooperation.

Voice control

The tone and volume of verbal communication can affect a patient's anxiety levels. Greenbaum et al. (1990) reported that an interaction with a dentist with a loud voice with a deep tone was rated as most pleasurable and was most effective in minimizing disruptive behaviour in children (compared to an interaction with a dentist with normal voice level).

Distraction

As noted earlier in this chapter, distraction can be used to reduce perceptions of pain. Distraction can also be used to reduce anxiety. Lahmann et al. (2008) conducted a randomized controlled trial to compare a brief relaxation technique, distraction (listening to music) and a control group (no intervention). They found that relaxation and distraction reduced anxiety compared to the control group. Distraction appeared to be most effective for those adults who were moderately anxious.

Modelling

Modelling is the term used to describe the form of learning whereby an individual learns how to perform or act via observing another individual. Just in the way that dental anxiety can be learnt via observation, dental anxiety can be reduced via observing a non-anxious patient. The 'model' should be similar in age, gender and level of anxiety to those who are learning for modelling to be most effective (Wardle 1982; Newton et al. 2012).

Memory reconstruction

When patients are anxious, they often only recall unpleasant or negative aspects of the dental visit. Memory reconstruction involves helping patients recall positive aspects of a dental visit that otherwise may be dismissed. Pickrell et al. (2007) asked children to smile whilst in the dental chair and took a photo to provide a record of this. The photo was sent to children prior to their next appointment to remind them of their previous visit. Along with additional tasks (e.g. children were asked to recall an example of how their behaviour had improved), the children were found to be subsequently less anxious at the second appointment.

Environmental change

The layout, smell and visual appearance of the dental practice can reduce patient's anxiety levels. For instance, exposure to positive images of the dental surgery (Fox & Newton 2006) and the smell of lavender (Kritsidima et al. 2010) have been shown to decrease anxiety prior to treatment.

11

Enhancing the sense of control

Dental anxiety can be reduced by increasing perceptions of control and reducing unpredictability. Ways to increase control are to offer choices (e.g. music selection, flavour of topical anaesthetic) and to encourage patients to use stop signals whereby the patient can signal the dentist (e.g. by raising their arm or pressing a button) to stop what the dentist is doing. Just learning that stop signals are available is enough to reduce anxiety (Corah 1973; Jackson & Lindsay 1995).

Provision of preparatory information

For those with moderate levels of anxiety, a further way of increasing a sense of predictability is the provision of preparatory information. Preparatory information can include *sensory information*, which provides warning as to the sensations the patient is likely to feel. *Procedural information* details the sequence of events that will (or may) occur, including what the dentist and dental nurse will be doing and why. *Behavioural information* includes the behaviours that the patient should engage in during (e.g. breathe steadily and focus on background music during administration of local anaesthetic) and after a procedure (e.g. rinse to clean mouth; avoid hot drinks until sensation is regained) to improve outcome or recovery (Vogele 2007).

Cognitive Behaviour Therapy

For patients with high levels of anxiety (who do not require urgent dental treatment), Cognitive Behaviour Therapy (CBT) may be a suitable option. CBT is the combination of cognitive therapies (talking therapy focusing on maladaptive thoughts and beliefs) and behavioural therapies (techniques that directly address, test and modify behaviours associated with anxiety). The aim of cognitive therapies is to challenge and alter maladaptive thoughts and to facilitate a new understanding that the feared stimuli are unlikely to be dangerous. For example, cognitive restructuring may aim to help a person lower their belief that 'I *will* choke on dental equipment during treatment' but instead believe 'I am *unlikely* to choke during treatment, especially if the dentist uses a rubber dam'. Cognitive therapy techniques include directly challenging beliefs, examining the evidence for and against the beliefs, and considering the costs of holding on to maladaptive beliefs.

A typical behavioural therapy is systematic desensitization. This is the process whereby patients are taught relaxation techniques and are then gradually exposed to the feared object or situation in a hierarchy of steps. The patient starts with the least fearful step of the hierarchy and only progresses to the next step when they are comfortable with the previous step. For instance, a person who is afraid of dental injections may start by looking at a photo of a dental needle, then move on to look at an actual needle and then watch a video of the steps of a dental injection. Once the patient can manage this, they may try tasting topical anaesthetic, have topic anaesthetic applied, and then have a capped needle held in the mouth for a short time. Following this they may repeat the final step, but with an uncapped needle, before they are able to receive an injection. By gradual, systematic and repeated exposure to the feared object, the patient becomes desensitized to it and thus is no longer afraid.

CBT is relatively brief (6–10 sessions) and has proven effectiveness for a range of psychological disorders, including dental anxiety (Mansell & Morris 2003; National Institute for Clinical Excellence 2004). CBT is usually carried out by a psychologist, although dental professionals can train in CBT techniques via specialist training (for further information, see Newton et al. 2012).

Discussion Points

- Why may techniques that reduce dental anxiety also reduce pain?
- Reconsider the case study in box 11.1. How could a dentist help to reduce Mrs Kilpatrick's dental anxiety?

In summary, dental anxiety is fairly common and may result in avoidance of dental visits and poorer oral health as well as having negative personal and social consequences. Possible causes of dental anxiety include learning from previous experience and learning via observation. Some measures of dental anxiety are general, while others measure specific components of dental anxiety (e.g. physiological, behavioural or cognitive elements). Techniques such as building rapport, distraction, modelling, memory reconstruction, environmental change, enhancing the sense of control, provision of preparatory information and Cognitive Behaviour Therapy can be used to reduce dental anxiety.

Conclusion

Dentists should be acutely aware of the importance of minimizing pain. Patients may enter the practice in pain and patients may expect the dental visit to be painful, perhaps to such an extent that they are fearful of visiting the dentist. Dental fear and anxiety can be the result of a painful or unpleasant procedure in the past (experienced by the patient themselves, or by others from whom they have learnt vicariously). Dental fear and anxiety may also be a contributor to the experience of pain, due to heightened expectations of pain or by exacerbating physiological responses.

Thus the dental practitioner must be competent in maximizing a patient's comfort and reducing anxiety before, during and after a dental procedure. There are many evidence-based non-pharmacological techniques that a dentist can use alongside pharmacological interventions. The type of intervention should be appropriate to the level of anxiety (or pain) and, to enable this, the dentist should use reliable and valid measurement tools in order to assess patient needs and to evaluate the success of their interventions.

11

Communication in the Dental Surgery

Koula Asimakopoulou and Tim Newton

IN THIS CHAPTER YOU WILL LEARN ABOUT:

▶ The purpose of communication in general
▶ Models of communicating information in healthcare settings
▶ The idea of patient-centred care
▶ Types of verbal and non-verbal communication
▶ Ways to break bad news

Introduction

This chapter describes some basic features and models of communication and care in healthcare settings. It discusses the idea of patient-centred communication and the implications this may have for the consultation. Commonly held assumptions about how much patients actually remember of what goes on in a consultation are discussed. The chapter finishes with a look at some practical issues surrounding verbal and non-verbal communication and makes suggestions on one particular aspect of communication: the giving of bad news.

What is communication?

Communication is a process that usually involves a sender of a message and a recipient through one or more channels. There could be several senders (e.g. several people taking the stage during a theatre performance) or one (e.g. a dentist giving advice). The message could be sent to several recipients at a time (e.g. a theatre audience) or one (e.g. a patient sitting in your dental chair). Senders and recipients could all be present at the same time as in any of the examples described above, or the communication could be taking place asynchronously, e.g. through email. Whatever the number of senders and recipients, or indeed the mode of communication, the aim of the process is to share information.

The *way* that information is shared is important. Often, communication is less about *what* is said and more about the *way* it is said. Gestures, posture, pitch, eye contact or lack of it, proximity, facial expression and the like often add helpful cues about the content of communication. The recipient's reaction to the communication may be telling; laughter after a joke tells the person telling the joke that the person hearing it enjoyed it. Polite laughter after a joke reveals that they possibly liked it but also that they are keen to make an apparently socially acceptable response. Lack of laughter where laughter was expected is also helpful in conveying a message. So communication is about transferring information between senders and recipients, using one or several channels, settings, verbal or non-verbal cues.

Box 12.1: Case Study

Mr Fox is a professional in his thirties who has had difficulties attending the dentist for the past 10 years as he suffers from dental anxiety. He's been able to have basic check-ups but hasn't seen a hygienist in years.

The last time Mr Fox had an appointment for a scale and polish, the whole event was rather negative. Mr Fox was told by his dentist he had to have an appointment with the hygienist but he was unsure what the appointment entailed. Upon entering the surgery, the hygienist introduced herself. Mr Fox was instructed to sit in the dentist's chair while the hygienist filled in some medical forms. Mr Fox got very flustered while he was waiting and kept wondering how painful the treatment was going to be. In the end, and before the hygienist could examine him, Mr Fox stood up, made an excuse about needing to be elsewhere, and left in a hurry.

He has now come back to the practice to see a different hygienist. The hygienist explains what her role is and what is likely to take place during the appointment. She explains about the need to take some baseline scores of his oral hygiene so that they can then monitor his improvement patterns in subsequent visits. She then shows Mr Fox the various instruments she proposes using and explains their function. Mr Fox is not too sure he likes the sound of the sonic scaler but feels too embarrassed to admit it.

Before the treatment commences, the hygienist tells Mr Fox that she will be using a numbing gel. Even though the numbing gel is applied, as soon as the hygienist uses the scaler, Mr Fox gestures for the procedure to be stopped. He claims that he can still feel pain. The hygienist points out that she has checked carefully that the affected areas have been numbed before proceeding; however, Mr Fox insists that the treatment is painful. The hygienist wants to understand better the pain that the patient says he is experiencing. A brief discussion follows which is focused on explaining that the numbing gel won't stop Mr Fox from experiencing pressure and vibration on his teeth and gums, but that pressure and vibration are probably different to pain. Mr Fox is given more examples that show how pressure is different to pain with the acknowledgement that excessive pressure might be perceived as pain. The hygienist asks the patient whether he feels they can try scaling again and promises to stop should the pressure turn to pain. He agrees.

The appointment ends with Mr Fox receiving a full scale and polish. The hygienist explains that Mr Fox needs to maintain oral hygiene by regular brushing and flossing and suggests that she sees him again in three months' time.

12

Here, you are unlikely to have ticked 1 or 2; instead, most people would agree that taking a patient who has previously failed to have treatment through a full scale and polish is probably a fairly good outcome of a consultation with a hygienist. As you read through the chapter, consider the various issues that arise and think again about your rating.

In healthcare settings, communication has been proposed to have three functions (Ong et al. 1995). The first is about creating a good inter-personal relationship. That is, for patients to feel they can trust and believe the content of the information a healthcare professional gives them, it is important that they can feel they can trust and have faith in the sender of the message. The second aspect of any communication episode, and the part where a lot of the time is often spent during a consultation, is that of exchanging information. Symptom reporting, pain intensity and duration, the patient's thoughts and feelings about the illness, and the dentist's ideas and explanation about the condition and prognosis all feature in this second aspect of the communication exchange, according to Ong et al. Finally, a third aspect of the communication episode in a healthcare setting is a discussion of possible treatment options, ways of managing the illness, treatment recommendations and so on.

These general principles are said to apply to communication taking place in any healthcare setting. The dental surgery, however, tends to differ from most other healthcare settings (Newton & Brenneman 1999). Here, the emphasis is on treatment, rather than on conversing about treatment, where the dentist is expected to perform the required treatment on the patient, often under time constraints. In addition, whilst treatment is taking place in the oral cavity, the patient, by definition, is excluded from any meaningful verbal communication. This is starkly at odds with a consultation with, for example, a medical General Practitioner, where more often than not, a patient may be able to engage in verbal communication even if treatment is being performed. Finally, whilst visits to any healthcare professional may well cause some anxiety in patients, dental visits are often associated with a lot of anticipatory anxiety, which in itself may influence the quality and quantity of communication taking place in the dental surgery.

The rest of this chapter considers work that has primarily taken place in general healthcare settings. When discussing such work, it is important to consider whether the findings are readily transferable to the dental surgery or whether they would need to be modified for such a setting.

In summary, communication consists of an interaction between a sender and a recipient of a message. In healthcare settings there is normally a very concrete reason for communication, usually revolving round the receipt of care. Medical and dental consultations have similarities but also substantial differences between them that will limit how well medical settings research translates into dental settings.

Models of communication in healthcare settings

Who is responsible for leading the communication in the dental setting? Do patients have expectations about what takes place in the dental surgery and where does their position lie in terms of how much or little they should speak, how and whether to voice their concerns, and who is responsible for deciding on what treatment to administer and how? Do these expectations differ from person to person? What is their impact on the outcome of the communication and the consultation? What happens when patient expectations clash with those of a dentist?

It is proposed that the answers to these questions will shape a consultation and also what gets communicated, by whom and at what point. For example, where a patient has learnt from experience that their role is to sit on the chair, answer a few questions, do as the dentist says and then leave, they will communicate different things to their dentist than people who see the dentist as an equal partner, someone who is there to share in their expertise on how the patient should look after their oral health. So, the patient's perception of their expected role at the dental surgery will influence what they tell the dentist and what they keep to themselves.

An example that demonstrates this situation clearly is seen in some work by Edwards et al. (2013). Their study sought to understand better why people with HIV or diabetes might not tell their dentist about this pre-existing condition. Patients attending sexual health or diabetes clinics were interviewed in depth about, amongst other things, disclosure of their condition to their dentist. Whilst several factors such as the patient's understanding of their diagnosis and their age were important, in particular, their experience of stigma, past reactions to their disclosing such information, general experience of healthcare and the extent to which they saw dentists as people they could trust were seen to be substantial determinants of disclosure behaviour.

It would seem that where patients anticipate that the dentist is someone in a position of power and authority and is likely to 'judge' them, their communication differs from a situation where they view themselves as consumers of healthcare advice and treatment (because, for example, they are buying a dental service from privately practising individuals).

12

Roter and Hall (1992) have written extensively on this issue. Their work is best summed up by their framework outlining four possible ways to understand the relationship between healthcare professionals and patients, and hence the communication between the two. In particular, they proposed four types of consultation model, each described below.

1 *The 'traditional' medical model.* This model proposes that the dentist knows what is best for the patient. The patient is seen to be a passive recipient of care, whose role is to listen to the expert professional. In this model, patients are expected to do what the dentist tells them and where they fail to do it, it is appropriate to brand them as 'non-compliant'. The dentist's role is that of an expert clinician; they know what is best in terms of dental care, they have the knowledge and skills to deliver it, and, as such, they are in a strong position to be an authority figure within their surgery. In this model, patient responsibility for the communication is really very low, whilst the dentist carries all of that responsibility.

2 *The 'patient as expert' model.* Here, it is proposed that although dentists might be technical experts, what is actually important is the expertise of the person presenting with the health problem. To take an analogy, if a car is taken for a service at a local garage, the garage technician might know how to tune the engine, but it is the overall experience as a driver that is important and should guide the exchange. So, in this model, patients are perceived as experts in their condition. This expertise arises from the fact that it is patients rather than dentists who have lived with the health problem and will have to live with the treatment consequences. They know what symptoms they are experiencing, how severe these are and what impact they have on their daily lives. They also know how well or not they can live with any treatment side-effects and consequences. Because of this expertise that, according to the model, only the patient possesses and can communicate, it is patients rather than dentists who should be responsible for leading the communication in the consultation. In this model, clinician responsibility for communication is low whilst patients are driving the communication.

3 *The consumerist model.* As the name would suggest, in this model the dental surgery and the consultation are seen as a marketplace exchange. Here the dentist provides a range of services which the patient, as the potential consumer of such services, may choose to purchase or not. In this model, dental care is seen as a consumer transaction. As such, it is the patient-purchaser who is primarily responsible for the verbal exchange during such a sale of goods and services, whilst the dentist has a more passive role.

4 *The transformed medical model.* This approach sees both dentists and patients as experts, albeit in different fields. The model acknowledges that dentists are technical experts who have the knowledge and skills to deliver expert healthcare. On the other hand, patients are seen as experts in their own life, their symptoms and the impact of those symptoms on their oral health. It is therefore proposed that patients can inform the consultation by bringing in information which will help the expert technician fit the clinical service they are about to provide to that particular patient, with their particular anxieties, feelings and activities of daily living. In this model, patients and dentists are seen as equals, where expertise and knowledge from both parties need to be combined in order to ensure that the work delivered will meet the psychosocial and clinical needs of the person seeking it. Here, responsibility for the communication episode is shared between the healthcare professional and the patient.

Clearly there is not a 'one size fits all' model which dentists should all ascribe to and adopt for ever more. Things that are beyond a dentist's personal control, such as the length of time they are given to spend with patients (and everyday practical issues such as the length of the queue in their waiting room), the sort of patient they are treating (e.g. a middle-class, middle-aged, professional as opposed to a working-class, of limited education, elderly woman with dementia and dental anxiety), the reason why they are seeing the patient (e.g. an urgent referral because the patient is in excruciating pain as opposed to a routine dental check-up), and the patient's experience of dentists and expectations of what their and the dentist's role might be in the surgery, might all constrain (or in some cases enable) dentists' choice of communication model.

That being said, a paper published in the *British Medical Journal* (Politi et al. 2013) cautioned against assuming that some patients do not feel able or do not wish to be involved in decisions to do with their health. Rather than questioning whether to involve them or not, they suggest that a more appropriate question would be to find out how much patients wish to be involved. This will partly be determined by how well the healthcare professional has prepared the patient for involvement by, amongst other things, making it explicit that the patients' preference for a treatment is valued and valuable.

We suggest clinicians start by acknowledging equipoise, recognizing underlying trade-offs between options, and offering treatment choices. They should discuss evidence-based information without assuming some patients will not want to engage in shared decision making. Once patients are informed, they can decide whether they would like more (or less) responsibility for their health decision. (Politi et al. 2013: 2)

The above extract clearly argues that, to the extent that all communication taking place in the dental surgery is directed at the best possible health outcome for patients, it is proposed that all such communication should be patient-centred. The next section explores what is meant by the concept of patient-centred communication and care.

> **In summary**, according to Roter and Hall, communication in the surgery can vary depending on the roles that the HCP and the patient assume. Some of these styles will be more paternalistic than others and will influence what gets communicated and how.

Patient-centred communication: a hierarchy

The Institute of Medicine has defined patient-centred care (PCC) as 'Providing care that is respectful of and responsive to individual patient preferences, needs, and values, and ensuring that patient values guide all clinical decisions' (Committee on Quality of Healthcare in America 2001). Thus, PCC is a mode of healthcare delivery that puts the patient at the forefront of all decision-making and treatment. PCC is a popular concept that has been associated with tangible benefits in physical and psychological outcomes (Inzucchi et al. 2012; Rathert et al. 2012) and is adopted by healthcare systems such as the National Health Service in the UK.

So what is PCC about? And how is dentist–patient communication related to it? There are several popular models of PCC in the literature (Mead & Bower 2000, 2002; Stewart et al. 2003) and it is beyond the scope of this chapter to take the reader through all of these. In brief, however, it has been proposed by researchers in the field (Asimakopoulou & Scambler 2013; Scambler & Asimakopoulou 2014) that PCC is about a consultation that considers the following four basic factors:

1 *The illness in its widest context*: for instance, a patient-centred consultation about the need for an extraction would need to explore not just the technical aspects of the procedure but the impact that the extraction is going to have on the person's overall life, from the need for a repeat appointment to the need to take pain-control medication that may interact with other medications, to the need to have someone look after the patient's children whilst the patient is at the dentist having the dental extraction.

2 *The patient as a whole person*: this is about the dentist focusing not just on the mouth but also on the person behind it. A consultation that is truly patient-centred looks at the oral health of the whole person. For example, a dental consultation about poor oral hygiene taking place with a middle-class professional who can afford to invest in floss and an electric toothbrush would focus

on different issues and run quite differently from a consultation taking place with an older person who relies on others for help with their oral hygiene routine.

3 *The ethos behind the relationship with your patient*: this component is about an understanding of the therapeutic alliance and the development of a relationship built on trust, compassion, empathy and shared humanity. These features are then seen as key to developing a long-term relationship that is going to be conducive to appropriate decision-making about possible treatments and their outcomes.

4 *Finding common ground with the view of sharing responsibility*: this is a process in which dentists and patients reach a 'mutual understanding and mutual agreement' (Stewart et al. 2000) in three important areas: problem definition, establishing the goals/priorities of treatment and identifying the roles to be assumed by the two partners. The aim is to achieve a common understanding of the health issue in question and, where there is disagreement or divergence, to reach a consensus. So, in the dental surgery, the type of situation that would be relevant would be a consultation where the patient is asking for a certain treatment to take place which, in the dentist's clinical opinion, is not the best available for them. In a PCC consultation, the divergence of opinion in treatment outcomes would be something to discuss with a view to achieving a consensus and mutual understanding.

Following on from these four factors, a 'hierarchy of patient-centred care' has been put forward (Asimakopoulou & Scambler 2013; Scambler & Asimakopoulou 2014) that a consultation could be more or less patient-centred based on the amount of choice that the dentist makes available to the patient. See figure 12.1 for the hierarchy of PCC.

> **Discussion Point**
>
> Think back to the case study at the beginning of this chapter. How patient-centred would you say the consultation was? At what level of the Scambler and Asimakopoulou PCC hierarchy above would you say the hygienist was practising?

It is likely that different people will assess the case study as quite different in terms of PCC. The main reason for that is that the PCC concept can vary in meaning from person to person and the literature so far has not given us a widely accepted and acceptable definition to endorse. However, if you think of PCC as not just about being 'nice' to patients (which is a basic feature of good quality care after all), but about information and choice, you may find it easier to rate the case study on the basis of that. Doing so is unlikely to place that consultation very high on the PCC hierarchy. The section that follows explains in detail features of the hierarchy.

12

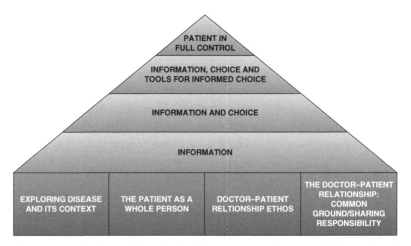

Figure 12.1 The four building blocks of patient-centred care and the hierarchy of patient-centred giving of information and choice

As shown in the figure, it is suggested that dentists need to give patients both information and choice about how to handle information and make a treatment choice, but also to support them in implementing this information with an ultimate aim of being in overall control of their own care. So, whilst at the most basic level PCC in the dental surgery will require the communication of some basic information to patients (Level 1: 'you will need an extraction'), at higher levels, patients will be presented with a choice between different treatment alternatives or oral healthcare routines (Level 2: 'you can have an extraction or you can choose not to have any treatment or you can have endodontic treatment'), be supported in exploring for themselves which option is best for their own unique circumstances (Level 3: 'the effects of the extraction for you as a person will be, A, B, C – but have you thought about X, Y, Z?') with the ultimate aim of enabling the patient to be in complete control over their decisions to do with their oral health regime (Level 4: 'You know all there is to know about all the different ways we have available to deal with this tooth. What do you think would suit you best given the pros and cons you have considered?'). If we look back at the case study, it is likely that we will conclude that, whilst the hygienist gave some information to the patient, namely about the difference between pain and pressure, the amount of choice available to him was not really explicit.

So far then, it has been argued that giving patients choice is a good, patient-centred thing to do. But is there any evidence that choice is actually a good thing for patients? In some now fairly dated but nevertheless relevant research, Lefer et al. (1962) made the same recommendation. They compared two groups of denture patients. Group A were offered a choice of either an individualized set of dentures made especially for them, or an 'average' set of dentures made to fit most people. Group B were not offered a choice, but were given a set of individualized dentures made especially for them. The group given a choice of denture

(Group A) were not only more satisfied with their dentures, but also less likely to complain about them or refuse to wear them. This was despite the fact that most of Group A chose the 'average' set. On the basis of these findings we suggest that giving patients choice is important.

It follows that a dental consultation will be more likely to be patient-centred if it is carried out in ways that will be conducive to patients feeling that they can talk to the dental team, that they can trust them, that the dental healthcare professional will listen and explore alternatives with them, and that, ultimately, both the dental team and patient are working towards the same, shared goal: the patient's best interests.

The following section considers some verbal and non-verbal behaviours that are helpful in being patient-centred in communicating with patients.

> **In summary**, patient-centred care is a method and philosophy of delivering care that puts the patient at the centre of all consultation and treatment. Whilst the concept is not particularly well defined, some attempts have been made to elaborate on it; it has been proposed that over and above a basic level of humanity that should be inherent in all healthcare consultations, patient-centred care is about offering patients information and choice at different levels, with the ultimate aim of enabling the patient to make the most appropriate decisions to do with their health, having evaluated all possible treatment options.

Practical issues I: verbal, paralinguistic and non-verbal communication

In order to understand communication better, psychologists choose to break it down into three categories. These examine:

- 'verbal communication': the exchanged utterances, in other words, what gets said;
- 'paralinguistic communication': those aspects of speech that are not words but which convey information, such as tone of voice, confirmatory noises;
- 'non-verbal communication': the behaviours and environmental factors that contribute to a communication exchange, but are not actual words.

The vast majority of research in this area is focused on verbal communication. However, all three communication categories are important and have a role to play in daily communication with patients. This section examines each one of these in turn.

12

Verbal communication: asking questions, giving information, checking understanding

Verbal communication is about what people actually say, that is, it is about the words and utterances they exchange. Verbal communication is usually about seeking and giving information with the purpose of helping the sender and recipient of the message understand each other, often in the form of asking questions.

Asking questions

Information-seeking questions can be 'open' (e.g. 'how are you?'), 'focused' (e.g. 'What sort of pain is it?') or 'closed' (e.g. 'Do you brush every day?'). Open questions allow maximum scope for the patient to engage with the dentist, as they do not in any obvious way restrict the information the patient delivers. Closed questions, on the other hand, invite a 'Yes' or 'No' response and, as such, are highly directive; here, patient involvement is limited in that the sort of information they offer has already been pre-defined by the person asking the question. Focused questions are potentially a happy medium where, although the patient is allowed some leeway in how much information they convey to their dentist, the dentist can limit the conversation to a specific topic. Obviously, there is a time and place for each; it is not suggested that only open questions should ever get asked or that patients are never directed. However, some questions (e.g. open) are more suited to some stages of the consultation. For example, starting with open questions when initiating the session, then moving to more focused or closed questions to obtain specific details about the patient's history.

Interestingly, there are three more categories of question that are relevant when considering verbal communication issues, mainly because they should be best avoided at all times. These are leading questions, that is, questions that imply a specific answer ('you don't really floss twice a day, do you?'); compound questions, which ask more than one question in one and can potentially confuse the patient (and the dentist!) ('Do you brush and floss daily' – where an answer of 'Yes' could be said to apply to one, but not the other of the two behaviours that are enquired about); and, finally, questions that contain jargon (e.g. 'you seem to be showing the typical symptomatology of chronic periodontitis, what do you think?').

Giving information

Giving information is not a simple matter of the dentist telling patients what they believe the patients should know. Bombarding patients with a lot of facts or planned actions, in the forlorn hope they will take all the information in and remember it, is neither patient-centred not conducive to care. This is because patients may not remember what was said in a consultation.

For example, it has been shown that most patients quickly forget the vast majority of what healthcare professionals tell them (Kessels 2003). In particular, in a study carried out with patients having a dental assessment (Misra et al. 2013), patients and the treating dentist were invited to write down, immediately after the end of the consultation, (i) the general issues they had discussed, (ii) any dental health advice given, (iii) the treatment the dentist had performed and (iv) all agreed future actions. The answers received from dentists and patients about the consultation were then compared. It was found that dentists generally remembered more of the consultation than patients, also reporting giving out more dental health education messages than patients remembered. Patients tended to remember what had brought them to clinic and quite a bit of detail about the technical procedures that the dentist performed, whilst psychosocial issues like, for example, pain and embarrassment were only very infrequently recalled as having been discussed by either dentists or patients. Worryingly, the area most patients recalled the least was 'agreed future actions'. This is quite concerning given that dentists' expectations are that having agreed actions, patients will go away and perform them! This study builds on previous work which clearly shows that most patients reliably forget most of what takes place in healthcare consultations. This means that communicating information which the dental team hope that patients will remember needs to be done methodically and carefully.

There are, generally, four stages that are involved in the process of giving information:

1 *Showing empathy/understanding*: Normally, people quickly dismiss information they are given unless the source of the information is one they trust, like and feel confident about (Wensing et al. 1998). Showing empathy and understanding is likely to put the dentist in a situation where their patient is more likely to want to listen to what they have to say rather than if they perceive the dentist as an indifferent professional with no time for them.

2 *Establish current knowledge*: This is about finding out what the patient already knows. Research into human memory tells us that people are more likely to remember information if (a) it makes sense to them and (b) it fits in with what they already know – their starting point (Bartlett 1932; Bartlett et al. 1984). Finding out what patients already know is thus helpful in that it assists dentists in 'pitching' the new information at an appropriate level. A second obvious advantage is that the process helps avoid telling patients things they already know (hence wasting both the patient's and the dental team's time). A third positive outcome of checking how much patients know first is that it gives dentists the chance

12

to correct any misconceptions patients may have by establishing whether what they know already is accurate or not.

3 *Chunking*: Giving information in a few small chunks is another useful skill. It is generally advisable to break down the information that needs to be delivered, whilst at the same time telling the patient that this is what the dentist is doing. Long narratives and explanations are generally not helpful when giving information. Categorizing the information about to be given and signposting, on the other hand ('there are three important things I would like to tell you. Firstly, . . .'), builds on the well-researched and evidenced principle that people find it easier to remember a limited number (normally five plus or minus two) of information chunks at any one time (Miller 1956). Chunking is thus likely to help patients recall the information later. Whilst chunking is a useful strategy, it should be obvious that an important aspect of information provision is to ensure that the information delivered matches the needs for information of each patient. Clearly, a highly educated, professional adult will have different information expectations and needs to a toddler and, as such, the content and complexity of the 'chunks' will need to be adapted to one's audience.

4 *Checking understanding*: The final stage of the information-giving sequence is to check patient understanding. This sounds easier than it actually is in practice as it may appear to be quite patronizing if the patient has fully understood. Rather than asking a closed question such as 'Do you understand?', the dentist's task is to test the patient's understanding. For example, the dentist could ask the patient 'Can you recap what I've just said so I can check that I have explained it properly?' This is one of those skills where the more one practises, the better one is likely to become at it. A technique that is often used is to ask patients to re-state in their own words the information they have been given, as if they were telling a friend. This will again need to be adapted to match the intellectual level of the patient the dentist is working with and their respective information needs.

Paralinguistic and non-verbal communication

This section outlines some of those communication behaviours that supplement verbal communication and can either aid or hinder a collaborative or consultative style of communication. Things like the dentist's vocal cues (e.g. tone, pitch, rate, volume, silence, effect and responsiveness) and confirmatory noises (e.g. 'hmmm', 'aha') convey to patients important information about the type of communication episode between them and the dentist. The dentist's posture (e.g. whether they speak to their patient whilst they are lying flat on a chair whilst the dentist is standing), the dentist's facial expression (e.g. raised eyebrows, smiles, frowns), the amount of eye contact, the amount of physical space between them and the patient, as well as environmental features such as furniture placement, lighting and so on, will all give patients ideas about the sort of dentist they might be as well as what the dentist's expectation are about the way patients behave in their surgery.

In a now dated but important study, Jackson (1978) found that patients made judgements on the technical ability of dentists based on the appearance of the dental surgery. In an experimental study, respondents were more likely to rate as clinically competent a dentist whose surgery appeared modern and clean. This effect correlated with the age of the dentist and was particularly strong if the dentist was young. Older dentists were assumed to have experience, which made up for their inadequate facilities, but a young dentist in an old-fashioned surgery was viewed as most incompetent. It would appear that patients read a lot into not only what dentists tell them, but also in how and where they convey the information.

> **In summary**, communication is not just about what gets said, it is also about the non-verbal signs people send to one another in any verbal exchange. Both verbal and non-verbal communication will shape the quality and quantity of information exchanged in the dental setting.

Practical issues II: putting it all together

Having established the medium for communication (verbal, non-verbal and paralinguistic channels) and our philosophy of care delivery (patient-centred), the question arises how to put together these components in a typical consultation.

The Calgary-Cambridge framework (Silverman et al. 2004) provides an overview of the key tasks that a healthcare professional seeks to achieve when communicating with their patients. This consists of a description of the process of the consultation (starting the session, gathering information, explanation and planning, and finally closing the consultation) together with two themes running throughout the consultation, that is, providing structure and building the relationship between patient and HCP. Not all consultations will include all the phases, but it should be obvious that a typical dental visit would include many of them. The tasks to achieve at each stage will call for the use of different skills – for example, when gathering information the focus will be on asking questions and active listening, whereas in the explanation and planning part of the consultation, there will be a shift to giving information and using strategies to encourage shared decision-making. The end of each phase of the consultation is probably a good point to use 'Chunking'.

Alongside the structure of the consultation, the model proposes that there are two tasks of which the clinician should be mindful – providing structure and building rapport.

12

1 **Providing structure**: Be aware of the structure of the consultation and make clear to the patient what is happening. Ensure that the stages progress satisfactorily.

2 **Building the relationship**: A relationship of trust and mutual respect will enable the dentist and their patient to work towards joint decisions about the most effective pathway of care. Three key skills help to build such relationships:
   - Developing rapport through showing an interest in the patient and a willingness to help.
   - Appropriate empathic responses.
   - Involving the patient in decision-making through seeking the patient's opinion of options, and offering the patient choices, as discussed above.

In summary, the Calgary-Cambridge framework provides a useful, practical overview of the key tasks that a healthcare professional seeks to achieve when communicating with their patients. This widely used model is helpful as it addresses not just the process, but also the structure and relational aspects of the consultation.

Practical issues III: communicating bad news

In the final section of this chapter, we address a very practical issue that often concerns the dental team both ethically and practically; that is, the giving of bad news to patients.

What is bad news? And how bad does bad news have to be in order to be considered truly bad news? These are some of the questions to consider when examining the skills required to communicate news to patients that is likely to be considered as 'bad news'. Such situations may arise when, for example, patients need to be told that they have a suspicious lesion in their mouth that will need to be investigated, or that they will need surgery to remove it. Similarly, telling patients that they will lose one or more of their teeth can be considered as news that can potentially be classified as 'bad'. Ultimately, whilst dentists may have a view on what might constitute bad news, the degree to which patients will also consider it as bad may vary; a fashion model who relies on a perfect smile for high self-esteem and their day-to-day job is likely to find the news of an extraction more upsetting than someone whose esteem and perhaps their livelihood do not depend on a perfect smile. So it is important to remember that what may or may not be considered as 'bad news' has quite a large subjective element to it.

A lot has been written in the medical field as to how best to give patients bad news (Minichiello et al. 2007; Fujimori & Uchitomi 2009; Jacobsen & Jackson 2009; McGuigan 2009), although the dental literature has not seen the same expansion. Work by Newton and Fiske, however, has been very helpful in outlining how best to communicate bad news in the dental surgery (Newton & Fiske 1999). According to these authors, there are three, sequential stages to be followed when bad news is communicated in the dental surgery. These stages involve preparatory work, discussing the actual situation and agreeing to review the situation. Within each one of these areas, there are some typical tasks that need to be performed so that the bad news can be given in the most sensitive, empathic way. The rest of this section examines these three areas in turn.

The preparation phase

Here, it is suggested that the dentist carefully considers three areas: (1) the information that is actually going to be communicated, (2) the setting in which the interaction is going to take place, and (3) the amount of available time.

Firstly, the information that is to be communicated to people needs to be clear, understandable and jargon-free. If given in writing, the writing needs to be legible and the text should have been assessed for readability. Drawings and illustrations may help to make the message clearer. The setting needs to be conducive to a consultation that is going to take place with empathy and sensitivity; phones ringing, people coming in and out of the room, an open door so that the conversation may be overheard should all be avoided (Newton & Fiske 1999). Instead, the consultation needs to take place in an area that is free from distractions and where the patient is likely to feel at ease. If the interaction would benefit from the presence of a chaperone or a patient advocate, these are issues to be considered and arranged for in advance, if at all possible. Time is a final important consideration here; it is important that the dental team have allowed plenty of time to communicate the bad news and that the patient knows how much time there is available. Equally important is to share with the patient how much time is available 'today'. Using the word 'today' signals to the patient the HCP's availability to revisit the issue at a future date, which is important in letting the patient know that the HCP is prepared and able to offer ongoing rather than one-off support.

Discussing the actual news

This stage involves starting the conversation, checking the patient's reaction and view of the bad news, deciding on what to do next, summarizing and finally closing the consultation. Here, the dentist may wonder where to start and how much to actually disclose; there is literature to suggest that different people want different amounts of information to be given to them concerning health news (Politi et al. 2013). For example, in a systematic review of studies examining cancer patients' preferences for information, Fujimori and Uchitomi (2009) found that younger, female and higher educated patients reported

12

wishing to receive as much detailed information as possible; Asian patients were found to have a strong preference for a family member to be present at the time the news was delivered, more than Western patients. Life expectancy conversations were not a preferred topic of conversation with the Asian groups, although Western patients had a preference for receiving such information. It is thus important to be aware of such socio-demographic preferences for information and to act accordingly.

Next, it is suggested that patients get asked how much they know about their condition and how much more they would like to know; so here it is important that the information that is communicated is matched to the patient's level of knowledge at that moment, that it is given in small chunks that the patient can comprehend, and that understanding and desire to hear more are assessed at frequent intervals (Newton & Fiske 1999). Giving time for silences so that the patient can take in what the dentist is telling them, as well as empathizing with the patient and acknowledging their surprise, if indeed they show it ('I think you did not expect to hear about this white patch in what should have been a routine check-up') are useful techniques to use here. Allowing strong emotions and accepting them (e.g. crying) rather than trying to reassure patients that you understand how they must feel (when you possibly do not) has been recommended as a way of dealing with patients who find the news overwhelming (Newton & Fiske 1999).

Within this stage, it is really important that enough time is put aside in the dental consultation to explore the patient's reaction to receiving the bad news. Was the news expected? Was it not? What do they expect to be the best and worst case scenarios? Allowing people to tell their dentist how they feel about the bad news is important in helping the empathic communication to carry on, but also it is an invaluable source of information for the dental team to assess how much the patient has taken in and how much more it is reasonable to present them with.

Finally, the next step here would be to jointly decide on the next steps and the way forward. For example, will a follow-up appointment be needed? Will the patient get referred elsewhere? Exploring the patient's support network and agreeing to review the conversation that has taken place is important; patients are unlikely to remember everything they have been told as part of the bad news, so it is vitally important that the consultation is followed up by another appointment within a week or so (Newton & Fiske 1999). A coherent, sensitive summary to close the consultation is the final task to undertake in this situation. The summary is likely to attempt to tie in the events that led the patient to come to the present consultation with the content of the consultation, and to focus on the support that is available and the next agreed steps. Telephone or email contacts in case patients have more questions should be given out at this stage.

Reviewing the consultation

It is important, at the end of a consultation in which patients have been presented with bad news, that the HCP takes time out to review the impact of the consultation on themselves. Here, Newton and Fiske suggest that dentists should consider what went well, what did not work that well and, finally, what aspects of the consultation they think they should change for future appointments of this nature. It is proposed that the person from the dental team who has given the bad news may consider seeking the support or advice of other colleagues who can guide and advise them on how best to handle these sensitive situations. With repeat exposure to such difficult situations it is likely that a set of behaviours, skills and techniques will be developed that will enhance the communicator's skill in giving bad news to patients.

In summary, giving bad news can be made easier on both the dental team and the patient by following a three-phase, stepped approach involving preparing the patient, giving the bad news and then reviewing the situation.

Discussion Points
1. What communication features make a consultation patient-centred?
2. How might patients be supported to remember important health advice given at a consultation?
3. What are the processes involved in breaking bad news?

Conclusion

Good communication in the dental surgery is of paramount importance. It is at the cornerstone of patient-centred care and an opportunity for the dental team to build a sound relationship with patients. Communication that matches the patient's expectations is important and has a role to play in any consultation. Depending on the model of care the dental team adopts, different communication styles will be required at different stages of the consultation.

12

The Dentist in Society

Sasha Scambler

> **IN THIS CHAPTER YOU WILL LEARN ABOUT:**
> ▶ The changing perceptions of dentistry and dentists
> ▶ Models of health service supply
> ▶ The history of dental services
> ▷ The rise and fall of dentistry in the National Health Service
> ▷ Professionalism and dentistry
> ▶ The provision and shape of dental services today
> ▶ The dental team

Introduction

The aim of this chapter is to explore the changing nature of the relationship between the dentist and society, the different roles that dentists and dental care more widely have occupied, and public perceptions of dentistry, dental services and oral health. Although there will necessarily be some historical detail about the ways in which dental services have been provided across time, this chapter is not interested in policy detail per se, but rather in the relationship between dentistry and society and the impact that changes in policy and provision of services has on wider society, the way that dentistry is perceived and the provision of dental care.

This chapter starts with a brief look at the way in which dentists and dentistry are portrayed in the media, literature and the arts and the potential effect of this on public perceptions of dentistry and dentists. What do we think of dentists? And does that affect the likelihood of us visiting a dentist? The chapter then focuses on the changing environment in which dental services are provided, starting with a brief outline of the main models of health service supply which is used as a means of understanding the context of a historical overview of dental care. The rise and fall of dentistry in the National Health Service in the UK is outlined to explore changing perceptions and use of dental care. The final part of the chapter focuses on the idea of professionalism in dentistry, the dental team and the shape of dental services today.

Changing perceptions of dentistry

Media representations of dentists and dentistry can be found throughout film, literature and other forms of media and, up until relatively recently, have been almost universally negative. Perhaps the most terrifying of all representations of the dentist was that portrayed in the 1976 film adaptation of William Goldman's *Marathon Man*, in which the main role is played by a dentist/murderer who causes his patients extreme pain, experiments on their mouths and kills. In a song from *Little Shop of Horrors* ('Dentist!'), the villain of the piece is a sadistic dentist called Scrivello who was encouraged to put his 'talent for causing things pain' to good use by his mother and become a dentist. And it's not just sadism or generally unpleasant personality characteristics that are highlighted. As early as 1924, the first ever motion picture, *Greed* by Eric von Stroheim, indicates an association between dentistry and greed. In this silent movie, a picture of a big gold tooth sways in the wind outside the dentist's office.

Negative images of dentists are also found in more recent films such as the Disney cartoon *Finding Nemo*, where the dentist captures Nemo the clownfish and plans to give him to his brace- and headgear-wearing, violent young niece as a present. Whilst the dentist himself is relatively benign, the dental surgery becomes a scene of threat and potentially violent death at the hands of the niece. A recent opinion piece by Schoon-Tong (2012) calls for more positive representations of dentists in the media. She suggests that negative images on social media reflect the way that dentists are portrayed in film and television and suggests the need to 'humanize and humorize dentistry'. Gideon (2013) goes further to suggest that if we want to reduce dental fear, which is well recognized as a barrier to dental attendance, we need to look at the portrayal of dentistry in the media with the aim of creating a more positive image.

More recently, some positive, or at least neutral, images of dentistry have started to emerge. In *Rameau's Niece*, a novel by Cathleen Schine, for example, the dentist is seen as a romantic, kindly figure and in Jane Smiley's novel *The Age of Grief*, a story of marriage and the nature of love, the main protagonists just happen to be dentists who met at dental school. The link between dentistry, oral hygiene and aesthetics is perhaps the most clear-cut area in which positive images are emerging, as demonstrated by television shows like Channel 4's *10 Years Younger*, in which dental makeovers feature heavily. In this context, the dentist is

13

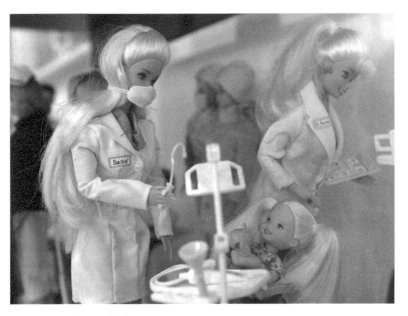

Image 13.1 Dentist Barbie
© Britta Pedersen/dpa/Corbis

part of a make-over team and oral health is seen as aesthetically important. This same theme is portrayed in the film *Pretty Woman*, where Julia Roberts' character is seen going into the bathroom, supposedly to snort cocaine, but actually flosses her teeth. Indeed, perhaps in the US, instead of the toothbrush, the icon of dentistry has become floss. These more positive images have started to challenge traditional negative images of dentistry and suggest that the way the profession is being perceived is beginning to change. We have even had the recent release of Dentist Barbie by Mattel!

Discussion Point

- The examples given above demonstrate the often negative ways in which dentists are portrayed in the media. How might these types of representation affect the likelihood of people attending the dentist and the incidence of dental fear?

It is not just in the media that attention is paid to public perceptions of dentists and dentistry. A number of papers have been published exploring public perceptions and experiences of dentistry and the implications of this for oral health and future dental care provision. Studies by Liddell and May (1984) and Liddell and Locker (1992), for example, suggested that levels of patient satisfaction with their dentist and dental treatment directly affected their willingness to seek further preventive or symptom-related dental care. Communication and interpersonal skills were found to be a key factor in decision-making about future care. This work built on a number of earlier studies which explored the ideal characteristics of a dentist from the perspective of patients. Two studies conducted in Europe (Van Groenestijn et al. 1980; Lahti et al. 1992) compiled a list of characteristics deemed particularly important, which included: professional skill, being trustworthy, friendliness, good communication and up-to-date knowledge. Similar studies conducted in the United States (Kriesberg & Treiman 1962; McKeithen 1966; Rankin & Harris 1985; Patterson 1993) echoed these characteristics, but also identified truthfulness, an awareness of the implication of cost and not telling patients off for poor oral hygiene, as particularly important.

In a study in 1995, DiMatteo et al. used the US Household Survey to explore 'public attitudes towards dentists'. A random sample of adults (aged 18+) were asked to rate dentists according to a range of criteria. Of the 647 respondents in the study, almost two-thirds had only a moderate amount of trust in their dentist at most, nearly 10 per cent had little or no respect for their dentist, whilst a further 48.5 per cent had a moderate amount of respect for them. Technical skill, ethical conduct, communication and a focus on prevention were deemed most important by patients in this study. This ties in with work by Borreani et al. (2008, 2010a, 2010b) which found that the character of the dentist, a perceived lack of empathy and poor communication skills were identified as barriers to accessing dental care amongst older people. In an earlier study, Finch et al. (1988) also identified impersonal treatment and being treated simply as a 'mouth' as barriers to dental service use. For a more detailed exploration of the impact of communication, and poor communication in particular, along with guidance on improving communication skills, see chapter 12. Suffice to say here that negative images of the dentist as a person, both through personal experiences and through images portrayed in the media, still have the potential to impact on dental service usage and therefore on oral health.

> **In summary**, there are now a multiplicity of images of dentistry in the media. Whilst there is a clear shift away from the worst images of psychopathic dentists towards a more positive link between the dentist, aesthetics and positive body image, research suggests that patients are still reticent about the positive characteristics displayed by their dentists, and poor communication and a lack of empathy, along with dental fear, are still identified as key barriers to dental attendance.

Models of health service supply

This chapter started with a brief overview of changing public perceptions of dentistry and dentists. As has been seen, the way in which dentists are viewed is not just reliant on how they are portrayed in the media but also on individual patient experiences, as highlighted in the studies above. Whilst individual experiences can be studied,

13

these experiences are often shaped by the context within which they have occurred. In this case it can be suggested that public perceptions of dentistry and dentists have been shaped, at least in part, by the way in which dental care has been provided over time, and that changes in public perception may reflect changes in ideology or service provision, including the development of pain relief and new, more effective prevention techniques. From this perspective the role of dentistry and dentists in society needs to be understood within the context of changing models of health service supply.

The concept of health and the different ways in which it can be understood was explored in some detail in the first chapter of this book. In the context of health policy, the concept of health can relate either to individuals and their specific circumstances or to the population as a whole. These two quotes illustrate the two viewpoints:

> health affects every aspect of life. Our ability to work, to play, to enjoy our families and to socialise with friends, all depend crucially on our physical wellbeing. Serious illnesses create enormous pain and suffering, even minor transient ailments can be depressing psychologically as well as debilitating physically. And ill-health which leads to death makes all other services of satisfaction irrelevant. (Le Grand 1982: 23)

The view of the need to focus on the health of the population as a whole is summed up by a Canadian health report which stated:

> Good health is the bedrock on which social progress is built. A nation of healthy people can do those things which make life worthwhile and as the level of health increases so does the potential for happiness. (Ministry of National Health and Welfare, Canada 1974)

Both of these quotes suggest different reasons why governments might seek to provide healthcare. It may be to protect individuals from the cost of healthcare or the devastating effects of loss of income through health problems, or it may be a way of ensuring that there is a constant supply of healthy people ready to provide the necessary workforce for the country. Health policy consists of statements of intent made by governments relating to the maintenance of good health in individuals or populations as a whole. It may relate to curing disease or to providing care for people unable to care for themselves either through age, disability or other social or health circumstances. The way in which policies are conceived or implemented depends on the particular view of the problem to be solved. Thus the way in which we understand health and disease will affect the way that we seek to deal with or solve issues around them.

Within health policy there can be any number of policy paradigms. Government policies may focus on the care or treatment of people who are ill on an individual level. Or they may focus on the maintenance and promotion of health in individuals or in populations. The focus of policy will have a profound effect on the problems to be identified, the services to be provided and the people who will be seen as the authorities on health issues. Table 13.1 illustrates the implications of a paradigm shift from an illness-based model to a preventive-based model of care.

Table 13.1 Illness and Health	
Illness	Health
Treatment	Prevention
Cure	Care
Disease	Behaviour producing disease
Individual	Population as unit of treatment
Illness as concern of medical profession	Health as business of everyone
Right to treatment	Duty to remain healthy

This shift can be seen in dentistry with the move from a symptomatic, treatment-based (initially extractions and then aspects of restoration) approach, to the public health approach, which is more common today with the provision of preventive care and oral health promotion and education. Paradigm shifts in the way we think about health and healthcare have an effect on the kind of care that we receive and that the government provides. The following section briefly outlines the three main models of health service provision. These are then explored further in the context of the history of dental care in the UK and beyond.

If it is assumed that all people will require some kind of healthcare at some point in their lives and that there is no such thing as perfect health, then access to the best possible healthcare for those who are ill is of fundamental importance. There are three main models of healthcare provision: the market model, the professional model and the bureaucratic model.

A market model

A market model assumes that healthcare is a product like any other. Where demand exists, then market forces will supply the goods required for a price. Market theory suggests that suppliers (either individuals or companies) will harness available technologies to provide healthcare commensurate with the demand from users for a price. Suppliers will advertise their wares. Competition will ensure that services are provided for a price, which ensures a margin of profit and that consumer needs are met. In theory, the consumer is in control, whilst the hidden hand of the market ensures that scarce resources are used in the most efficient way through matching supply with demand. In this context, the market has the authority to determine resource allocation.

13

As will be seen, this is the model that was prevalent prior to the professionalization of dentistry in the late nineteenth century.

The professional model

The development of medical sciences in the nineteenth century led to the implementation of two other models of healthcare supply. Both the bureaucratic model and the professional model assume that medical care is too important and that medical knowledge is too specialized for it to be treated as a market good. The professional model places authority of care in the hands of the expert – in this case the dentist, although the same model can be applied to medicine. Dental care is based on technical and expert knowledge. Therefore the general public must be protected from those who do not have the necessary expertise. This may include the authority to determine training and qualifications and to judge what is in the best interests of the patients. This approach is essentially paternalistic. The dental profession remains dominant in determining the shape of the healthcare system, although modern state arrangements may ensure that the whole population has access to the doctors.

The bureaucratic model

In this model, the state takes over the role of determining health policy. This system tends to be encouraged by the democratic system as the government is seen to represent the interests of the population as a whole. Healthcare tends to have a high value and the emphasis in this model is on the rights of citizenship. The state becomes involved in distributional issues such as ensuring access to services according to the criteria of equity, allocation of resources, management of services and prioritizing of services. The benefits to the collectivity as well as to the individual are stressed.

Despite the gradual introduction of a co-payment system in dentistry from 1951, until the 1980s the main models of healthcare in the UK were the bureaucratic and professional models, with the market model being introduced into general medicine in the 1980s through the internal market and the purchaser/provider split. The implications of the different shifts in ideology (from the disease model to the health model, cure to prevention, institutional care to community-based care and so forth) and the different modes of health service supply can be seen in the history of dental services in the UK over the past few centuries.

In summary, healthcare can be organized and funded in a variety of ways. The type, or combination, of health system models adopted will depend on the policy paradigm underlying it. Health can be seen in a variety of ways: as an individual or a society level issue, involving treating disease or maintaining health. The paradigm adopted shapes the model utilized.

A brief history of dental services in the UK

The changing models of health service supply and changing policy paradigms can be charted through a social history of dentistry. It is useful, therefore, to briefly explore the history of dentistry to provide a context for current service provision and the place and role of dentistry and dentists in contemporary society. This can relate to oral health outcome measures such as disease levels, but also to service use, patient satisfaction and wider public perceptions of dentistry and dentists.

Early dentistry

It is suggested that there is evidence of dentistry taking place as far back as 7000 BC in the Indus Valley Civilization, and the ancient Egyptian 'Hesy Re' is thought by many to be the first person identified as a dental practitioner (Hussain & Khan 2014). It was not until the Middle Ages, however, that a distinct group of people can be identified as dental practitioners. Prior to the early 1200s, members of the clergy carried out healing roles, which included tooth extraction, and it is suggested that wigmakers, blacksmiths, jewellers and apothecaries may also have carried out tooth extractions as a sideline to their main areas of business (British Dental Association 2012a). A Guild of Barbers was established in France in 1210 AD, evolving into two distinct groups: surgeons (educated to perform complex surgical procedures) and barber-surgeons (lay people who performed routine procedures like blood-letting and tooth extraction). In the UK, reference was made to 'tooth drawrers' and it wasn't until 1462 that the first charter for barbers was drawn up, later merging with the group known as surgeons.

The first known book focusing entirely on dentistry was published in Germany by Artzney Buchlein in 1530 and was called *Little Medicinal Book for All Kinds of Diseases and Infirmities of the Teeth* (American Dental Association, referenced in Hussain & Khan 2014). This was followed by the first book about dental treatment written in English, *The Operator for the Teeth*, written by Charles Allen in 1685. What is interesting about the emergence of the 'operators for the teeth' in the seventeenth century is that they did not just extract teeth but also made dentures, usually from elephant, walrus or hippopotamus ivory. According to the museum of the British Dental Association, the term 'dentist' first emerged in eighteenth-century France and was adopted in Britain in the 1750s. This coincided with the division of the body, with specialist groups laying claim to various parts of the body (Porter 1997). The mouth was one area of the body claimed by specialists. At this time the demand for dental services started to grow, most likely because of the increase in sugar consumption, and advertisements could be found for dentists, offering a range of services including 'restorative techniques and treatment of gum diseases . . . scaling, fillings, dentures

13

and even tooth whitening' (British Dental Association 2012b). Early dentistry clearly fell within a market model. Services developed to meet the needs of the population, and prices were set according to the level of need and the willingness and ability of different sectors of the population to pay for services. This led to piecemeal services with different tiers of care according to cost and the ability to pay.

By the end of the nineteenth century, there was an established group of people practising as dentists and treating an ever-expanding middle-class population. Most learned their trade through apprenticeships and there were no controls in place to ensure quality or guard against malpractice. Whilst the occasional formal lecture on dentistry was offered from the end of the 1800s, it was not until 1858 that the Dental Hospital

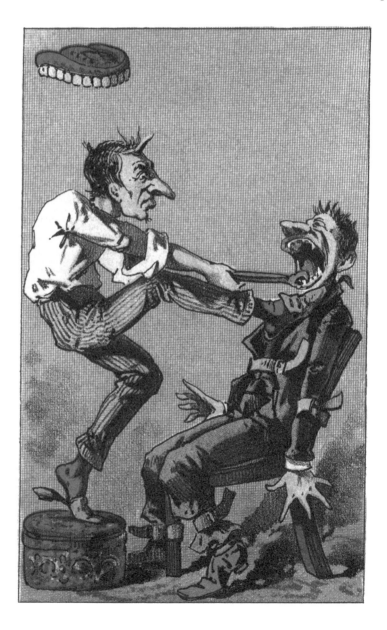

Image 13.2 A nineteenth-century cartoon depiction of 'tooth-drawing'.

of London was opened, with the National Dental Hospital opening its doors the following year. Both hospitals had teaching schools attached and this heralded the start of the formalization of dental training. By the late nineteenth century, a number of surgical colleges were offering diplomas in dentistry (British Dental Association 2012c).

The emergence of a dental profession

It was not until the 1870s that an attempt was made to regulate the practice of dentistry with the establishment of the Dental Reform Committee. This resulted in the Dentists Act of 1878, two decades after the first dental school was set up in London to provide a formal training route for people wanting to call themselves dentists (British Dental Association 2012c). This Act required anyone who wished to practise as a dentist to undertake the London Dental School (LDS) course and register on the Dentists Register which was set up in 1879. Whilst a positive move for dentistry, and the birth of dentistry as a profession, regulation was not initially a good move for women who wished to practise as dentists, as they were refused entry into the first dental schools and it was not until 1895 that the first female dentist qualified in Edinburgh. The first women were admitted into English dental schools almost two decades later.

Whilst the 1878 Dentists Act restricted those who were able to call themselves dentists, it did not actually regulate the practice of dentistry per se, and unqualified practitioners outnumbered qualified dentists for many more decades. The British Dental Association was set up in 1880 and was the official body representing legally practising dentists. One of its main roles was to prosecute illegally practising dentists (British Dental Association 2012c). It was not until the 1921 Dentists Act that it became illegal to practise dentistry without being a registered dentist who had undergone formal training.

General and local anaesthesia were developed in the nineteenth century and, following this, there was a rapid growth in technology, knowledge about oral health and dental disease and materials that could be used to protect and restore teeth in the early twentieth century. Whilst treatments and materials were improving, however, there was still limited access to dental care, particularly amongst poorer people. A certain amount of free or low-cost care was available in the large voluntary hospitals, but this was limited. There were also a number of 'approved societies' which provided dental care along with medical care for workers, but families and children were not covered under these schemes. The emergence of dentistry as a profession heralded the introduction of some protection against substandard care for patients but did not bring with it wider access or universal care. The late nineteenth and early twentieth centuries thus saw a move towards a professional model of care, with supply (and therefore prices) controlled by the profession of dentistry under the auspices of the British Dental Association.

13

The rise and fall of NHS dentistry

The case has been made that the establishment of the National Health Service in the UK was a direct result of positive state intervention in many areas of national life during the Second World War. The idea of free healthcare was not a new one; however, the issue of public levels of health and disease was brought to a head during the Boer War (1899–1901). The government was forced to intervene when it was discovered that as many as one in three recruits into the army were unfit to serve because of ill-health. The early twentieth century was characterized by international tension and a rise in the power of socialism across Europe. Social reforms were introduced by the government of the time to appease the working classes and stop the spread of socialism. The UK government introduced pensions in 1908, and in 1911 the National Health Insurance scheme (NHI) was introduced. The NHI covered manual workers between the ages of 16 and 65 whose earnings were below taxable level and provided funds for sickness; accident and disability benefits in cash; and access to GP services free of charge. Limited dental care was also provided. The system was set up simply to provide a healthy workforce and armed services should they be needed.

The introduction of National Insurance in 1911 had made some difference, but financial barriers to the use of health services remained because NHI was available to less than half the population and it did not cover the dependants of the insured workers. In addition, specialists, GPs, dentists and hospital beds were unevenly distributed across the country, there were wide variations in the standards of services and the GP services were uncoordinated. By the latter half of the 1930s, popular support was growing for the idea that everyone should have access to good quality care. The establishment of the NHS in Britain may be seen, in many ways, as a direct outcome of the Second World War – although clearly the context of healthcare in Britain at the time also played a part. The Second World War promised new and equal conditions for all, the victorious nation expected a change (Mays 2008). As a result, a national universally available healthcare system, administered by the state rather than the insurance industry, was a central plank in Beveridge's famous blueprint for a post-war welfare state (Beveridge Report 1942). The aims of the health service were:

> To ensure that everyone in the country – irrespective of means, age, sex and occupation – shall have equal opportunity to benefit from the best and most up-to-date medical and allied services available. To provide, therefore, for all who want it, a comprehensive service covering every branch of medical and allied activity.
>
> To divorce the case of health from questions of personal means or other factors irrelevant to it; to provide the service free of charge (apart from certain possible charges in respect of appliances) and to encourage a new attitude to

health – the easier obtaining of advice early, the promotion of good health rather than only the treatment of bad. (Ministry of Health 1944: 47)

The need for an attitude change in dental care from symptomatic to preventive care was also highlighted by Beveridge. In terms of overall control, finance and access, the system had changed dramatically from a system based on a professional model to one reflecting both a professional and bureaucratic model. The NHS was open to the whole population solely on the basis of healthcare need. It was free at the point of use and funded almost entirely from general tax revenues of the central government. The goal was to secure equality of access throughout the country to a comprehensive range of modern health services. There were three branches of dentistry included in the NHS: a general dental practice (GDP) service with GDPs mainly working as contractors from local surgeries; a community service (predominantly special care); and a hospital-based dental service (Health Committee Publication 2008).

Once it had been established, the NHS immediately proved both popular with the public and 'financially attractive to the vast majority of medical practitioners' (Mays 2008). Original funding plans had assumed that costs would stabilize relatively quickly once initial unmet need had been addressed. They had not accounted, however, for the popularity of the NHS which, in combination with rising public expectations, inflation and post-war development in medical technology and drugs, drove up the price of the service (Mays 2008). The huge public demand for dentures, nicknamed the 'denture dash' (British Dental Association 2012d) at the start of the NHS meant that within the first nine months of the NHS, 33 million artificial teeth had been supplied. To limit public spending, charges were introduced for spectacles and dentures and eventually for prescriptions.

Unlike general medical services, dental services provided by general dental practitioners continued to be a mix of private and NHS care, with the subsidized charges for NHS dentures introduced in 1951, being followed by charges (co-payments) to cover routine dental care up to a preset limit (Boyle 2008). Charges were made according to an itemized list of treatments. By 2006, over 400 treatments were separately itemized for charges. Whilst early NHS dentistry focused on treating a backlog of dental disease and decay, by the 1970s the focus was shifting towards public health measures such as fluoridation and oral health education, which have resulted in an increasing number of older people retaining their teeth into old age. In 1992 the Health Committee (cited in Health Committee Publication 2008) stated that the way dental services were provided had been largely unchanged over the past four decades. Dentists working for the General Dental Service as GDPs were largely able to establish their practices where they wished and choose which services to make available to their patients.

In 1990 the Department of Health introduced registration for dental services with the aim of increasing continuity of care, but this

13

resulted in an overspend of £190 million which the government then tried to recoup by reducing the amount paid to dentists for each item of treatment by 7 per cent (Department of Health 2000c). This led to dentists restricting the number of NHS patients they accepted (Rhodes & Gregory 1995) and led to a significant decrease in the availability of NHS dental care (Hancock et al. 1999) and a subsequent increase in the number of people accessing private dentistry. Interestingly, the fall in NHS dentistry and accompanying rise in private dentistry has coincided with a fall in levels of satisfaction with dentistry amongst the general public (Judge et al. 1997). According to Calnan et al. (2000), the main source of dissatisfaction was the lack of access to NHS dental care and perceived costs of private treatment. This ties in with a study by Borreani et al. (2010a) which found that access to NHS care was seen as a citizenship right amongst older people, a major cause of discontent where a lack of NHS dental care was perceived.

Similar findings from a study by Calnan et al. (2000) on patient attitudes towards private and NHS dental care found that, whilst patients were dissatisfied with their ability to access NHS services, once they had gained access there was little difference in reported satisfaction levels between private and NHS patients in relation to the quality of technical care received and the ability of the dentist to relieve symptoms. Interestingly, whilst respondents in this study expressed higher satisfaction with certain aspects of private dentistry, the majority did not perceive private dentistry as the preferred option, again linking the egalitarian nature of NHS dentistry with citizenship rights. Whilst we still have both a professional model and a bureaucratic model of health service supply at work in UK dentistry at the moment, we are moving inexorably away from the bureaucratic model towards a professional/market partnership model.

In summary, there is evidence that dental care has been around from at least 7000 BC. The provision of dental care can be categorized in three stages. The earliest form of documented dental care involved primarily extractions, the creation of replacement teeth and the treatment of dental pain. From the seventeenth century, dental care became more organized with different groups performing dental services. It was not until the end of the nineteenth century that dentistry became a profession, however, the first step towards dentistry as we know it today.

Professionalism and dentistry

The emergence of dentistry as a profession is outlined above and is an important milestone in understanding the development of modern dental practice. In common with medicine, dentistry was able to develop as a largely unaccountable, self-regulated profession due to the combination of a 'highly regarded body of expertise and skills with a high degree of cohesion and a tradition of forceful political organization' (Langan 1998: 10). Sociological work suggests that a distinct body of knowledge is the epistemological foundation for the establishment of any profession (Crinson 2008). Whilst the dental and medical professions are long established, it is only relatively recently that there has been more of a focus on professionalism and what it means to be and/or act as a professional within a healthcare setting. The importance of professionalism as a concept in dentistry can be seen in the fact that it forms one of four key domains in which all dental students in the UK must demonstrate their competence in order to be accepted, on completion of the Bachelor of Dental Sciences degree, as a qualified dentist (General Dental Council 2011).

There is widespread agreement that the concept of professionalism is an important one for healthcare professionals, although, perhaps ironically, it is also accepted that there is no agreed definition of what professionalism is in this context (Hafferty & Levinson 2008). The lack of an agreed, universal definition leads to a situation where dentists are required to demonstrate qualities of professionalism without clear guidance on what this actually means, either in theory or in practice. There has been an attempt to create a definition of professionalism for dentistry (Welie 2004; Trathen & Gallagher 2009), building on work that has been undertaken in medicine, but there are clear differences in terms of the relationship between care and business and the exchange of money in dentistry that are not so apparent in the still largely tax-funded National Health Service that provides the vast majority of medical care in the UK. This makes direct comparisons between medicine and dentistry as professions difficult (Trathen 2013).

Definitions that have been suggested to date vary between broad definitions of professionalism and lists of attributes required by those seeking to engender professionalism. Examples of the former type of definition are included in the work of Welie (2004) in dentistry and Nath et al. (2006) in medicine. Interestingly, both definitions include putting the patient's interests before those of the dentist/doctor even where doing so is 'not in one's own best financial, social or physical interest'. Examples of the latter type of definition tend to be the work of professional groups. The Royal College of Physicians Working Party, for example, offers a list of attributes doctors are expected to display in their day-to-day work, incorporating: integrity, compassion, altruism, continuous improvement, excellence, and working in partnership with members of the wider healthcare team. They go on to suggest that these attributes form the basis of the moral contract between doctors and society *(Royal College of Physicians Working Party 2005)*. Current work by Trathen et al. (forthcoming) is looking to address this and explore how dentists understand the concept of professionalism and what this means in practice.

What ties together approaches to professionalism across different healthcare professional groups is the fact that professionalism itself

13

is heralded as something to be idealized and pursued. This in itself is interesting, as few people seem willing to tie themselves to a concrete definition of what this means. There is a significant body of research within sociology that explores professionalism as a concept and its use by healthcare professionals, which offers an insight into why it is that the concept is so popular in healthcare and possibly why there is little urgency to tie down a universal definition.

Sociologists working in this area are particularly interested in how professions are formulated and in the social roles that they perform. Freidson (2001) set out an 'ideal type' profession to act as a starting point. He suggests that professions are occupations and, like any other type of occupation, attract an income which is dependent on the place of that occupation within the marketplace. The ideal professional occupation is associated with the possession of 'specialised skills rooted in a knowledge base founded upon abstract concepts and formal learning' (Crinson 2008: 253). Importantly, however, this expert body of knowledge and skills must be linked to an acceptance that the group who are best placed to regulate the use of this expertise are members of the profession itself and that the profession is trusted to police itself by the general public. The state then provides the legitimation and legal support required to ensure that only those with the required professional status are allowed to perform that particular occupation. This has the effect of providing members of the profession with an elevated status and a protected income stream by making the work that they do exclusive to them.

From this perspective, professionalism has very little to do with the duty that professionals have towards those that they serve. Professionalism here is about protecting the interests of professionals and securing status and economic position through establishing legitimate and legitimated social position. Larson (2013) describes this as setting up a monopoly or 'sheltered' market. Macdonald (1995) takes this further to suggest that the result of the establishment of a legitimate monopoly of skills and expertise is the 'exclusivization' of the occupation performed by the profession through:

- legislation
- permitting entry only through educational institutions
- a requirement of formal testing and regulation.

Macdonald (1995) goes on to suggest that knowledge and skills can be considered as cultural capital (Bourdieu 1986) when they allow access to an exclusive field of practice. This form of cultural capital brings with it both power and social status. It is also worth noting that the route to achieving the cultural capital in this case is through higher education, which itself is subject to inequality. In this way a profession may both seek to protect itself in its current form and control those who seek to enter the profession in the future, thus perpetuating existing power and class relations and maintaining the status quo.

Discussion Point

- Referring back to the brief history of dentistry provided in the previous section, reflect on how the development of dentistry as a profession might be understood as a process of establishing a monopoly of skills and expertise to ensure economic status and market position.
- What are the implications of this for patient care?

Once a profession has established itself, it may over the course of time get embroiled in jurisdictional boundary disputes as different professions vie for occupational territory (Abbott 1988). This can be seen in the recent work undertaken by the General Dental Council in fighting for the right for dentists to be the exclusive providers of tooth whitening and thus making it illegal for beauticians to provide the service. The General Dental Council states that they have a duty to ensure patient safety and that this can only be done if such treatments are provided by an appropriately qualified and regulated dental team. And yet it is worth noting that unregulated beauty salons routinely use peroxides on hair which are stronger than those used in home teeth-whitening kits. From this perspective, professionalism could be seen as inherently protectionist.

Thus, sociologists would suggest that a focus on professionalism and professional boundaries amongst dentists, at an organizational and regulatory level, if not so much amongst individual dentists them-selves, is as much to do with dentistry protecting itself and retaining a monopoly for dental practice, as it is in seeking to provide a quality standard of care for patients. Retaining the monopoly is essential if dentists wish to maintain their current income levels, and recent research by Crossley and Mubarik (2002), amongst others, shows that a high income is one of the most frequently cited criteria undergradu-ate dental students give as a reason for choosing to pursue a career in dentistry.

In summary, there is currently significant interest within the dental profession in being seen to display attributes of professionalism, yet there is not currently a universal definition of what these attributes are and how they might be measured in practice. One possible way of understanding the preoccupation with professionalism is as a means of protecting the monopoly on skills and expertise that gives dentistry its status – and the associated financial benefits – within society.

Dental services today

The role of dentists in society today, the perceptions that people have about oral health and dentists and the shape of dental provision can only be understood in light of the sociohistorical context in which dental care has developed. This chapter has sought to outline three

13

contextual strands which help us to understand where we are today. These are:

- Changing perceptions and media presentations of dentistry and dentists – which can be understood in relation to the development of the profession; improvements in technology, skills and materials (particularly pain relief techniques); and the emergence of cosmetic dentistry in relation to aesthetics and identity. Interpersonal skills and communication remain key areas of concern in relation to patient satisfaction, however, and are addressed in some detail in chapter 12.
- Different models of health service supply, which can be mapped to the historical development of dental care – taking dental care in the UK as an example, we have seen how the provision of care has moved from a market model to a professional model and then to a professional/bureaucratic model. The rise in private care and the associated fall in NHS dentistry suggests that we are now moving, inexorably, towards a professional/market model of care.
- The focus on professionalism and self-regulation within dentistry, which can be seen as a mechanism for protecting patients from poorly skilled or unscrupulous dentists and/or as a way of ensuring a market monopoly of dental care and maintaining prices.

The most recent research and policy documentation talks about the dental team (e.g. in the most recent guidance on dental education from the General Dental Council, 'Preparing for Practice – Dental Team Learning Outcomes for Registration, GDC 2011, which combined dental and allied outcomes for the first time) and explores issues around skill mix in the dental surgery. The suggestion is that the team approach will better meet the needs of patients, ensuring a more holistic approach to oral healthcare. There seems little doubt, however, that the dentists remain in charge. Indeed, allied professional groups – dental nurses, dental hygienists, dental therapists, orthodontic therapists, dental technicians and clinical dental technicians/denturists – are also required to register with the General Dental Council in order to practise. Again this can be seen as the desire to protect patients and/ or extend the monopoly of the professional/market model of dental healthcare, and is probably a mixture of the two.

Dentistry in a risk society

The final area to touch on briefly concerns the way dental care has changed over time. The history presented above shows the move from extractions to treatment and restoration to prevention. This ties in with the development of medical/dental knowledge and wider trends within medicine. In his seminal work on changing medical knowledge and paradigm shifts, Jewson (1976) suggested that the place of the patient

1. **Bedside Medicine** – pre-scientific medicine, the physician had a close relationship with the paying patient. This involved visiting the patient's home and understanding the complaints, symptoms and circumstances of each individual patient.
2. **Hospital Medicine** – at the birth of modern medicine the study of the physical body and build-up of case studies of normal and abnormal bodies was seen as key. Patients were removed from their home environment to the hospital, where their bodies could better be studied.
3. **Laboratory Medicine** – By the twentieth century the physical body was deemed less important than the underlying molecular processes that underlie normal functioning of the body. The patient's body and experiences became of secondary importance and diagnoses were made through the analysis of specimens and treated pharmacologically.
4. **Surveillance Medicine** – the success of biomedicine in treating infectious disease, the growth of population level surveys and the belief that health is not the same as an absence of disease created the conditions for surveillance medicine. Medicine is no longer solely interested in illness or disease but also in risks associated with poor health.

Figure 13.1 The four phases of medicine

in medicine can be charted across time. Jewson suggested three distinct phases shaped by medical knowledge, the medical gaze and the place of the patient. The fourth phase is a more contemporary addition, reflecting the emergence of surveillance medicine and the assessment of risk (Armstrong 1995). The four phases (drawn from Higgs 2008a) are presented in figure 13.1.

An analysis of the history of dental care suggests the same broad pattern can be seen, at least in relation to the move from direct clinical care to a focus on prevention and surveillance. Interestingly, however, the argument can be made that direct patient contact and physical examination remained at the heart of dental care and the move to laboratory medicine was less obvious – although clearly present in the use of X-rays and other diagnostic tools. Furthermore, the market relationship between dentists and their patients has remained, even in the era of NHS dentistry, through the co-payment system. The move towards surveillance dentistry is clear to see, in the large-scale population-level data that is collected on oral health, the wealth of research on the social determinants of oral health, the common risk factor approach to oral healthcare and the focus on prevention. Again, however, it can be argued that surveillance has long been a part of dentistry in a systematic way through recall appointments and the emphasis on routine dental check-ups and that medicine is only now catching up with this approach to healthcare.

13

In summary, medical/dental knowledge and the associated ways of practising have changed over time. In line with similar work in medicine, surveillance and public health dentistry are now established as the way forward as levels of decay, dental disease and edentulism fall and the focus becomes the maintenance of oral health rather than the treatment of oral disease.

A final word . . .

Being aware of the sociohistorical context within which the profession of dentistry has developed and changing public perceptions of dentists and dentistry may allow dentists and allied professionals to better understand the wider implications of the work that they do. Alongside this, the research presented in the previous chapters in this book help to build a picture not just of the wider context of oral health, taking a holistic approach to understanding patients, but also of individual factors and the implications of psychological research and models in better understanding patients' responses to, and perceptions of, dentistry.

References

Abbott, A. (1988) *The System of the Professions: An Essay on the Division of Expert Labour*. Chicago, IL: University of Chicago Press.

Acheson, D. (1998) *Independent Inquiry into Inequalities in Health*. London: The Stationery Office.

Ackernecht, E.W. (1947) The role of medical history in medical education. *Bulletin of the History of Medicine*, 21, 135–45.

Aday, L.A. and Andersen, R. (1974) A framework for the study of access to medical care. *Health Services Research*, 9, 208–20.

Adult Dental Health Survey 1998 (1998) London: The Stationery Office.

Adult Dental Health Survey 2009 (2009) Leeds: Health and Social Care Information Centre.

Age Concern Policy Unit (2008) The Age Agenda 2008. Available at: http://www.globalaging.org/elderrights/world/2008/ageagenda.pdf.

AgeUK (2013) Later life in the United Kingdom. Factsheet, updated monthly. Available at: AgeUK.org.uk

Agostoni, E., Frigerio, R. and Santoro, P. (2005) Atypical facial pain: clinical considerations and differential diagnosis. *Neurological Sciences*, s2, 71–4.

Ahmed, B., Gilthorpe, M. and Bedi, R. (2008) Agreement between normative and perceived orthodontic need amongst deprived multiethnic school children in London. *Clinical Orthodontics and Research*, 4, 65–71.

Ajzen, I. (1985) From intentions to actions: a theory of planned behavior. In Kuhland, J. and Beckman, J. (eds) *Action-Control: From Cognition to Behavior*. Heidelberg: Springer.

Albert, B. (2006) *In or Out of the Mainstream: Lessons from Research on Disability and Development Cooperation*. Leeds: Disability Press.

Alder, B., Porter, M., Abraham, C. and van Teijlingen, E. (2004) *Psychology and Sociology Applied to Medicine*. London: Churchill Livingstone.

Aleksejuniene, J., Holst, D., Eriksen, H.M. and Gjermo, P. (2002) Psychosocial stress, lifestyle and periodontal health. *Journal of Clinical Periodontology*, 29, 326–35.

Allen, F. (2003) Assessment of oral health related quality of life. *Health and Quality of Life Outcomes*, 1, 40.

Allison, P., Franco, E., Black, M. and Feine, J. (1998) The role of professional diagnostic delays in the prognosis of upper aerodigestive tract carcinoma. *Oral Oncology*, 34, 147–53.

Allison, P.J., Faulks, D. and Hennequin, M. (2001) Dentist-related barriers to treatment in a group of individuals with Down syndrome in

France: implications for dental education. *Journal of Disability and Oral Health*, 2, 18–26.

American Psychiatric Association (2000) *Diagnostic and Statistical Manual of Mental Disorders*, 4th rev. edn. Washington, DC: American Psychiatric Association.

Anantharaman, D., Marron, M., Lagiou, P. et al. (2011) Population attributable risk of tobacco and alcohol for upper aerodigestive tract cancer. *Oral Oncology*, 47, 725–31.

Andersen, B.L., Cacioppo, J.T. and Roberts, D.C. (1995) Delay in seeking a cancer diagnosis: Delay stages and psychophysiological comparison processes. *British Journal of Social Psychology*, 34, 33–52.

Andersen, R.M. (1995) Revisiting the behavioural model and access to medical care: does it matter? *Journal of Health and Social Behavior*, 36, 1–10.

Andersen, R.S., Paarup, B., Vedsted, P., Bro, F. and Soendergaard, J. (2010) 'Containment' as an analytical framework for understanding patient delay: a qualitative study of cancer patients' symptom interpretation processes. *Social Science & Medicine*, 71, 378–85.

Antoni, M., Wimberly, S., Lechner, S., Kazi, A., Sifre, T., Urcuyo, K. and Carver, C. (2006) Reduction of cancer-specific thought intrusions and anxiety symptoms with a stress management intervention among women undergoing treatment for breast cancer. *American Journal of Psychiatry*, 163, 1791–7.

Arber, S. and Ginn, J. (1993) Gender and inequalities in health in later life. *Social Science & Medicine*, 36, 33–46.

Armfield, J.M. (2010) Development and psychometric evaluation of the Index of Dental Anxiety and Fear (IDAF-4C+). *Psychological Assessment*, 22, 279–87.

Armfield, J.M., Slade, G.D. and Spencer, A.J. (2008) Cognitive vulnerability and dental fear. *BMC Oral Health*, 8, 2.

Armitage, C.J. and Conner, M. (2001) Efficacy of the theory of planned behaviour: a meta-analytic review. *British Journal of Social Psychology*, 40, 471–99.

Armstrong, D. (1995) The rise of surveillance medicine. *Sociology of Health and Illness*, 17, 393–404.

Asch, S.E. (1955) Opinions and social pressure. *Scientific American*, 193, 31–5.

Asimakopoulou, K. and Scambler, S. (2013) The role of information and choice in patient-centred care in diabetes: a hierarchy of patient-centredness. *European Diabetes Nursing*, 10, 58–62.

Awojobi, O., Scott, S.E. and Newton, T. (2012) Patients' perceptions of oral cancer screening in dental practice: a cross-sectional study. *BMC Oral Health*, 12, 55.

Babu, S., Bhat, R.V., Kumar, P.U., Sesikaran, B., Rao, K.V., Aruna, P. and Reddy, P.R. (1996) A comparative clinico-pathological study of oral submucous fibrosis in habitual chewers of pan masala and betelquid. *Journal of Toxicology and Clinical Toxicology*, 34, 317–22.

Bakri, I., Douglas, C.W. and Rawlinson, A. (2013) The effects of stress on periodontal treatment: a longitudinal investigation using clinical and biological markers. *Journal of Clinical Periodontology*, 40, 955–961.

Bandura, A. (1977) *Social Learning Theory*. Englewood Cliffs, NJ: Prentice-Hall.

Bandura, A. (1998) Health promotion from the perspective of social cognitive theory. *Psychology & Health*, 13, 623–49.

Barker, T. (1994) Role of health beliefs in patient compliance with preventive dental advice. *Community Dentistry and Oral Epidemiology*, 22, 327–30.

Barnard, H. and Turner, C. (2011) *Poverty and Ethnicity: A Review of the Evidence*. London: Joseph Rowntree Foundation.

Baron, R.A. and Byrne, D. (2003) *Social Psychology*. Boston, MA: Allyn and Bacon.

Barratt, J. (1997) The cost and availability of healthy food choices in Southern Derbyshire. *Journal of Human Nutrition and Dietetics*, 10, 63–9.

Barsky, A.J. and Borus, J.F. (1995) Somatization and medicalisation in the era of managed care. *Journal of the American Medical Association*, 274, 1931–4.

Bartlett, D. (1998) *Stress, Perspectives and Processes*. Buckingham: Open University Press.

Bartlett, E.E., Grayson, M., Barker, R., Levine, D.M., Golden, A. and Libber, S. (1984) The effects of physician communications skills on patient satisfaction; recall, and adherence. *Journal of Chronic Diseases*, 37, 755–64.

Bartlett, F. (1932) *Remembering*. Cambridge: Cambridge University Press.

Bartley, M. (2004) *Health Inequality: An Introduction to Theories, Concepts and Methods*. Cambridge: Polity.

Bartley, M. and Blane, D. (2008) Inequality and social class. In Scambler, G. (ed.) *Sociology as Applied to Medicine*, 6th edn. London: Elsevier.

Bedi, R., Lewsey, J.D. and Gilthorpe, M.S. (2000) Changes in oral health over ten years amongst UK children aged 4–5 years living in a deprived multiethnic area. *British Dental Journal*, 189, 88–92.

Bell, G., Large, D. and Barclay, S. (1999) Oral health care in diabetes mellitus. *Dental Update*, 26, 322–30.

Berggren, U. and Meynert, G. (1984) Dental fear and avoidance: causes symptoms and consequences. *Journal of American Dental Association*, 109, 247–51.

Berkman, L.F., Glass, T., Brissette, I. and Seeman, T.E. (2000) From social integration to health: Durkheim in the new millennium. *Social Science & Medicine*, 51, 843–57.

Bernstein, D., Kleinknecht, R. and Alexander, L. (1979) Antecedents of dental fear. *Journal of Public Health Dentistry*, 39, 113–24.

Beveridge Report (1942) Interdepartmental Committee on Social Insurance and Allied Services. Cmnd 6404. London: HMSO.

Bickenbach, J.E. (2009) Disability, culture and the UN Convention. *Disability and Rehabilitation*, 31, 1111–24.

Bickenbach, J.E. (2012) The International Classification of Functioning, Disability and Health and its relationship to disability studies. In Watson, N., Roulstone, A. and Thomas, C. (eds) *Routledge Handbook of Disability Studies*. London: Routledge, pp. 51–66.

Bickenbach, J.E., Chatterji, S., Badley, E.M. and Ustun, T.B. (1999) Models of disablement, universalism and the international classification of impairments, disabilities and handicaps. *Social Science & Medicine*, 48, 1173–87.

Bircher, J. (2005) Towards a dynamic definition of health and disease. *Medicine, Health Care and Philosophy*, 8, 335–41.

Black Report (1980) *Inequalities in Health: Report of a Research Working Group*. London: DHSS.

Bollard, M. (2002) Health promotion and learning disability. *Learning Disability Practice*, 5, 31–7.

Bond, J., Peace, S., Dittmann-Kohli, F. and Westerhof, G. (2007) *Aging in Society*, 3rd edn. London: Sage.

Bond, R. and Smith, P.B. (1996) Culture and conformity: a meta-analysis of studies using Asch's (1952, 1956) line judgment task. *Psychological Bulletin*, 119, 111–27.

Borreani, E., Wright, D., Scambler, S. and Gallagher, J. (2008) Minimising barriers to dental care in older people. *BMC Oral Health*, 8, 7.

Borreani, E., Jones, K., Scambler, S. and Gallagher J. (2010a) Informing the debate on oral healthcare for older people: a qualitative study of older people's views on oral health and oral healthcare. *Gerodontology*, 27, 11–18.

Borreani, E., Jones, K., Wright, D., Scambler, S. and Gallagher, J. (2010b) Improving access to dental care for older people. *Dental Update*, 37, 301–2.

Boundouki, G., Humphris, G. and Field, A. (2004) Knowledge of oral cancer, distress and screening intentions: longer term effects of a patient information leaflet. *Patient Education & Counseling*, 53, 71–7.

Bourdieu, P. (1986) The forms of capital. In Biggart, N.W. (ed.) *Readings in Economic Sociology*. Oxford: Blackwell Publishers, pp. 280–91.

Boyle, S. (2008) The health system in England. *Eurohealth*, 14, 1–2.

British Dental Association (2012a) Barber-surgeons and toothdrawers. Available at: https://www.bda.org/museum/the-story-of-dentistry/ancient-modern/barber-surgeons-and-toothdrawers

British Dental Association (2012b) The first dentists. Available at: https://www.bda.org/museum/the-story-of-dentistry/ancient-modern/the-first-dentists

British Dental Association (2012c) Development of the profession. Available at: https://www.bda.org/museum/the-story-of-dentistry/ancient-modern/development-of-the-profession

British Dental Association (2012d) Dentistry for all. Available at: https://www.bda.org/museum/the-story-of-dentistry/ancient-modern/dentistry-for-all

Broadbent, E. and Petrie, K.J. (2007) Symptom perception. In Ayers, S., Baum, A., McManus, C., Newman, S., Wallston, K., Weinman, J. and West, R. (eds) *Cambridge Handbook of Psychology, Health and Medicine*, 2nd edn. Cambridge: Cambridge University Press, pp. 219–23.

Brown, J.L. and Vanable, P.A. (2008) Cognitive–behavioral stress management interventions for persons living with HIV: a review and critique of the literature. *Annals of Behavioral Medicine*, 35, 26–40.

Brummett, B.H., Mark, D.B., Siegler, I.C., Williams, R.B., Babyak, M.A., Clapp-Channing, N.E. and Barefoot, J.C. (2005) Perceived social support as a predictor of mortality in coronary patients: effects of smoking, sedentary behaviour and depressive symptoms. *Psychosomatic Medicine*, 67, 40–5.

Buljevac, D., Hop, W.C., Reedeker, W., Janssens, A.C., van der Meche, F.G., van Doorn, P.A. and Hintzen, R.Q. (2003) Self-reported stressful life events and exacerbations in multiple sclerosis: prospective study. *British Medical Journal*, 328, 646.

Bunde, J. and Martin, R. (2006) Depression and prehospital delay in the context of myocardial infarction. *Psychosomatic Medicine*, 68, 51–7.

Burkhart, N.W., Burker, E.J., Burkes, E.J. and Wolfe, L. (1996) Assessing the characteristics of patients with oral lichen planus. *Journal of the American Dental Association*, 127, 648, 651–6.

Caldwell, M. and Miaskowski, C. (2002) Mass media interventions to reduce help-seeking delay in people with symptoms of acute myocardial infarction: time for a new approach? *Patient Education and Counseling*, 46, 1–9.

Calnan, M., Silvester, S., Manley, G. and Taylor-Gooby, P. (2000) Doing business in the NHS: exploring dentists' decisions to practise in the public and private sectors. *Sociology of Health & Illness*, 22, 742–64.

Cancer Research UK (2011) Oral cancer incidence statistics. Available at: http://info.cancerresearchuk.org/cancerstats/types/oral/incidence/

Cannon, W.B. (1914) The emergency function of the adrenal medulla in pain and the major emotions. *American Journal of Physiology*, 33, 356–72.

Care Quality Commission (2009) Statistics on accessing primary care. Available at: www.cqc.org.uk

Carlisle, L. (2015) The Gender Shift, the demographics of women in dentistry. What impact will it have? American Dental Association Survey Centre. Available at: http://www.spiritofcaring.com/public/488.cfm

Carstairs, V. and Morris, R. (1991) *Deprivation and Health in Scotland*. Aberdeen: Aberdeen University Press.

Chadwick, E. (1842) *Report on the Sanitary Condition of the Labouring Population of Great Britain*. Edinburgh: Edinburgh University Press.

Chandna, S. and Bathia, M. (2011) Oral manifestations of thyroid disorders and its management. *Indian Journal of Endocrinology and Metabolism*, 15, S113–16.

Charlton, J.I. (1998) *Nothing About Us Without Us: Disability, Oppression and Empowerment*. Berkeley, CA: University of California Press.

Chaudhary, S. (2004) Psychosocial stressors in oral lichen planus. *Australian Dental Journal*, 49, 192–5.

Chen, M. and Land, K.C. (1986) Testing the health belief model: LISREL analysis of alternative models of causal relationships between health beliefs and preventive dental behavior. *Social Psychology Quarterly*, 49, 45–60.

Cheng, C. and Cheung, M.W.L. (2005) Cognitive processes underlying coping flexibility: differentiation and integration. *Journal of Personality*, 73, 859–86.

Chesney, M., Folkman, S. and Chambers, D. (1996) Coping effectiveness training for men living with HIV: preliminary findings. *International Journal of STD & AIDS*, 7, 75–82.

Chida, Y. and Steptoe, A. (2009) Cortisol awakening response and psychosocial factors: a systematic review and meta-analysis. *Biological Psychology*, 80, 265–78.

Chida, Y. and Vedhara, K. (2009) Adverse psychosocial factors predict poorer prognosis in HIV disease: a meta-analytic review of prospective investigations. *Brain Behaviour and Immunity*, 23, 434–45.

Chida, Y., Hamer, M., Wardle, J. and Steptoe, A. (2008) Do stress-related psychosocial factors contribute to cancer incidence and survival? *Nature Clinical Practice Oncology*, 5, 466–75.

Christensen, L.B., Jeppe-Jensen, D. and Petersen, P.E. (2003) Self-reported gingival conditions and self-care in the oral health of Danish women during pregnancy. *Journal of Clinical Periodontology*, 30, 949–53.

Cioffi, D. (1991) Beyond attentional strategies: a cognitive-perceptual model of somatic information. *Psychological Bulletin*, 109, 25–41.

Cioffi, D. (1996) Making public the private: possible effects of expressing somatic experience. *Psychology & Health*, 11, 203–22.

Cohen, F., Kemeny, M.E., Kearney, K.A., Zegans, L.S., Neuhas, J.M. and Conant, M.A. (1999) Persistent stress as a predictor of genital herpes recurrence. *Archives of Internal Medicine*, 159, 2430–6.

Cohen, S. (2004) Social relationships and health. *American Psychologist*, 59, 676–84.

Cohen, S. (2005) Keynote Presentation at the Eight International Congress of Behavioural Medicine: the Pittsburgh common cold studies: psychosocial predictors of susceptibility to respiratory infectious illness. *International Journal of Behavioural Medicine*, 12, 123–31.

Cohen, S., Kamarack, T. and Mermelstein, R. (1983) A global measure of perceived stress. *Journal of Health and Social Behaviour*, 24, 385–96.

Cohen, S., Tyrrell, D.A.J. and Smith, A.P. (1991) Psychological stress and susceptibility to the common cold. *New England Journal of Medicine*, 325, 606–12.

Cohen, S., Tyrrell, D.A.J. and Smith, A.P. (1993) Negative life events, perceived stress, negative affect and susceptibility to the common cold. *Journal of Personality and Social Psychology*, 64, 131–40.

Cohen, S., Frank, E., Doyle, W.J., Skoner, D.P., Rabin, B.S. and Gwaltney, J.M. Jr. (1998) Types of stressors that increase susceptibility to the common cold in healthy adults. *Health Psychology*, 17, 214–23.

Cohen, S.M., Fiske, J. and Newton, J.T. (2000) The impact of dental anxiety on daily living, *British Dental Journal*, 189, 385–90.

Colgrove, J. (2002) The McKeown Thesis: A historical controversy and its enduring influence. *American Journal of Public Health*, 92, 725–9.

Comfort, A. (1960) Discussion session 1. Definition and universality of aging. In Strehler, L. (ed.) *The Biology of Aging*. Washington, DC: American Institute of Biological Sciences, pp. 3–13.

Committee on Quality of Healthcare in America (2001) *Crossing the Quality Chasm: A New Health System for the 21st Century*. Washington, DC: National Academies Press.

Conner, M. and Norman, P. (2005) *Predicting Health Behaviour*. London: Open University Press.

Corah, N. (1973) Effect of perceived control on stress reduction in pedodontic patients. *Journal of Dental Research*, 52, 1261–4.

Corner, J., Hopkinson, J. and Roffe, L. (2006) Experience of health changes and reasons for delay in seeking care: a UK study of the months prior to the diagnosis of lung cancer. *Social Science & Medicine*, 62, 1381–91.

Cornford, C.S. and Cornford, H.M. (1999) 'I'm only here because of my family': a study of lay referral networks. *British Journal of General Practice*, 49, 617–20.

Cornwell, J. (1984) *Hard-Earned Lives: Accounts of Health and Illness from East London*. London: Tavistock.

Costa, P.T. and McCrae, R.R. (1980) Somatic complaints in males as a function of age and neuroticism: a longitudinal analysis. *Journal of Behavioral Medicine*, 3, 245–57.

Coulson, N. and Buchanan, H. (2002) Student attendance at dental checkups: an application of the Transtheoretical Model. *Health Education Journal*, 61, 309–19.

Covello, V.T. and Peters, R.G. (2002) Women's perceptions of the risks of age-related diseases, including breast cancer: reports from a 3-year research study. *Health Communication*, 14, 377–95.

Covington, P. (1996) Women's oral health issues: an exploration of the literature. *Probe*, 30, 173–7.

Cracknell, R. and Gay, O. (2013) Women in Parliament: Making a Difference since 1918. Commons Briefing Papers RP13-65.

Craig, R. and Mindell, J. (eds) (2007) *Health Survey for England 2005: The Health of Older People.* London: Information Centre.

Crawford, R. (1987) Cultural influences on prevention and emergence of a new health consciousness. In Weinstein, N. (ed.) *Taking Care: Understanding and Encouraging Self-Protective Behaviour.* Cambridge: Cambridge University Press.

Crawford, A.N. and Lennon, M.A. (1992) Dental attendance patterns among mothers and their children in an area of social deprivation. *Community Dental Health,* 9, 289–94.

Crinson, I. (2008) The health professions. In Scambler, G. (ed.) *Sociology as Applied to Medicine,* 6th edn. London: Elsevier, pp. 252–64.

Crombie, I.K., Irvine, L., Elliott, L. and Wallace, H. (2005) *Closing the Health Inequalities Gap: An International Perspective.* Copenhagen: World Health Organisation Regional Office for Europe.

Croog, S., Baume, R. and Nalbandian, J. (1994) Pain response after psychological preparation for periodontal surgery. *Journal of American Dental Association,* 125, 1353–60.

Crossley, M.L. and Mubarik, A. (2002) A comparative investigation of dental and medical student's motivation towards career choice. *British Dental Journal,* 193, 471–3.

Croucher, R., Marcenes, W.S., Torres, M.C., Hughes, F. and Sheiham A. (1997) The relationship between life-events and periodontitis: a case-control study. *Journal of Clinical Periodontoly,* 24, 39–43.

Croyle, R.T. and Sande, G.N. (1988) Denial and confirmatory search: paradoxical consequences of medical diagnosis. *Journal of Applied Social Psychology,* 18, 473–90.

Cumella, S., Ransford, N., Lyons, J. and Burnham, H. (2000) Need for oral care among people with intellectual disability not in contact with community dental services. *Journal of Intellectual Disability Research,* 44, 45–52.

Cummings, E. and Henry, W.E. (1961) *Growing Old: The Process of Disengagement.* New York: Basic Books.

Dahl, K.E., Wang, N.J. and Ohrn, K. (2012) Does oral health matter in people's daily life? Oral health-related quality of life in adults 35–47 years of age in Norway. *International Journal of Dental Hygiene,* 10, 15–21.

Dahlgren, G. and Whitehead, M. (1991) Policies and strategies to promote social equity in health. Stockholm: Institute of Futures Studies.

Daly, B., Watt, R., Batchelor, P. and Treasure, E. (2002) *Essential Dental Public Health.* Oxford: Oxford University Press.

Davey Smith, G., Bartley, M. and Blane, D. (1990) The Black Report on socioeconomic inequalities in health 10 years on. *British Medical Journal,* 301, 373–7.

Davidson, P., Rams, T.E. and Andersen, R.M. (1997) Socio-behavioural determinants of oral hygiene practices among USA ethnic and age groups. *Advancing Dental Research*, 11, 245–53.

de Jongh, A. and Ter Horst, G. (1993) What do anxious patients think? An exploratory investigation of anxious dental patients' thoughts. *Community Dentistry & Oral Epidemiology*, 21, 221–3.

de Jongh, A., Muris, P., Ter Horst, G., Van Zuuren, F.J. and De Wit, C. (1994) Cognitive correlates of dental anxiety. *Journal of Dental Research*, 73, 561–6.

de Nooijer, J., Lechner, L., Candel, M. and de Vries, H. (2004) Short- and long-term effects of tailored information versus general information on determinants and intentions related to early detection of cancer. *Preventive Medicine*, 38, 694–703.

de Zwart, F. (2000) The logic of affirmative action: caste, class and quotas in India. *Acta Sociologica*, 43, 235–49.

Department for Business, Enterprise and Regulatory Reform. Employment Market Analysis and Research (2010) *Fair Treatment at Work Survey, 2008*. [data collection]. UK Data Service. SN: 6382. Available at: http://dx.doi.org/10.5255/UKDA-SN-6382-1.

Department of Education (2011) *National Pupil Database 2010–11*. London: Department of Education.

Department of Health (1994) *An Oral Health Strategy for England*. London: Department of Health.

Department of Health (1999) *Our Healthier Nation – Reducing Health Inequalities: An Action Report*. London: Department of Health.

Department of Health (2000a) *National Service Framework for Coronary Heart Disease: Modern Standards and Service Models*. London: Department of Health.

Department of Health (2000b) *The NHS Plan*. London: Department of Health.

Department of Health (2000c) *Modernising NHS Dentistry: Implementing the NHS Plan*. London: Department of Health.

Department of Health (2003) *Tackling Health Inequalities: A Programme for Action*. London: Department of Health.

Department of Health (2005) *Choosing Better Oral Health: An Oral Health Plan for England*. London: Department of Health.

Department of Health (2007) *Valuing Oral Health: A Good Practice Guide for Improving the Oral Health of Disabled Children and Adults*. London: Department of Health.

Department of Health (2008) *National NHS Patient Survey Programme: Survey of Adult Inpatients 2008*. London: Department of Health.

Department of Health (2010) *Fair Society, Healthy Lives: A Strategic Review of Health Inequalities in England Post-2010*. London: Department of Health.

Department of Health (2012) *Liberating the NHS: No Decision About Me Without Me*. London: Department of Health.

Department of Health (2014) *Delivering Better Oral Health: An Evidence-Based Toolkit for Prevention.* London: Public Health England.

Department of Health, Social Services and Public Safety (2004) Dental Branch Annual Report 2003/2004. Available at: http://www.dhs spsni.gov.uk/dental-report03-04.pdf.

Department for Work and Pensions (2011) Households below average income: an analysis of the income distribution 1994/95–2009/10. London: DWP.

Department for Work and Pensions (2012) *Family Resources Survey, UK, 2010–11.* Available at: http://research.dwp.gov.uk/asd/frs/.

Descartes, R. (1986) *A Discourse on Method: Meditations and Principles.* Guernsey: Everyman Classic.

Dhawan, N. and Bedi, R. (2001) Transcultural oral health care: 6. The oral health of minority ethnic groups in the United Kingdom – a review. *Dental Update*, 28, 30–4.

Dickerson, S.S. (2008) Emotional and physiological responses to social evaluative threat. *Social and Personality Psychology Compass*, 213, 1362–78.

Di Matteo, M.R. (2004) Variations in patients' adherence to medical reccomendations: a quantitative review of 50 years of research. *Medical Care*, 42, 200–9.

DiMatteo, M.R., McBride, C.A., Shugars, D.A. and O'Neil, E.H. (1995) Public attitudes towards dentists: a US household survey. *Journal of the American Dental Association*, 126, 1563–70.

Doblhammer, G. and Kytir, J. (2001) Compression or expansion of morbidity? Trends in healthy-life expectancy in the elderly Austrian population between 1978 and 1998. *Social Science & Medicine*, 52, 385–91.

Dohrenwend, B.P. (2006) Inventorying stressful life events as risk factors for psychopathology: toward resolution of the problem of intracategory variability. *Psychological Bulletin*, 132, 477–95.

Dolan, T. (1993) Identification of appropriate outcomes for an ageing population. *Special Care in Dentistry*, 13, 35–9.

Dougall, A. and Fiske, J. (2008) Access to special care dentistry, part 1. Access. *British Dental Journal*, 204, 605–16.

Downer, M. (1994) Caries prevalence in the UK. *International Dental Journal*, 176, 209–14.

Drever, F. and Whitehead, M. (eds) (1999) *Health Inequalities*. London: The Stationery Office.

Eadie, D., MacKintosh, A.M., MacAskill, S. and Brown A. (2009) Development and evaluation of an early detection intervention for mouth cancer using a mass media approach. *British Journal of Cancer*, 101, S73–S79.

Edwards, D.M. and Merry, A.J. (2002) Disability Part 2: Access to dental services for disabled people: a questionnaire survey of dental practices in Merseyside. *British Dental Journal*, 193, 253–5.

Edwards, J., Palmer, G., Osbourne, N. and Scambler, S. (2013) Why individuals with HIV or diabetes do not disclose their medical history to the dentist: a qualitative analysis. *British Dental Journal*, 215, E10.

Elstad, J. (1998) The psycho-social perspective on social inequalities in health. *Sociology of Health and Illness*, 20, 598–618.

Engel, G.L. (1977) The need for a new medical model: a challenge for biomedicine. *Science*, 196, 129–36.

Enkling, N., Marwinski, G. and Johren, P. (2006) Dental anxiety in a representative sample of residents of a large German city. *Clinical Oral Investigations*, 10, 84–91.

ESRC Centre on Dynamics of Ethnicity (2013a) Ethnic inequalities in labour market participation. In *Dynamics of Diversity: Evidence from the 2011 Census*. Manchester: University of Manchester and Joseph Rowntree Foundation.

ESRC Centre on Dynamics of Ethnicity (2013b) Which ethnic groups have the poorest health? Ethnic health inequalities 1991 to 2011. In *Dynamics of Diversity: Evidence from the 2011 Census*. Manchester: University of Manchester and Joseph Rowntree Foundation.

Everson, S.A., Kauhanen, J., Kaplan, G.A., Goldberg, D.E., Julkunen, J., Tuomilehto, J. and Salonen, J.T. (1997) Hostility and increased risk of mortality and acute myocardial infarction: the mediating role of behavioural risk factors. *American Journal of Epidemiology*, 146, 142–52.

Ewles, L. and Simnett, I. (1999) *Promoting Health: A Practical Guide*. London: Bailliere Tindall.

Feldman, P.J., Cohen, S., Lepore, S.J., Matthews, K.A., Kamarck, T.W. and Marsland, A.L. (1999) Negative emotions and acute physiological responses to stress. *Annals of Behavioural Medicine*, 21, 216–22.

Feldner, M.T. and Hekmat, H. (2001) Perceived control over anxiety-related events as a predictor of pain behaviours in a cold pressor task. *Journal of Behaviour Therapy & Experimental Psychology*, 32, 191–202.

Finch, H., Keegan, J. and Ward, K. (1988) *Barriers to the Receipt of Dental Care – A Qualitative Research Study*. London: Social and Community Planning Research.

Finestone, H.M., Alfeeli, A. and Fisher, W.A. (2008) Stress-induced physiologic changes as a basis for the biopsychosocial model of chronic musculoskeletal pain: a new theory? *The Clinical Journal of Pain*, 24, 767–75.

Finkelstein, V. (1993) Disability: a social challenge or an administrative responsibility? In J. Swain, J., Finkelstein, V., French, S. and Oliver, M. (eds) *Disabling Barriers – Enabling Environments*. London: Sage.

Fiske J. (2006) Special care dentistry. *British Dental Journal*, 200, 61.

Fiske, S. and Taylor, S.E. (1991) *Social Cognition*. New York: McGraw-Hill.

Fitzpatrick, R. (2008) Society and changing patterns of disease. In Scambler, G. (ed.) *Sociology As Applied to Medicine*, 6th edn. London: Elsevier, pp. 3–17.

Floyd, D.L., Prentice-Dunn, S. and Rogers, R.W. (2000) A meta-analysis of research on protection motivation theory. *Journal of Applied Social Psychology*, 30, 407–29.

Folkins, C.H., Lawson, K.D., Opton Jr, E.M. and Lazarus, R.S. (1968) Desensitization and the experimental reduction of threat. *Journal of Abnormal Psychology*, 73, 100–13.

Fox, C. and Newton, J.T. (2006) A controlled trial of the impact of exposure to positive images of dentistry on anticipatory dental fear in children. *Community Dentistry Oral Epidemiology*, 34, 455–9.

Freeman, R., Main, J.R. and Burke, F.J. (1995) Occupational stress and dentistry: theory and practice. Part I. Recognition. *British Dental Journal*, 178, 214–17.

Freidson, E. (2001) *Professionalism, the Third Logic.* Chicago, IL: University of Chicago Press.

Freire, M., Sheiham, A. and Hardy, R. (2001) Adolescents' sense of coherence, oral health status, and oral health related behaviours. *Community Dentistry and Oral Epidemiology*, 29, 204–12.

Freire, M., Hardy, R. and Sheiham, A. (2002) Mothers' sense of coherence and their adolescent children's oral health status and behaviours. *Community Dental Health*, 19, 24–31.

French, T., Weiss L., Waters, M., Tesoriero, J., Finkelstein, R. and Agins, B. (2005) Correlation of a brief perceived stress measure with nonadherence to antiretroviral therapy over time. *Journal of Acquired Immune Deficiency Syndrome*, 38, 590–7.

French, T., Tesoriero, J. and Agins, B. (2011) Changes in stress, substance use and medication beliefs are associated with changes in adherence to HIV antiretroviral therapy. *AIDS and Behavior*, 15, 1416–28.

Frere, C.L., Crout, R., Yorty, J. and McNeil, D.W. (2001) Effects of audiovisual distraction during dental prophylaxis. *Journal of the American Dental Association*, 132, 1031–8.

Fries, J.F. (1980) Aging, natural death, and the compression of morbidity. *New England Journal of Medicine*, 303, 130–5.

Fujimori, M. and Uchitomi, Y. (2009) Preferences of cancer patients regarding communication of bad news: a systematic literature review. *Japanese Journal of Clinical Oncology*, 39, 201–16.

Galipeault, J.P. (2003) as cited in Townsend, E. (2003) Reflections on power and justice in enabling occupation. *The Canadian Journal of Occupational Therapy*, 70, 74–157.

Gallagher, J.E. and Fiske, J. (2007) Special care dentistry: a professional challenge. *British Dental Journal*, 202, 619–29.

General Dental Council (2008) GDC opens new Specialist List in Special Care Dentistry. 5 October. Available at: http://www.odonti.com/dental-professionals/news/uk-gdc-opens-new-specialist-list-in-special-care-dentistry/tn-p--4.html

General Dental Council (2011) Preparing for Practice – Dental Team Learning Outcomes for Registration. Available at: https://www.gdc-uk.org/Newsandpublications/Publications/Publications/GDC%20Learning%20Outcomes.pdf.

General Dental Council (2013) Annual report and accounts 2013. Available at: http://www.gdc-uk.org/Newsandpublications/Publications/Publications/GDC%20AR%202013%20FINAL%20WEB.pdf

General Household Survey (2005) London: Office of Population Censuses and Surveys.

Gideon (2013) What society thinks you do. Dental Buzz, 11 September. Available at: http://www.dentalbuzz.com/2013/09/11/what-society-thinks-you-do/

Gijsbers van Wijk, C.M.T. and Kolk, A.M. (1997) Sex differences in physical symptoms: the contribution of symptom perception theory. *Social Science & Medicine*, 45, 231–46.

Gijsbers van Wijk, C.M.T., Huisman, H. and Kolk, A.M. (1999) Gender differences in physical symptoms and illness behavior: a health diary study. *Social Science & Medicine*, 49, 1061–74.

Glaser, R. (2005) Stress associated immune dysregulation and its importance for human health: a personal history of psychoneuro-immunology. *Brain, Behaviour and Immunity*, 19, 3–11.

Glaser, R. and Kiecolt-Glaser, J. (2005) Stress-induced immune dysfunction: implications for health. *Nature Reviews Immunology*, 5, 243–51.

Godfrey, H. (2005) Understanding pain, part 1: Physiology of pain. *British Journal of Nursing*, 14, 846–52.

Godson, J.H. and Williams, S.A. (1996) Oral health and related behaviours among three year old children born to first and second generation Pakistani mothers in Bradford, UK. *Community Dental Health*, 13, 27–33.

Gollwitzer, P.M. (1993) Goal achievement: the role of intentions. *European Review of Social Psychology*, 4, 141–85.

Goss, N. (2007) Editorial. *Journal of Disability and Oral Health*, 8, 98.

Gray, M., Morris, A.J. and Davies, J. (2000) The oral health of South Asian five-year-old children in deprived areas of Dudley compared with White children of equal deprivation and fluoridation status. *Community Dental Health*, 17, 243–5.

Greenbaum, P.E., Turner, C., Cook, E.W. and Melamed, B.G. (1990) Dentists' voice control: effects on children's disruptive and affective behaviour. *Health Psychology*, 9, 546–58.

Grimsby, G., Finstam, J. and Jette, A. (1988) On the application of the WHO handicap classification in rehabilitation. *Scandinavian Journal of Rehabilitation Medicine*, 20, 93–8.

Haefner, D.P. (1974) The health belief model and preventive dental behavior. In Becker, M.H. (ed.), *The Health Belief Model and Personal Health Behavior*. Thorofare, NJ: C.B. Slack, pp. 93–105.

Hafferty, F.W. and Levinson, D. (2008) Moving beyond nostalgia and motives: towards a complexity science view of medical professionalism. *Perspectives in Biology and Medicine*, 51, 599–615.

Hall, M., Baum, A., Buysse, D., Prigerson, H.G., Kupfer, D.J. and Reynolds, C.F. (1998) Sleep as a mediator of the stress-immune relationship. *Psychosomatic Medicine*, 60, 48–51.

Hallberg, U. and Klingberg, G. (2005) Medical health care professionals' assessments of oral health needs in children with disabilities: a qualitative study. *European Journal of Oral Sciences*, 113, 363–8.

Hancock, M., Calnan, M. and Manley, G. (1999) Private or NHS General Dental Service care in the United Kingdom? A study of public perceptions and experiences. *Journal of Public Health Medicine*, 21, 415–20.

Haralambos, M. and Holborn, M. (2000) Social stratification. In Haralambos, M. and Holborn, M. (eds) *Sociology: Themes and Perspectives*. London: Collins, pp. 22–126.

Hardeman, W., Johnston, M., Johnston, D., Bonetti, D., Wareham, N. and Kinmonth, A.L. (2002) Application of the theory of planned behaviour in behaviour change interventions: a systematic review. *Psychology & Health*, 17, 123–58.

Haynes, R.B., Taylor, D.W. and Sackett, D.L. (1979) *Compliance in Health Care*. Baltimore, MD: Johns Hopkins University Press.

Health Committee Publication (2008) Health – Fifth Report. Available at: http://www.publications.parliament.uk/pa/cm200708/cmselect/cmhealth/289/28902.htm

Health and Social Care Information Centre (HSIC) (2012) *NHS Dental Statistics for England: 2011–2012*. London: HSIC. Available at www.hscic.gov.uk/catalogue/PUB07163

Health Poverty Action Group (2014) The Determinants of Health: Factors that Determine Good or Poor Health. Available at: http://www.healthpovertyaction.org/policy-and-resources/the-determinants-of-health/

Hedges, J.R., Mann, N.C., Meischke, H., Robbins, M., Goldberg, R. and Zapka, J. (1998) Assessment of chest pain onset and out-of-hospital delay using standardized interview questions: The REACT Pilot Study. Rapid Early Action for Coronary Treatment (REACT) Study Group. *Academic Emergency Medicine*, 5, 773–80.

Heider, F. (1958) *The Psychology of Interpersonal Relations*. New York: John Wiley & Sons.

Helgesson, O., Cabrera, C., Lapidus, L., Bengtsson, C. and Lissner, L. (2003) Self-reported stress levels predict subsequent breast cancer in a cohort of Swedish women. *European Journal of Cancer Prevention*, 12, 377–81.

Higgs, P. (2008a) The limits and boundaries to medical knowledge. In Scambler, G. (ed.) *Sociology as Applied to Medicine*, 6th edn. London: Elsevier, pp. 193–204.

Higgs, P. (2008b) Later life, health and society. In Scambler, G. (ed.) *Sociology as Applied to Medicine*, 6th edn. London: Elsevier, pp. 176–90.

Hill, K.B., White, D.A., Morris, A.J., Hall, A.C, Goodwin, N. and Burke, F.J. (2003) National evaluation of personal dental services: a qualitative investigation into patients' perceptions of dental services. *British Dental Journal*, 195, 654–6.

Hill, K.B., Chadwick, B., Freeman, R., O'Sullivan, I. and Murray, J.J. (2013) Adult Dental Health Survey 2009: relationships between dental attendance patterns, oral health behaviour and the current barriers to dental care. *British Dental Journal*, 214, 25–32.

Hills, J., Brewer, M., Jenkins, S., Lister, R., Lupton, R., Machin, S., Mills, C., Modood, T., Rees, T. and Riddell, S. (2010) *An Anatomy of Economic Inequality in the UK: Report of the National Equality Panel*. London: Government Equalities Office/Centre for Analysis of Social Exclusion.

Holmes, T.H. and Rahe, R.H. (1967) The social readjustment rating scale. *Journal of Psychosomatic Research*, 11, 213–18.

Holtzman, J.M., Berkey, A.B. and Mann, J. (1990) Predicting utilization of dental services by the aged. *Journal of Public Health Dentistry*, 50, 164–71.

Home Office (2011) British Crime Survey 2010–11. London: Home Office.

Honkala, S. and Al-Ansari, J. (2005) Self-reported oral health, oral hygiene habits, and dental attendance of pregnant women in Kuwait. *Journal of Clinical Periodontology*, 32, 809–14.

Hughes, B. and Paterson, K. (1997) The social model of disability and the disappearing body: towards a sociology of impairment. *Disability and Society*, 12, 325–40.

Hull, P. and Humphris, G. (2010) Anxiety reduction via brief intervention in dentally anxious patients: a randomised controlled trial. *Social Science & Dentistry*, 1, 108–17.

Humphrey, C. (1999) *Population Studies Course Book, Sociology*. Royal Free & University College Medical School.

Humphris, G.M. and Ling, M.S. (2000) *Behavioural Sciences for Dentistry*. Edinburgh: Churchill Livingstone.

Humphris, G.M., Mair, L., Lee, G.T.R. and Birch, R.H. (1991) Dental anxiety, pain and uncooperative behaviour in child dental patients. *Anxiety Research*, 4, 61–77.

Humphris, G.M., Morrison, T. and Lindsay, S.J.E. (1995) The Modified Dental Anxiety Scale: UK norms and evidence for validity. *Community Dental Health*, 12, 143–50.

Humphris, G.M., Blinkhorn, A., Freeman, R., Gorter, R., Hoad-Reddick, G., Murtomaa, H., O'Sullivan, R. and Splieth, C. (2002) Psychological stress in undergraduate dental students: baseline results from seven European dental schools. *European Journal of Dental Education*, 6, 22–9.

Humphris, G.M., Clarke, H.M. and Freeman, R. (2006) Does completing a dental anxiety questionnaire increase anxiety? A randomised controlled trial with adults in general dental practice. *British Dental Journal*, 201, 33–35.

Hussain, A. and Khan, F.A. (2014) History of dentistry. *Archives of Medicine & Health Sciences*, 2, 106–10.

ICM Research (2008) *Pain and Dignity Survey*. London: ICM.

International Women's Democracy Centre (2008a) A timeline of women's suffrage for selected countries. Available at: http://www.iwdc.org/resources/suffrage.htm

International Women's Democracy Centre (2008b) Fact sheet: Women's political participation. Available at: http://www.iwdc.org/resources/fact_sheet.htm

Inzucchi, S.E., Bergenstal, R.M., Buse, J.B., Diamant, M., Ferrannini, E., Nauck, M., Peters, A.L., Tsapas, A., Wender, R. and Matthews, D.R. (2012) Management of hyperglycaemia in type 2 diabetes: a patient-centered approach. Position statement of the American Diabetes Association (ADA) and the European Association for the Study of Diabetes (EASD). *Diabetologia*, 55, 1577–96.

Iso, H., Date, C., Yamamoto, A., Toyoshima, H., Tanabe, N., Kikuchi, S., Kondo, T., Watanabe, Y., Wada, Y., Ishibashi, T., Suzuki, H., Koizumi, A., Inaba, Y., Tamakoshi, A. and Ohno, Y. (2002) Perceived mental stress and mortality from cardiovascular disease among Japanese men and women. *Circulation*, 106, 1229–36.

Jackson, C. and Lindsay, S. (1995) Reducing anxiety in new dental patients by means of a leaflet. *British Dental Journal*, 179, 163–7.

Jackson, E. (1978) Patients' perceptions of dentistry. In Weinstein, P. (ed.) *Advances in Behavioral Research in Dentistry*. Seattle, WA: University of Washington, Department of Community Dentistry.

Jacobsen, J. and Jackson, V.A. (2009) A communication approach for oncologists: understanding patient coping and communicating about bad news, palliative care, and hospice. *Journal of the National Comprehensive Cancer Network*, 7, 475–80.

JACSCD (2003) *A Case of Need: Special Care Dentistry*. London: Joint Advisory Committee for Special Care Dentistry.

Janssens, T., Verleden, G., De Peuter, S., Van Diest, I. and Van den Bergh, O. (2009) Inaccurate perception of asthma symptoms: a cognitive-affective framework and implications for asthma treatment. *Clinical Psychology Review*, 29, 317–27.

Jarman, B. (1983) Identification of underprivileged areas. *British Medical Journal*, 286, 1705–8.

Jarvis, M. and Wardle, J. (2006) Social patterning of individual health behaviours: the case of cigarette smoking. In Marmot, M. and Wilkinson, R. (eds) *Social Determinants of Health*. Oxford: Oxford University Press, pp. 224–37.

Jensen, M., Brant-Zawadzki, M., Obuchowski, N., Modic, M.T., Malkasian, D. and Ross, J.S. (1994) Magnetic resonance imaging of the lumbar spine in people without back pain. *The New England Journal of Medicine*, 331, 69–73.

Jewson, N. (1976) The disappearance of the sick man from medical cosmology. *Sociology*, 10, 225–44.

Johnson, R. and Baldwin, D.C. (1968) Relationship of maternal anxiety to the behaviour of young children undergoing dental extraction. *Journal of Dental Research*, 47, 801–5.

Jones, C.J., Smith, H. and Llewellyn, C. (2014) Evaluating the effectiveness of health belief model interventions in improving adherence: a systematic review. *Health Psychology Review*, 8, 253–69.

Jones, E.E. and Davis, K.E. (1965) From acts to dispositions: the attribution process in social psychology. In Berkowitz, K.E. (ed.) *Advances in Experimental Social Psychology*. New York: Academic Press.

Jones, E.E. and Harris, V.A. (1967) The attribution of attitudes. *Journal of Experimental Social Psychology*, 3, 1–24.

Jones, E.E. and Nisbett, R.E. (1971) *The Actor and the Observer: Divergent Perceptions of the Causes of Behavior*. New York: General Learning Press.

Judge, K., Mulligan, J. and New, B. (1997) The NHS: new prescriptions needed? In Jowell, R., Curtice, J., Park, A., Brook, L., Thompson, K. and Bryson, C. (eds) *British Social Attitudes: 14th Report*. Aldershot: Ashgate.

Kagan, J. and Havemann, E. (1976) *Psychology: An Introduction*. New York: Harcourt Brace Jovanovich.

Kainth, A., Hewitt, A., Sowden, A., Duffy, S., Pattenden, J., Lewin, R., Watt, I. and Thompson, D. (2004) Systematic review of interventions to reduce delay in patients with suspected heart attack. *Emergency Medicine Journal*, 21, 506–8.

Kaplan, J.R., Pettersson, K., Manuck, S.B. and Olsson, G. (1991) Role of sympathoadrenal medullary activation in the initiation and progression of atherosclerosis. *Circulation*, 84, 23–32.

Kasl, S.V. (1987) Methodologies in stress and health: past difficulties, present dilemmas and future directions. In Kasl, S.V. and Cooper, C.L. (eds) *Stress and Health: Issues in Research Methodology*. Chichester: John Wiley & Sons, pp. 307–18.

Kaur, R., Lopez, V. and Thompson, D.R. (2006) Factors influencing Hong Kong Chinese patients' decision making in seeking early treatment for acute myocardial infarction. *Research in Nursing & Health*, 29, 636–46.

Kaye, J. and Lightman, S. (2005) Psychological stress and endocrine axes. In Vedhara, K. and Irwin, M. (eds) *Human Psychoneuroimmunology*. New York: Oxford University Press, pp. 25–52.

Kegeles, S.S. (1963) Why people seek dental care: a test of a conceptual formulation. *Journal of Health and Human Behavior*, 4, 166–73.

Kelley, H.H. (1973) The process of causal attribution. *American Psychologist*, 28, 108–28.

Kemeny, M.E. and Schedlowski, M. (2007) Understanding the interaction between psychological stress and immune-related diseases: a stepwise progression. *Brain Behaviour and Immunity*, 21, 1009–18.

Kenny, D.T. (2007) Stress management. In Ayers, S., Baum, A., McManus, C., Newman, S., Wallston, K., Weinman, J. and West, R. (eds) *Cambridge Handbook of Psychology, Health and Medicine*. Cambridge: Cambridge University Press, pp. 403–7.

Kent, G. and Croucher, R. (1998) *Achieving Oral Health: The Social Context of Dental Care*, 3rd edn. Oxford: Wright (Reed Educational & Professional Publishing).

Kessels, R.P. (2003) Patients' memory for medical information. *Journal of the Royal Society of Medicine*, 96, 219–22.

Kiecolt-Glaser, J.K. and Glaser, R. (1988) Methodological issues in behavioural immunology research with humans. *Brain, Behaviour and Immunity*, 2, 67–78.

Kiecolt-Glaser, J.K., Marucha, P.T., Malarkey, W.B., Mercado, A.M. and Glaser, R. (1995) Slowing of wound healing by psychological stress. *The Lancet*, 346, 1194–6.

Kiecolt-Glaser, J.K., Loving, T.J., Stowell, J.R., Malarkey, W.B., Lemeshow, S., Dickinson, S.L. and Glaser, R. (2005) Hostile marital interactions, proinflammatory cytokine production and wound healing. *Archives of General Psychiatry*, 62, 1377–84.

Kirsh, I. (2007) Placebos. In Ayers, S., Baum, A., McManus, C., Newman, S., Wallston, K., Weinman, J. and West, R. (eds) *Cambridge Handbook of Psychology, Health and Medicine*, 2nd edn. Cambridge: Cambridge University Press.

Koch, R. (1882) Die Atiologic der Tuberkulose. *Berliner Klinische Wochenschrift*, 15, 221–30.

Kolk, A., Hanewald, G., Schagen, S. and Gijsbers van Wijk, C. (2003) A symptom perception approach to common physical symptoms. *Social Science & Medicine*, 57, 2343–54.

Komaroff, A.L. (2001) Symptoms: in the head or in the brain? *Annals of Internal Medicine*, 134, 783–5.

Korte, S.M., Koolhaas, J.M., Wingfield, J.C. and McEwen, B.S. (2005) The Darwinian concept of stress: benefits of allostasis and costs of allostatic load and the trade-offs in health and disease. *Neuroscience and Biobehavioural Reviews*, 29, 3–38.

Kotecha, M., Arthur, S., Coutinho, S., Bartlett, A., Frew, C., Gilroy, J. and Lisa Taylor, L. (2013) *Understanding Pensioner Poverty and Material Deprivation – A Synthesis of Findings*. London: DWP.

Kriegbaum, M., Christensen, U., Lund, R., Prescott, E. and Osler, M. (2008) Job loss and broken partnerships: do the number of stressful life events influence the risk of ischemic heart disease in men? *Annals of Epidemiology*, 18, 743–5.

Krieger, N. (2001) A glossary of social epidemiology. *Journal of Epidemiology and Community Health*, 55, 693–700.

Kriesberg, L. and Treiman, B.R. (1962) Dentists and the practice of dentistry as viewed by the public. *Journal of the American Dental Association*, 64, 58–73.

Kritsidima, M., Newton, T. and Asimakopoulou, K. (2010) The effects of lavender scent on dental patient anxiety levels: a cluster randomised controlled trial. *Community Dentistry and Oral Epidemiology*, 38, 83–7.

Kudielka, B.M., Buske-Kirschbaum, A., Hellhammer, D.H. and Kirschbaum, C. (2004) HPA axis responses to laboratory psychosocial stress in healthy elderly adults, younger adults and children: impact of age and gender. *Psychoneuroendocrinology*, 29, 83–98.

Kuhner, M.K. and Raetzke, P.B. (1989) The effect of health beliefs on the compliance of periodontal patients with oral hygiene instructions. *Journal of Periodontology*, 60, 51–6.

Labonté, R. (1993) Health promotion and empowerment: practice frameworks. Issues in Health Promotion no 3. Centre for Health Promotion, University of Toronto.

Lahmann, C., Schoen, R., Henningsen, P., Ronel, J., Muehlbacher, M., Loew, T., Tritt, K., Nickel, M. and Doering, S. (2008) Brief relaxation versus music distraction in the treatment of dental anxiety: a randomized controlled clinical trial. *Journal of American Dental Association*, 139, 317–24.

Lahti, S., Tuutti, H., Hausen, H. and Kaariainen, R. (1992) Dentist and patient opinions about the ideal dentist and patient – developing a compact questionnaire. *Community Dentistry and Oral Epidemiology*, 20, 229–34.

Langan, M. (1998) The contested concept of need. In Langan, M. (ed.) *Welfare: Needs, Rights and Risks*. London: Routledge, pp. 3–37.

Langford, A. and Johnson, B. (2009) Social inequalities in adult female mortality by the National Statistics Socio-economic Classification, England and Wales, 2001–03. *Health Statistics Quarterly*, 42.

Larson, M.S. (2013) *The Rise of Profesionalism: Monopolies of Competence and Sheltered Markets*. New Brunswick, NJ: Transaction Publishers.

Laslett, P. (1989) *A Fresh Map of Life: The Emergence of the Third Age*. London: Weidenfeld and Nicolson.

Lautch, H. (1971) Dental phobia. *British Journal of Psychiatry*, 119, 151–8.

Lavin, D. and Groarke, A. (2005) Dental floss behavior: a test of the predictive validity of the theory of planned behavior and the effects of implementation intentions. *Psychology, Health and Medicine*, 10, 243–52.

Lazarus, R.S. and Alfert, E. (1964) Short-circuiting of threat by experimentally altering cognitive appraisal. *The Journal of Abnormal and Social Psychology*, 69, 195–205.

Lazarus, R.S. and Folkman, S. (1984) *Stress, Appraisal and Coping*. New York: Springer.

Le Grand, J. (1982) *The Strategy of Equality: Redistribution and the Social Services*. London: Allen & Unwin.

Le Moal, M. (2007) Historical approach and evolution of the stress concept: a personal account. *Psychoneuroendocrinology*, 32, S3–S9.

Leaker, D. (2008) The gender pay gap. *Economic & Labour Market Review*, 2(4), 19–24.

Lefer, L., Pleasure, M.A. and Rosenthal, L.A. (1962) A psychiatric approach to the denture patient. *Journal of Psychosomatic Research*, 6, 199–207.

Leventhal, H. and Diefenbach, M. (1991) The active side of illness cognition. In Skelton, J.A. and Croyle, R.T. (eds) *Mental Representations in Health and Illness*. New York: Springer-Verlag, pp. 247–72.

Leventhal, H. and Tomarken, A. (1987) Stress and illness: perspectives from health psychology. In Kasl, S.V. and Cooper, C.L. (eds) *Stress and Health: Issues in Research Methodology*. Chichester: John Wiley & Son, pp. 27–55.

Leventhal, H., Forster, R. and Leventhal, E. (2007) Self-regulation of health threats, affect and the self: lessons from older adults. In Aldwin, C.M., Park, C.L. and Spiro, A. (eds) *Handbook of Health Psychology and Aging*. New York: Guilford Press, pp. 341–66.

Liddell, A. and Locker, D. (1992) Dental visit satisfaction in a group of adults aged 50 years and over. *Journal of Behavioural Medicine*, 15, 415–27.

Liddell, A. and Locker, D. (1997) Gender and age differences in attitudes to dental pain and dental control. *Community Dentistry and Oral Epidemiology*, 25, 314–18.

Liddell, A. and May, B. (1984) Patients' perception of dentists' positive and negative attributes. *Social Science & Medicine*, 19, 839–42.

Locker, D. (1983) *Disability and Disadvantage: The Consequences of Chronic Illness*. London: Tavistock.

Locker, D. (1988a) Measuring oral health: a conceptual framework. *Community Dental Health*, 5, 3–18.

Locker, D. (1988b) The symptom iceberg in dentistry: treatment seeking in relation to oral and facial pain. *The Journal of the Canadian Dental Association*, 54, 271–4.

Locker, D. (1989) *An Introduction to Behavioural Science and Dentistry*. London: Tavistock/Routledge.

Locker, D. (2008) Social determinants of health and disease. In Scambler, G. (ed.) *Sociology As Applied to Medicine*, 6th edn. London: Elsevier, pp. 18–37.

Lovallo, W.R. (2005) *Stress and Health: Biological and Psychological Interactions*, 2nd edn. London: Sage Publications.

Lukes, S. (1974) *Power: A Radical View*. London: Macmillan.

Lundqvist, E.N., Wahlin, Y.B., Bergdahl, M. and Bergdahl J. (2006) Psychological health in patients with genital and oral erosive lichen planus. *Journal of the European Academy of Dermatology and Venereology*, 20, 661–6.

Lupien, S.J. and McEwen, B.S. (1997) The acute effects of corticosteroids on cognition: integration of animal and human model studies. *Brain Research Reviews*, 24, 1–26.

Macdonald, K.M. (1995) *The Sociology of the Professions*. London: Sage.

MacEntee, M.I., Stolar, E. and Glick, N. (1993) Influence of age and gender on oral health and related behaviour in an independent elderly population. *Community Dentistry and Oral Epidemiology*, 21(4), 234–9.

MacEntee, M.I., Hole, R. and Stolar, E. (1997) The significance of the mouth in old age. *Social Science & Medicine*, 45, 1449–58.

Mansell, W. and Morris, K. (2003) The Dental Cognitions Questionnaire in CBT for dental phobia in an adolescent with multiple phobias. *Journal of Behavior Therapy & Experimental Psychiatry*, 34, 65–71.

Marcenes, W.S. and Sheiham, A. (1992) The relationship between work stress and oral health status. *Social Science & Medicine*, 35, 1511–20.

Marcenes, W., Muirhead, V.E., Murray, S., Redshaw, P., Bennett, U. and Wright, D. (2013) Ethnic disparities in the oral health of three- to four-year-old children in East London. *British Dental Journal*, 215, E4.

Marucha, P.T., Kiecolt-Glaser, J.K. and Favagehi, M. (1998) Mucosal wound healing is impaired by examination stress, *Psychosomatic Medicine*, 60, 362–5.

Maslach, C., Jackson, S.E. and Leiter, M.P. (1996) *MBI: The Maslach Burnout Inventory: Manual*. Palo Alto, CA: Consulting Psychologists Press.

Matthews, K.A. and Gump, B.B. (2002) Chronic work stress and marital dissolution increase risk of post trial mortality in men from the Multiple Risk Factor Intervention Trial. *Archives of Internal Medicine*, 162, 309–15.

Mattin, D. and Smith, J. (1991) The oral health status, dental needs and factors affecting utilisation of dental services in Asians aged 55 years and over, resident in Southampton. *British Dental Journal*, 199, 369–72.

Mausner, J. and Kramer, S. (1985) *Epidemiology: An Introductory Text*. Philadelphia, PA: W.B. Saunders.

Mays, N. (2008) Origins and development of the National Health Service. In Scambler, G. (ed.) *Sociology as Applied to Medicine*, 6th edn. London: Elsevier.

McDonald, S. (2013) Lots in the health psychology mix. *The Psychologist*, 26, 792–3.

McEwen, B.S. (1998) Protective and damaging effects of stress mediators. *New England Journal of Medicine*, 338, 171–9.

McGregor, B.A. and Antoni, M.H. (2009) Psychological intervention and health outcomes among women treated for breast cancer: a review of stress pathways and biological mediators. *Brain, Behavior, and Immunity*, 23, 159–66.

McGuigan, D. (2009) Communicating bad news to patients: a reflective approach. *Nursing Standard*, 23, 51–6; quiz 57.

McKay, J.C. and Quinonez, C.R. (2012) The feminization of dentistry: implications for the profession. *Journal of the Canadian Dental Association*, 78: c1.

McKeithen, E.J. (1966) The patient's image of the dentist. *Journal of the American College of Dentistry*, 33, 87–107.

McKeown, T. (1976) *The Role of Medicine: Dream, Mirage or Nemesis?* Oxford: Blackwell.

McNeil, D.W., Sorrell, J.T. and Vowles, K.E. (2006) Emotional and environmental determinants of dental pain. In Mostofsky, D.I., Forgione, A.G. and Giddon, D.B. (eds) *Behavioural Dentistry*. Copenhagen: Blackwell Munksgaard.

Mead, N. and Bower, P. (2000) Patient-centredness: a conceptual framework and review of the empirical literature. *Social Science & Medicine*, 51, 1087–110.

Mead, N. and Bower, P. (2002) Patient-centred consultations and outcomes in primary care: a review of the literature. *Patient Education and Counseling*, 48, 51–61.

Mechanic, D. (1975) Sociocultural and socio-psychological factors affecting personal responses to psychological disorder. *Journal of Health and Social Behavior*, 16, 393–404.

Mechanic, D. (1979) Correlates of physician utilization: why do major multivariate studies of physician utilization find trivial psychosocial and organizational effects? *Journal of Health & Social Behaviour*, 20, 387–96.

Melville, R.B.M., Pool, M.D., Jaffe, C.E., Gelbier, S. and Tulley, J.W. (1981) A dental service for handicapped children. *British Dental Journal*, 20, 259–61.

Melzack, R. (1975) The McGill pain questionnaire: major properties and scoring methods. *Pain*, 1, 279–99.

Melzack, R. and Wall, P.D. (1965) Pain mechanisms: a new theory. *Science*, 50, 971–9.

Mengel, R., Bacher, M. and Flores-de-Jacoby, L. (2002) Interactions between stress, interleukin-1β, interleukin-6 and cortisol in periodontally diseased patients. *Journal of Clinical Periodontology*, 29, 1012–22.

Merskey, H. and Bogduk, N. (1994) *Classification of Chronic Pain*, 2nd edn. Seattle, WA: IASP Press.

Mesfin, M., Newell, J., Walley, J., Gessessew, A. and Madeley, R. (2009) Delayed consultation among pulmonary tuberculosis patients: a cross sectional study of 10 DOTS districts of Ethiopia. *BMC Public Health*, 9, 53.

Michie, S. and West, R. (2012) Behaviour change theory and evidence: a presentation to government. *Health Psychology Review*, 7, 1–22.

Michie, S., Johnston, M., Abraham, C., Lawton, R., Parker, D. and Walker, A. (2005) Making psychological theory useful for implementing evidence based practice: a consensus approach. *Quality & Safety in Health Care*, 14, 26–33.

Milgram, S. (1963) Behavioral study of obedience. *Journal of Abnormal and Social Psychology*, 67, 371–8.

Milgrom, P., Vignesha, H. and Weinstein, P. (1992) Adolescent dental fear and control: prevalence and theoretical implications. *Behaviour Research and Therapy*, 30, 367–73.

Miller, G.A. (1956) The magical number seven plus or minus two: some limits on our capacity for processing information. *The Psychological Review*, 63, 81–97.

Miller, G. and Cohen, S. (2005) Infectious disease and psychoneuroimmunology. In Vedhara, K. and Irwin, M. (eds) *Human Psychoneuroimmunology*. New York: Oxford University Press, pp. 219–42.

Miller, W.R. and Rollnick, S. (2002) *Motivational Interviewing: Preparing People for Change*. New York, Guildford Press.

Milne, S., Sheeran, P. and Orbell, S. (2000) Prediction and intervention in health-related behavior: a meta-analytic review of protection motivation theory. *Journal of Applied Social Psychology*, 30, 106–43.

Minichiello, T.A., Ling, D. and Ucci, D.K. (2007) Breaking bad news: a practical approach for the hospitalist. *Journal of Hospital Medicine*, 2, 415–21.

Ministry of Health (1944) *A National Health Service*, Cmnd 6502. London: HMSO.

Ministry of National Health and Welfare, Canada (1974) *A New Perspective on the Health of Canadians: a working document*. Available at: http://www.phac-aspc.gc.ca/ph-sp/pdf/perspect-eng.pdf.

Mishler, E. (1981) The machine metaphor in medicine. In *Social Contexts of Health, Illness and Patient Care*. Cambridge: Cambridge University Press.

Misra, S., Daly, B., Dunne, S., Millar, B., Packer, M. and Asimakopoulou, K. (2013) Dentist–patient communication: what do patients and dentists remember following a consultation? Implications for patient compliance. *Patient Prefer Adherence*, 7, 543–9.

Mitsonis, C.I., Zervas, I.M., Mitropoulos, P.A., Dimopoulos, N.P., Soldatos, C.R., Potagas, C.M. and Sfagos, C.A. (2008) The impact of stressful life events on risk of relapse in women with multiple sclerosis: a prospective study. *European Psychiatry*, 23, 497–504.

Mohamadi Hasel, K., Besharat, M.A., Abdolhoseini, A., Alaei Nasab, S. and Niknam, S. (2013) Relationships of personality factors to perceived stress, depression, and oral lichen planus severity. *International Journal of Behavioural Medicine*, 20, 286–92.

Moles, D.R., Fedele, S., Speight, P.M. and Porter, S.R. (2007) The unclear role of ethnicity in health inequalities: the scenario of oral cancer incidence and survival in the British South Asian population. *Oral Oncology*, 43, 831–4.

Monroe, S. (2008) Modern approaches to conceptualizing and measuring human life stress. *Annual Review of Clinical Psychology*, 4, 33–52.

Mora, P.A., Robitaille, C., Leventhal, H., Swigar, M. and Leventhal, E.A. (2002) Trait negative affect relates to prior-week symptoms, but not to reports of illness episodes, illness symptoms, and care seeking among older persons. *Psychosomatic Medicine*, 64, 436–49.

Mowrer, O.H. (1939) A stimulus-response analysis of anxiety and its role as a reinforcing agent. *Psychological Review*, 46, 553–66.

Mullen, B. and Suls, H. (1982) The effectiveness of attention and rejection of coping styles: a meta-analysis of temporal differences. *Journal of Psychosomatic Research*, 26, 43–9.

Nath, C., Schmidt, R. and Gunel, E. (2006) Perceptions of professionalism vary most with educational rank and age. *Journal of Dental Education*, 70, 825–34.

National Institute for Clinical Excellence (2004) *Anxiety: Management of Anxiety (Panic Disorder, with or without Agoraphobia, and Generalised Anxiety Disorder) in Adults in Primary, Secondary and Community Care*. London: NICE.

Nazroo, J. (1997) *The Health of Britain's Ethnic Minorities: Findings from a National Survey*. London: Policy Studies Institute.

Nazroo, J. (2003) The structuring of ethnic inequalities in health: economic position, racial discrimination and racism. *American Journal of Public Health*, 93, 277–84.

Nazroo, J., Falaschetti, E., Pierce, M. and Primatesta, P. (2009) Ethnic inequalities in access to and outcomes of healthcare: analysis of the health survey for England. *Journal of Epidemiology and Community Health*, 63, 1022–7.

Neugarten, B. (1984) Interpretive social science and research on aging. In Rossi, A. (ed.) *Gender and the Life Course*. Chicago, IL: Aldine.

Newman, E., Connor, D.B. and Conner, M. (2007) Daily hassles and eating behaviour: the role of cortisol reactivity status. *Psychoneuroendocrinology*, 32, 125–32.

Newton, J.T. and Brenneman, D.L. (1999) Communication in Dental Settings Scale (CDSS): preliminary development of a measure to assess communication in dental settings. *British Journal of Health Psychology*, 4, 277–84.

Newton, J.T. and Buck, D.J. (2000) Anxiety and pain measures in dentistry: a guide to their quality and application. *Journal of the American Dental Association*, 131, 1449–57.

Newton, J.T. and Fiske, J. (1999) Breaking bad news: a guide for dental healthcare professionals. *British Dental Journal*, 186, 278–81.

Newton, J.T., Buck, D. and Gibbons, D.E. (2001) Workforce planning in dentistry: the impact of shorter and more varied career patterns. *Community Dental Health*, 18, 236–41.

Newton, J.T., Asimakopoulou, K., Daly, B., Scambler, S. and Scott, S. (2012) The management of dental anxiety: time for a sense of proportion? *British Dental Journal*, 213, 271–4.

Ng, D.M. and Jeffery, R.W. (2003) Relationships between perceived stress and health behaviours in a sample of working adults. *Health Psychology*, 22, 638–42.

Nicolau, B., Marcenes, W., Hardy, R. and Sheiham, A. (2003) A life-course approach to assess the relationship between social and psychological circumstances and gingival status in adolescents. *Journal of Clinical Periodontology*, 30, 1038–45.

Nielsen, N., Kristensen, T., Schnohr, P. and Gronbaek, M. (2008) Perceived stress and cause-specific mortality among men and women: results from a perspective cohort study. *American Journal of Epidemiology*, 168, 481–91.

Nowjack-Raymer, R. & Gift, H.C. (1990) Contributing factors to maternal and child oral health. *Journal of Public Health Dentistry*, 50(6), 370–8.

Nunn, J. (2007) Prevalence of dental erosion and the implications for oral health. *European Journal of Oral Sciences*, 104, 156–61.

Nuttall, N., Freeman, R., Beavan-Seymour, C. and Hill, K. (2011) Access and barriers to care – a report from the Adult Dental Health Survey 2009. In O'Sullivan, I. and Lader, D. (eds) *Adult Dental Health Survey 2009*. Leeds: The Health and Social Care Information Centre, Dental and Eye Care Team.

O'Connor, D.B., Jones, F., Conner, M., McMillan, B. and Ferguson, E. (2008) Effects of daily hassles and eating style on eating behaviour. *Health Psychology*, 27, S20–S31.

O'Donovan, A. and Hughes, B.M. (2008) Access to social support in life and in the laboratory: combined impact on cardiovascular reactivity to stress and state anxiety. *Journal of Health Psychology*, 13, 1147–56.

Office for National Statistics (2001) *Social Trends 31*. London: ONS.

Office for National Statistics (2004) Age-standardised mortality rate by NS-SEC: men aged 25–64, England and Wales 2001–03. London: ONS.

Office for National Statistics (2005a) General practice research database. London: ONS.

Office for National Statistics (2005b) Focus on ethnicity and identity. London: ONS.

Office for National Statistics (2006) Facts about men and women in Great Britain. London: ONS.

Office for National Statistics (2007) NHS Dental Statistics, 2007–08, annual report. NHS Information Centre. London: ONS.

Office for National Statistics (2008) Large differences in infant mortality by ethnic group. News Release, June. London: ONS.

Office for National Statistics (2009a) National population projections, 2008-based projections. London: ONS.

Office for National Statistics (2009b) Chapter 7: Health. *Social Trends* 39. London: HMRC.

Office for National Statistics (2010) Limiting longstanding illness or disability of those aged 65–74 by income. General Lifestyle Survey, accessed through poverty.org.

Office for National Statistics (2011a) Census, Key statistics for local authorities in England and Wales. London: ONS.

Office for National Statistics (2011b) Opinions Survey 2011. London: ONS.

Office for National Statistics (2012a) Ethnicity and national identity in England and Wales 2011. London: ONS. Available at: http://www.ons.gov.uk/ons/rel/census/2011-census/key-statistics-for-local-authorities-in-england-and-wales/rpt-ethnicity.html.

Office for National Statistics (2012b) Labour Market Status of Disabled People. In *Labour Force Survey*. London: ONS.

Office for National Statistics (2013a) Key statistics and quick statistics for local authorities in the United Kingdom. London: ONS.

Office for National Statistics (2013b) What does the 2011 census tell us about older people? ONS 2011 Census Analysis. London: ONS.

Office for National Statistics (2013c) Estimates of the very old (including centenarians), England and Wales, 2002–2012. London: ONS. Available at: http://www.ons.gov.uk/ons/rel/mortality-ageing/estimates-of-the-very-old--including-centenarians-/2002-2012/index.html.

Office of Population Censuses and Surveys (2002) Living in Britain. General Household Survey. London: HMSO.

Ogden, J. (2007) *Health Psychology: A Textbook*, 4th edn. Maidenhead: Open University Press.

Ogden, J. (2012) *Health Psychology: A Textbook*, 5th edn. Maidenhead: Open University Press.

olde Hartman, T.C., Borghuis, M.S., Lucassen, P.L., van de Laar, F.A., Speckens, A.E. and van Weel, C. (2009) Medically unexplained symptoms, somatisation disorder and hypochondriasis: course and prognosis: a systematic review. *Journal of Psychosomatic Research*, 66, 363–77.

Oliver, C. and Barnes, C. (2012) *The New Politics of Disablement*, 2nd edn. Basingstoke: Palgrave Macmillan.

Oliver, C.H. and Nunn, J.H. (1995) The accessibility of dental treatment to adults with physical disabilities aged 16–64 in the North East of England. *Special Care Dentistry*, 15, 97–101.

Oliver, M. (1990) *The Politics of Disablement*. Basingstoke: Macmillan.

Ong, L.M.L., De Haas, C.J.M., Hoos, A.M. and Lammes, F.B. (1995) Doctor–patient communication: a review of the literature. *Social Science & Medicine*, 40, 903–18.

Oosterink, F.M.D., de Jongh, A. and Hoogstraten, J. (2009) Prevalence of dental fear and phobia relative to other fear and phobia subtypes. *European Journal of Oral Sciences*, 117, 135–43.

Orgogozo, J.M. (1994) The concepts of impairment, disability and handicap. *Cerebrovascular Disease*, 4, 2–6.

Owens, J., Mistry, K. and Dyer, T. (2011) Access to dental services for people with learning disabilities: quality care? *Journal of Disability and Oral Health*, 12, 17–27.

Pacak, K. and Palkovits, M. (2001) Stressor specificity of central neuroendocrine responses: implications for stress-related disorders. *Endocrine Reviews*, 22, 502–48.

Parliamentary Office of Science and Technology (2007) Ethnicity and Health. Postnote no. 276. London: POST.

Pasero, C. and McCaffery, M. (1999) *Pain: Clinical Manual*. St Louis, MO: Mosby.

Patterson, C.W. (1993) Pricing and the perception of health care service quality. *Journal of the American Dental Association*, 124, 132–7.

Patton, L.L. (2001) Ability of HIV/AIDS patients to self-diagnose oral opportunistic infections. *Community Dentistry and Oral Epidemiology*, 29, 23–9.

Pavlov, I.P. (1927) *Conditional Reflexes*. London: Oxford University Press.

Paykel, E.S. (1997) The interview for recent life events. *Psychological Medicine*, 27, 301–10.

Pearce, N. (1996) Traditional epidemiology, modern epidemiology and public health. *American Journal of Public Health*, 86, 678–83.

Penchansky, R. and Thomas, J.W. (1981) The concept of access: definition and relationship to consumer satisfaction. *Medical Care*, 19, 127–40.

Pennebaker, J.W. (1982) *The Psychology of Physical Symptoms*. New York: Springer.

Pennebaker, J.W. and Brittingham, G.L. (1982) Environmental and sensory cues affecting the perception of physical symptoms. In Baum, A., Taylor, S.E. and Singer, J.E. (eds) *Advances in Environmental Psychology IV*. Hillsdale, NJ: Lawrence Erlbaum Associates, pp. 115–36.

Pennebaker, J.W. and Skelton, J.A. (1981) Selective monitoring of physical sensations. *Journal of Personality and Social Psychology*, 41, 213–23.

Peretz, B. and Gluck, G. (2005) Magic trick: a behavioural strategy for the management of strong-willed children. *International Journal of Paediatric Dentistry*, 15, 429–36.

Petersen, P.E. and Yamamoto, T. (2005) Improving the oral health of older people: the approach of the WHO Global Oral Health

Programme. *Community Dentistry and Oral Epidemiology*, 33, 81–92.

Petersen, P.E., Kjøller, M., Christensen, L.B. and Krustrup, U. (2004) Changing dentate status of adults, use of dental health services, and achievement of national dental health goals in Denmark by the year 2000. *Journal of Public Health Dentistry*, 64(3), 127–35.

Petti, S. and Scully, C. (2007) Oral cancer knowledge and awareness: primary and secondary effects of an information leaflet. *Oral Oncology*, 43, 408–15.

Phillipson, C. (1982) *Capitalism and the Construction of Old Age.* London: Macmillan.

Pickrell, J.E., Heima, M., Weinstein, P., Coolidge, T., Coldwell, S.E., Skaret, E., Castillo, J. and Milgrom, P. (2007) Using memory restructuring strategy to enhance dental behaviour. *International Journal of Paediatric Dentistry*, 17, 439–48.

Pisinger, C., Vestbo, J., Borch-Johnsen, K. and Jorgensen, T. (2005) It is possible to help smokers in early motivational stages to quit: the Inter99 study. *Preventive Medicine*, 40, 278–84.

Pitts, M., Woolliscroft, J., Cannon, S., Johnson, I. and Singh, G. (2000) Factors influencing delay in treatment seeking by first-time attenders at a genitourinary clinic. *International Journal of STD & AIDS*, 11, 375–8.

Platt, L. (2011) JRF Programme Paper: Poverty and Inequality – Inequality within ethnic groups. London: Joseph Rowntree Foundation.

Plauth, M., Jenss, H. and Meyle, J. (1991) Oral manifestations of Crohn's disease: an analysis of 79 cases. *Journal of Clinical Gastroentorology*, 13, 29–37.

Politi, M.C., Dizon, D.S., Frosch, D.L., Kuzemchak, M.D. and Stiggelbout, A.M. (2013) Importance of clarifying patients' desired role in shared decision making to match their level of engagement with their preferences. *British Medical Journal*, 347, f7066.

Porter, R. (1997) *The Greatest Benefit to Mankind: A Medical History of Humanity from Antiquity to the Present.* London: HarperCollins.

Poulton, R., Caspi, A., Milne, B.J., Thomson, W.M., Taylor, A., Sears, M.R. and Moffitt, T.E. (2002) Association between children's experience of socioeconomic disadvantage and adult health: a life-course study. *Lancet*, 360, 1640–5.

Pradhan, A., Slade, G.D. and Spencer, A.J. (2009) Factors influencing caries experience among adults with physical and intellectual disabilities. *Community Dentistry and Oral Epidemiology*, 37, 143–54.

Pratelli, P. and Gelbier, S. (1998) Dental services for adults with a learning disability: care managers' experiences and opinions. *Community and Dental Health*, 15, 281–5.

Prochaska, J. and DiClemente, C. (1984) *The Transtheoretical Approach: Crossing Traditional Boundaries of Therapy.* Homewood, IL: Dow-Jones-Irwin.

Prochaska, T.R., Funch, D. and Blesch, K.S. (1990) Age patterns in symptom perception and illness behavior among colorectal cancer patients. *Behavior, Health & Aging*, 1, 27–39.

Prochaska, J.O., Redding, C.A. and Evers, K.E. (2002) The transtheoretical model and stages of change. In Glanz, K., Rimer, B.K. and Lewis, F.M. (eds) *Health Behavior and Health Education: Theory Research and Practice*. San Fransisco, CA: Jossey-Bass.

Pyle, M.A., Jasinevicius, T.R. and Sheehan, R. (1999) Dental student perceptions of the elderly: measuring negative perceptions with projective tests. *Special Care in Dentistry*, 19, 40–6.

Rabin, B. (2007) Stress: a system of the whole. In Ader, R. (ed.) *Psychoneuroimmunology*, 4th edn. London: Elsevier Academic Press, pp. 709–21.

Rankin, J.A. and Harris, M.B. (1985) Patients' preferences for dentists' behaviors. *Journal of the American Dental Association*, 110, 323–7.

Rathert, C., Wyrwich, M.D. and Boren, S.A. (2012) Patient-centered care and outcomes: a systematic review of the literature. *Medical Care Research and Review*, 70, 351–79.

Redford, M. (1993) Beyond pregnancy gingivitis: bringing a new focus to women's oral health. *Journal of Dental Education*, 57, 742–8.

Registrar General (1990) *Mortality Statistics*. London: ONS.

Renz, A.N.P.J. and Newton, J.T. (2009) Changing the behavior of patients with periodontitis. *Periodontology 2000*, 51, 252–68.

Reynolds, C.F., Frank, E., Perel, J.M., Imber, S.D., Cornes, C., Miller, M.D., Mazumdar, S., Houck, P.R., Dew, M.A., Stack, J.A., Pollock, B.G. and Kupfer, D.J. (1999) Nortriptyline and interpersonal psychotherapy as maintenance therapies for recurrent major depression: a randomised controlled trial in patients older than 59 years. *Journal of the American Medical Association*, 281, 39–45.

Rhodes, J. and Gregory, S. (1995) Biting the bullet: what drove dentistry into the private sector. *The Health Service Journal*, 33(6), 707–16.

Rief, W. and Broadbent, E. (2007) Explaining medically unexplained symptoms – models and mechanisms. *Clinical Psychology Review*, 27, 821–41.

Robinson, I. (1989) Reconstructing lives: negotiating the meaning of multiple sclerosis. In Anderson, R. and Bury, M. (eds) *Living with Chronic Illness: The Experience of Patients and their Families*. London: Hyman Unwin.

Robinson, P. (2010) Hospital readmissions and the 30 day threshold. CHKS Market Intelligence report. Available at: http://www.chks.co.uk/userfiles/files/CHKS%20Report%20Hospital%20read missions.pdf.

Robinson, P.G., Bhavnani, V., Kham, F.A., Newton, T., Pitt, J., Thorogood, N., Gelbier, S. and Gibbons, D. (2000) Dental caries and treatment experience of adults from minority ethnic communities living in the South Thames region, UK. *Community Dental Health*, 17, 41–7.

Robinson, P.G., Patrick, A. and Newton, T. (2011) *Modelling the Dental Workforce Supply in England*. Sheffield: University of Sheffield.

Rogers, R.W. (1975) A protection motivation theory of fear appeals and attitude change. *Journal of Psychology*, 91, 93–114.

Rogers, R.W. (1983) Cognitive and physiological processes in fear appeals and attitude change: a revised theory of protection motivation. In Cacioppo, J. and Petty, R. (eds) *Social Psychophysiology*. New York: Guilford Press.

Rogers, S.N. (1991) Dental attendance in a sample of pregnant women in Birmingham, UK. *Community Dental Health*, 8, 361–8.

Rohleder, N., Wolf, J.M., Herpfer, I., Fiebich, B.L., Kirschbaum, C. and Lieb, K. (2006) No response of plasma substance P but delayed increase of IL-1 receptor antagonist to acute psychological stress. *Life Sciences*, 78, 3082–9.

Rosania, A.E., Low, K.G., McCormick, C.M. and Rosania, D.A. (2009) Stress, depression, cortisol, and periodontal disease. *Journal of Periodontology*, 80, 260–6.

Rosengren, A., Orth-Gomer, K., Wedel, H. and Wilhelmsen, L. (1993) Stressful life events, social support and mortality in men born in 1933. *British Medical Journal*, 307, 1102–5.

Rosenstock, I.M. (1966) Why people use health services. *The Milbank Memorial Fund Quarterly*, 44, 94–127.

Rosenstock, I.M. (1990) The health belief model: explaining health behavior through expectancies. In Glanz, K., Lewis, F.M. and Rimer, B.K. (eds) *Health Behavior and Health Education: Theory, Research and Practice*. San Franscisco, CA: Jossey-Bass.

Ross, L. (1977) The intuitive psychologist and his shortcomings: distortions in the attribution process. In Berkowitz, K.L. (ed.) *Advances in Experimental Social Psychology*. New York: Academic Press.

Roter, D.L. and Hall, J.A. (1992) *Doctors Talking with Patients/Patients Talking with Doctors: Improving Communication in Medical Visits*. Westport, CT: Auburn House.

Rouleau, T., Harrington, A.L., Brennan, M.T., Hammond, F.M., Hirsch, M.A. and Bockenek, W.L. (2009) Disabled persons' receipt of dental care and barriers encountered. *Oral Surgery, Oral Medicine, Oral Pathology, Oral Radiology, and Endodontology*, 108, e17–e18.

Royal College of Physicians Working Party (2005) Doctors in society. Medical professionalism in a changing world. *Clinical Medicine*, 5: S5–40.

Royce, R.A., Seña, A., Cates, W. Jr. and Cohen, M.S. (1997) Sexual transmission of HIV. *New England Journal of Medicine*, 336, 1072–8.

Rozanski, I., Blumenthal, J.A., Davidson, K.W., Saab, P.G. and Kubzansky, L. (2005) The epidemiology, pathophysiology and management of psychosocial risk factors in cardiac practice. *Journal of the American College of Cardiology*, 45, 637–51.

Rudat, K. (1994) *Black and Minority Ethnic Groups in England: Health and Lifestyles*. London: Health Education Authority.

Russell, N.J. (2011) Milgram's obedience to authority experiments: origins and early evolution. *British Journal of Social Psychology*, 50, 140–62.

Sabbah, W., Tsakos, G., Sheiham, A. and Watt, R.G. (2009) The role of health-related behaviors in the socioeconomic disparities in oral health. *Social Science & Medicine*, 68, 298–303.

Sage, N., Sowden, M., Chorlton, E. and Edeleanu, A. (2008) *CBT for Chronic Illness and Palliative Care: A Workbook and Toolkit*. Chichester: John Wiley & Sons.

Sakki, T.K., Knuuttila, M.L. and Anttila, S.S. (1998) Lifestyle, gender and occupational status as determinants of dental health behaviour. *Journal of Clinical Periodontology*, 25, 566–70.

Salovey, P., Rothman, A.J., Detweiler, J.B. and Steward, W.T. (2000) Emotional states and physical health. *American Psychologist*, 55, 110–21.

Sanders, A.E. and Spencer, A.J. (2005) Why do poor adults rate their oral health poorly? *Australian Dental Journal*, 50, 161–7.

Sapolsky, R.M. (2004) *Why Zebras Don't Get Ulcers*, 3rd edn. New York: Henry Holt & Co.

Sarafino, E.P. (2002) *Health Psychology: Biopsychosocial Interactions*, 4th edn. New York: John Wiley & Sons.

Scambler, A. (2002) *Sociology As Applied to Dentistry*. London: St Bartholomews and the Royal London School of Medicine and Dentistry.

Scambler, A. (2008) Women and health. In Scambler, G. (ed.) *Sociology As Applied to Medicine*, 6th edn. London: Elsevier.

Scambler, A., Scambler, G. and Craig, D. (1981) Kinship and friendship networks and women's demand for primary care. *Journal of the Royal College of General Practitioners*, 26, 746–50.

Scambler, G. (ed.) (2008) *Sociology as Applied to Medicine*, 6th edn. London: Elsevier.

Scambler, G. and Hopkins, A. (1986) Being epileptic: Coming to terms with stigma. *Sociology of Health and Illness*, 8, 26–43.

Scambler, S. (2005) Exposing the limitations of disability theory: The case of juvenile Batten disease. *Social Theory and Health*, 3, 144–64.

Scambler, S. (2014) Beyond social determinants: a neo-Marxist approach to understanding the causes of the social determinants of inequalities in oral health. *Social Science and Dentistry*, 3, 27–33.

Scambler, S. and Asimakopoulou, K. (2014) A model of patient-centred care – turning good care into patient-centred care. *British Dental Journal*, 217, 225–8.

Scambler, S., Lowe, E., Zoitopoulos, L. and Gallagher, J.E. (2010) Dentistry and disability. Pacesetters Group Final Report. London: King's College London and King's College Hospital NHS Foundation Trust.

Schoon-Tong, J.G. (2012) Dentists in the media: why can't we be the good guys? *Dear Doctor – Dentistry and Oral Health Magazine*, 2. Available at: http://www.deardoctor.com/articles/dentists-in-the-media/

Schulman, S. and Smith, A.M. (1963) The concept of 'health' among Spanish-speaking villagers in New Mexico and Colorado. *Journal of Health and Human Behavior*, 4, 226–34.

Scott, A., March, L. and Stokes, M.L. (1998) A survey of oral health in a population of adults with developmental disabilities: comparison with a National Health survey of the general population. *Australian Dental Journal*, 43, 257–61.

Scott, S.E. and Walter, F. (2010) Studying help-seeking for symptoms: the challenges of methods and models. *Social and Personality Psychology Compass*, 4, 531–47.

Scott, S.E., Rizvi, K., Grunfeld, E.A. and McGurk, M. (2010) Pilot study to estimate the accuracy of mouth self-examination in an at-risk group. *Head & Neck*, 32, 1393–401.

Scott, S.E., Weinman, J. and Grunfeld, E.A. (2011) Developing ways to encourage early detection and presentation of oral cancer: what do high-risk individuals think? *Psychology & Health*, 26, 1392–405.

Scott, S.E, Khwaja, M., Low, E.L, Weinman, J. and Grunfeld, E.A. (2012) A randomised controlled trial of a pilot intervention to encourage early presentation of oral cancer in high risk groups. *Patient Education & Counseling*, 88, 241–8.

Scott, S.E., Walter, F.M., Webster, A., Sutton, S. and Emery, J. (2013) The model of pathways to treatment: conceptualization and integration with existing theory. *British Journal of Health Psychology*, 18, 45–65.

Scully, C., Dios, P.D. and Kumar, N. (2007) *Special Care in Dentistry: Handbook of Oral Healthcare*. London: Churchill Livingstone.

Segerstrom, S.C. and Miller, G.E. (2004) Psychological stress and the human immune system: a meta-analytic study of 30 years of inquiry. *Psychological Bulletin*, 130, 601–30.

Self, A. and Zealey, L. (2007) *Social Trends No. 37*. Basingstoke: Palgrave Macmillan.

Seligman, M.E.P. (1971) Phobias and preparedness. *Behavior Therapy*, 2, 307–20.

Selye, H. (1956) *The Stress of Life*. New York: McGraw-Hill.

Sentell, T., Shumway, M. and Snowden, L. (2007) Access to mental health treatment by English language proficiency and race/ethnicity. *Journal of General Internal Medicine*, 22, 289–93.

Shah, B., Ashok, L. and Sujatha, G.P. (2009) Evaluation of salivary cortisol and psychological factors in patients with oral lichen planus. *Indian Journal of Dental Research*, 20, 288–92.

Shaw, O. (1975) Dental anxiety in children. *British Dental Journal,* 139, 134–9.

Sheiham, A. and Watt, R.G. (2000) The common risk factor approach: a rational basis for promoting oral health. *Community Dentistry and Oral Epidemiology,* 28, 399–406.

Shipley, B.A., Weiss, A., Der, G., Taylor, M.D. and Deary, I.J. (2007) Neuroticism, extraversion and mortality in the UK Health and Lifestyle survey: a 21-year prospective cohort study. *Psychosomatic Medicine,* 69, 923–31.

Sideridis, G.D. (2006) Coping is not an 'either' 'or': the interaction of coping strategies in regulating affect, arousal and performance. *Stress and Health,* 22, 315–27.

Siegler, V., Langford, A. and Johnson, B. (2008) Regional differences in male mortality inequalities using the National Statistics Socio-economic Classification, England and Wales, 2001–03. *Health Statistics Quarterly 40.* London: ONS.

Silverman, J., Kurtz, S. and Draper, J. (2004) *Skills for Communicating with Patients,* 2nd edn. Oxford: Radcliffe Publishing.

Sisson, K. (2007) Theoretical explanations for social inequalities in oral health. *Community Dentistry and Oral Epidemiology,* 35, 81–8.

Skinner, B.F. (1938) *The Behavior of Organisms: An Experimental Analysis.* Acton, MA: Copley.

Smith, L.K., Pope, C. and Botha, J.L. (2005) Patients' help-seeking experiences and delay in cancer presentation: a qualitative synthesis. *Lancet,* 366, 825–31.

Smith, R. (2008) The end of disease and the beginning of health. BMJ Blogs, 8 July. Available at: http://blogs.bmj.com/bmj/2008/07/08/richard-smith-the-end-of-disease-and-the-beginning-of-health/

Sniehotta, F.F. (2009a) An experimental test of the theory of planned behavior. *Applied Psychology: Health and Well-Being,* 1, 257–70.

Sniehotta, F.F. (2009b) Towards a theory of intentional behaviour change: plans, planning, and self-regulation. *British Journal of Health Psychology,* 14, 261–73.

Sniehotta, F., Araujo Soares, V. and Dombrowski, S. (2007) Randomized controlled trial of a one-minute intervention changing oral self-care behavior. *Journal of Dental Research,* 86, 641–5.

Spangler, G., Pekrun, R., Kramer, K. and Hofmann, H. (2002) Students emotions, physiological reactions and coping in academic exams. *Anxiety, Stress and Coping,* 15, 413–32.

Steele, J. (2009) NHS Dental Services in England, an independent review led by Professor Jimmy Steele. London: Department of Health.

Steele, J. and Lader, D. (2004) Social Factors and Oral Health in Children. Children's Dental Health in the UK, 2003. London: Office for National Statistics.

Steele, J., Walls, A.W., Ayatollahi, S.M. and Murray, J.J. (1996) Major clinical findings from a dental survey of elderly people in three different English communities. *British Dental Journal,* 180, 17–23.

Steptoe, A. (2000) Health behaviour and stress. In Fink, G. (ed.) *Encyclopedia of Stress, Vol. 2.* New York: Academic Press, pp. 322–5.

Steptoe, A. and Ayers, S. (2005) Stress, health and illness. In Sutton, S., Baum, A. and Johnston, M. (eds) *The SAGE Handbook of Health Psychology*. London: Sage Publications, pp. 169–96.

Steptoe, A. and Brydon, L. (2005) Psychoneuroimmunology and coronary heart disease. In Vedhara, K. and Irwin, M. (eds) *Human Psychoneuroimmunology*. New York: Oxford University Press.

Steptoe, A., Wardle, J., Pollard, T.M., Canaan, L. and Davies, G.J. (1996) Stress, social support and health related behaviour: a study of smoking, alcohol consumption and physical exercise. *Journal of Psychosomatic Research*, 41, 171–80.

Stewart, M., Brown, J.B., Donner, A., McWhinney, I.R., Oates, J., Weston, W.W. and Jordan, J. (2000) The impact of patient-centered care on outcomes. *The Journal of Family Practice*, 49, 796–804.

Stewart, M., Brown, J.B., Weston, W.W., McWhinney, I.R., McWilliam, C.L. and Freeman, T.R. (2003) *Patient-Centred Medicine: Transforming the Clinical Method*. Oxford: Radcliffe Medical Press.

Stoller, E.P. and Forster, L.E. (1994) The impact of symptom interpretation on physician utilization. *Journal of Aging and Health*, 6, 507–34.

Strayer, M.S., DiAngelis, A.J. and Loupe, M.J. (1986) Dentists' knowledge of aging in relation to perceived elderly patient behaviour. *Gerodontics*, 2, 223–7.

Strehler, B.L. (1962) *Time, Cells, and Aging*. New York: Academic Press.

Studen-Pavlovich, D. and Elliott, M.A. (2001) Eating disorders in women's oral health. *Dental Clinician North America*, 45, 491–511.

Suglia, S.F., Ryan, L., Laden, F., Dockery, D.W. and Wright, R.J. (2008) Violence exposure, a chronic psychosocial stressor, and childhood lung function. *Psychosomatic Medicine*, 70, 160–9.

Suresh, R., Jones, K.C., Newton, J.T. and Asimakopoulou, K. (2012) An exploratory study into whether self-monitoring improves adherence to daily flossing among dental patients. *Journal of Public Health Dentistry*, 72, 1–7.

Sutherland, S. (1999) *With Respect to Old Age: Long-Term Care – Rights and Responsibilities*. A Report by the Royal Commission on Long-Term Care. Cm. 4192-1. London: HMSO.

Sutton, S. (2001) Back to the drawing board? A review of applications of the transtheoretical model to substance use. *Addiction*, 96, 175–86.

Swain, J., Finklestein, V., French, S. and Oliver, M. (eds) (1993) *Disabling Barriers – Enabling Environments*. London: Sage.

Tada, A. and Hanada, N. (2004) Sexual differences in oral health behaviour and factors associated with oral health behaviour in Japanese young adults. *Public Health*, 118, 104–9.

Taylor, S. and Field, D. (2003) *Sociology of Health and Health Care*. Oxford: Blackwell Publishing.

Thomas, J. and Clinton, F. (1963) Effects of group size. *Psychological Bulletin*, 60, 371–84.

Thorndike, E.L. (1901) Animal intelligence: an experimental study of the associative processes in animals. *Psychological Review: Monograph Supplements*, 2, 1–109.

Thrash, W., Marr, J. and Boone, S. (1982) Continuous self-monitoring of discomfort in the dental chair and feedback to the dentist. *Journal of Behavioural Assessment*, 4, 273–84.

Tinetti, M.E. and Fried, T. (2004) The end of the disease era. *American Journal of Medicine*, 116, 179–85.

Todd, J.E. and Lader, D. (1991) *Adult Dental Health 1998*. London: HMSO.

Towner, E. (1993) The history of dental health education: a case study of Britain. In Schou, L. and Blinkhorn, A. (eds) *Oral Health Promotion*. Oxford: Oxford University Press, pp. 1–23.

Townsend, P. (1981) The structured dependency of the elderly: the creation of social policy in the twentieth century. *Ageing and Society*, 1, 5–28.

Townsend, P. and Whitehead, M. (eds) (1988) *Inequalities in Health: the Black Report*. London: Penguin.

Trathen, A. (2013) Internal Report. King's College London.

Trathen, A. and Gallagher, J.E. (2009) Dental professionalism: definitions and debate. *British Dental Journal*, 206, 249–53.

Trathen, A., Scambler, S. and Gallagher, J. (forthcoming) Professionalisms and the business of dentistry: multiple-archetype model.

Tsigos, C. and Chrousos, G.P. (2002) Hypothalamic-pituitary-adrenal axis, neuroendocrine factors and stress. *Journal of Psychosomatic Research*, 53, 865–71.

Tudor-Hart, J. (1971) The inverse care law. *The Lancet*, 297, 405–12.

Turk, D.C. and Burwinkle, T. (2007) Pain: a multidimensional approach. In Ayers, S., Baum, A., McManus, C., Newman, S., Wallston, K., Weinman, J. and West, R. (eds) *Cambridge Handbook of Psychology, Health and Medicine*, 2nd edn. Cambridge: Cambridge University Press.

Turk, D.C. and Okifuji, A. (2001) Pain terms and taxonomies of pain. In Loeser, J.D., Butler, S.D., Chapman, C.R. and Turk, D.C. (eds) *Bonica's Management of Pain*, 3rd edn. Philadelphia, PA: Lippincott Williams & Wilkins.

Turrell, G. (1998) Socioeconomic differences in food preference and their influence on healthy food purchasing choices. *Journal of Human Nutrition and Dietetics*, 11, 135–49.

Turris, S.A. and Finamore, S. (2008) Reducing delay for women seeking treatment in the emergency department for symptoms of potential cardiac illness. *Journal of Emergency Nursing*, 34, 509–15.

Tversky, A. and Kahneman, D. (1974) Judgment under uncertainty; heursitics and biases. *Science*, 185, 1124–31.

Uchino, B.N. (2006) Social support and health: a review of physiological processes underlying links to disease outcomes. *Journal of Behavioural Medicine*, 29, 377–87.

United Nations (2006) *Convention on the Rights of Persons with Disabilities*. New York: United Nations.

United Nations (2007) *World Population Prospects: The 2006 Revision*. New York: United Nations.

United Nations Development Program (UNDP) (2006) *Human Development Report*. New York: Oxford University Press.

UPIAS (1976) *Fundamental Principles of Disability*. London: Union of the Physically Impaired Against Segregation.

Van Daele, T., Hermans, D., Van Audenhove, C. and Van den Bergh, O. (2013) Stress reduction through psychoeducation: a meta-analytic review. *Health Education and Behavior*, 39, 474–85.

Van Groenestijn, M.A., Mass-de Waal, C.J., Mileman, P.A. and Swallow, J.N. (1980) The ideal dentist. *Social Science and Medicine*, 14A, 541–6.

Vassend, O. (1993) Anxiety, pain and discomfort associated with dental treatment. *Behaviour, Research & Therapy*, 31, 659–66.

Vedhara, K. and Nott, K. (1996) The assessment of the emotional and immunological consequences of examination stress. *Journal of Behavioural Medicine*, 19, 467–78.

Victor, C. (1991) *Health and Health Care in Later Life*. Milton Keynes: Open University Press.

Vogele, C. (2007) Surgery. In Ayers, S., Baum, A., McManus, C., Newman, S., Wallston, K., Weinman, J. and West, R. (eds) *Cambridge Handbook of Psychology, Health and Medicine*, 2nd edn. Cambridge: Cambridge University Press.

Wagner, J., Arteaga, S., D'Ambrosio, J., Hodge, C., Ioannidou, E., Pfeiffer, C.A. and Reisine, S. (2008) Dental students' attitudes toward treating diverse patients: effects of a cross-cultural patient-instructor program. *Journal of Dental Education*, 72, 1128–34.

Walburn, J., Vedhara, K., Hankins, M., Rixon, L. and Weinman, J. (2009) Psychological stress and wound healing in humans: a systematic review and meta-analysis. *Journal of Psychosomatic Research*, 67, 253–71.

Walker, A. (1981) Towards a political economy of old age. *Ageing and Society*, 1, 73–94.

Walter, F.M., Humphrys, E., Tso, S., Johnson, M. and Cohn, S. (2010) Patient understanding of moles and skin cancer, and factors influencing presentation in primary care: a qualitative study. *BMC Family Practice*, 11, 62.

Wanless, D. (2004) *Securing Good Health for the Whole Population: Final Report*. Norwich: HMSO.

Waplington, J., White, D.A. and Clarke, J.R. (1998) A comparison of the social backgrounds and dental health of patients attending community dental services and general dental services and non-registered patients. *Community Dental Health*, 15, 93–6.

Wardle, J. (1982) Management of dental pain. Paper presented at British Psychological Society, York.

Watson, S.L., Shively, C.A., Kaplan, J.R. and Line, S.W. (1998) Effects of chronic social separation on cardiovascular disease risk factors in female cynomolgus monkeys. *Atherosclerosis*, 137, 259–66.

Watt, R.G. (2007) From victim blaming to upstream action: tackling the social determinants of oral health inequalities. *Community Dentistry and Oral Epidemiology, 35, 1–11.*

Watt, R.G. (2012) Social determinants of oral health inequalities: implications for action. *Community Dentistry and Oral Epidemiology*, 40, 44–8.

Watt, R.G. and Sheiham, A. (1999a) Inequalities in oral health: a review of the evidence and recommendations for action. *British Dental Journal*, 187, 6–12.

Watt, R.G. and Sheiham, A. (1999b) The authors respond. *British Dental Journal*, 187, 238.

Weinstein, N.D. (1980) Unrealistic optimism about future life events. *Journal of Personality and Social Psychology*, 39, 806–20.

Weinstein, N.D. (1982) Unrealistic optimism about susceptibility to health problems. *Journal of Behavioral Medicine*, 5, 441–60.

Weinstein, N.D. (1984) Why it won't happen to me: perceptions of risk factors and susceptibility. *Health Psychology*, 3, 431–57.

Weinstein, N.D. (1987) Unrealistic optimism about susceptibility to health problems: conclusions from a community-wide sample. *Journal of Behavioural Medicine*, 10, 481–500.

Welie, J.V. (2004) Is dentistry a profession? Part 1. Professionalism defined. *Journal of the Canadian Dental Association*, 70, 529–32.

Wensing, M., Jung, H.P., Mainz, J., Olesen, F. and Grol, R. (1998) A systematic review of the literature on patient priorities for general practice care. Part 1: Description of the research domain. *Social Science & Medicine*, 47, 1573–88.

Wessa, M., Rohleder, N., Kirschbaum, C. and Flor, H. (2006) Altered cortisol awakening response in posttraumatic stress disorder. *Psychoneuroendocrinology*, 31, 209–15.

West, R. (2006) *Theory of Addiction*. Oxford: Blackwell.

White, C., Glickman, M., Johnson, B. and Corbin, T. (2007) Social inequalities in adult male mortality by the National Statistics Socio-Economic Classification, England and Wales, 2001–03. *Health Statistics Quarterly*, 36, 6–23.

White, C., Edgar, G. and Siegler, V. (2008) Social inequalities in male mortality for selected causes of death by the National Statistics Socio-economic Classification, England and Wales, 2001–03. *Health Statistics Quarterly*, 38, 19–32.

White, S. (2007) *Equality*. Cambridge: Polity.

Wilkinson, R. and Pickett, K. (2009a) *The Spirit Level: Why Equal Societies Almost Always Do Better*. London: Penguin Books.

Wilkinson, R. and Pickett, K. (2009b) The Equality Trust Resource Page. http://www.equalitytrust.co.uk.

Williams, S. (1999) Is anybody there? Critical realism, chronic illness and the disability debate. *Sociology of Health and Illness*, 21, 797–819.

Wills, T.A. and Ainette, M.G. (2007) Social support and health. In Ayers, S., Baum, A., McManus, C., Newman, S., Wallston, K., Weinman, J. and West, R. (eds) *Cambridge Handbook of Psychology, Health and Medicine*. Cambridge: Cambridge University Press, pp. 202–7.

Wilson, G. (2000) *Understanding Old Age: Critical and Global Perspectives*. London: Sage.

Wong, H.M., Humphris, G.M. and Lee, G.T. (1998) Preliminary validation and reliability of the Modified Child Dental Anxiety Scale. *Psychological Reports*, 83, 1179–86.

World Health Organization (1948) Preamble to the Constitution of the World Health Organization as adopted by the International Health Conference, New York, 19–22 June, 1946; signed on 22 July 1946 by the representatives of 61 States (Official Records of the World Health Organization, no. 2, p. 100) and entered into force on 7 April 1948.

World Health Organization (1980) *International Classification of Impairments, Disabilities, and Handicaps (ICIDH)*. Geneva: WHO.

World Health Organization (2001) *International Classification of Functioning, Disability and Health (ICF)*. Geneva: WHO.

World Health Organization (2002) *Towards a Common Language for Functioning, Disability and Health*. Geneva: WHO.

World Health Organization (2003) *Adherence to Long-Term Therapies – Evidence for Action*. Available at: http://apps.who.int/medicinedocs/en/d/Js4883e/6.1.html.

World Health Organization (2011a) *Global Health and Ageing*. Geneva: WHO.

World Health Organization (2011b) *World Report on Disability*. Geneva: WHO.

World Health Organization (2014) International Classification of Functioning, Disability and Health (ICF) framework to facilitate interprofessional education and collaborative practice. Available at: http://www.who.int/hrh/news/2014/hrh_icf_framework/en/

World Health Organization (2015) Poverty and health. Available at: http://www.who.int/hdp/poverty/en/

Yinger, J.M. (1986) Intersecting strands in the theorisation of race and ethnic relations. In Rex, J. and Mason, D. (eds) *Theories of Race and Ethnic Relations*. Cambridge: Cambridge University Press, pp. 20–41.

Zadik, Y., Levin, L., Shmuly, T., Sandler, V. and Tarrasch, R. (2012) Recurrent aphthous stomatitis: stress, trait anger and anxiety of patients. *Journal of the Californian Dental Association*, 40, 879–83.

Zakrzewska, J. (1996) Women as dental patients: are there any gender differences? *International Dental Journal*, 46, 548–57.

Zborowski, M. (1952) Cultural components in responses to pain. *Journal of Social Issues*, 8, 16–30.

Zimbardo, P.G. (2007) *The Lucifer Effect: Understanding How Good People Turn Evil*. New York: Random House.

Zola, I.K. (1973) Pathways to the doctor – from person to patient. *Social Science & Medicine*, 7, 677–89.

Index

Page numbers in *italics* denote tables/figures